Careers in Chiropractic Health Care

Exploring a Growing Field

Cheryl Hawk, DC, PhD, CHES, Editor

Foreword by John Weeks

D0081996

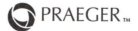

PRAEGER™

An Imprint of ABC-CLIO, LLC

Santa Barbara, California • Denver, Colorado

Library of Congress Cataloging-in-Publication Data

Names: Hawk, Cheryl, editor.
Title: Careers in chiropractic health care : exploring a growing field / Cheryl Hawk, editor ; foreword by John Weeks.
Description: Santa Barbara, California : Praeger, an imprint of ABC-CLIO, LLC, [2017] | Includes bibliographical references and index.
Identifiers: LCCN 2016059849 (print) | LCCN 2017000122 (ebook) | ISBN 9781440837487 (alk. paper) | ISBN 9781440837494 (eBook)
Subjects: | MESH: Chiropractic | Chiropractic—education | Career Choice
Classification: LCC RZ236 (print) | LCC RZ236 (ebook) | NLM WB 905.7 | DDC 615.5/340711—dc23
LC record available at https://lccn.loc.gov/2016059849

ISBN: 978-1-4408-3748-7
EISBN: 978-1-4408-3749-4

21 20 19 18 17   1 2 3 4 5

This book is also available as an eBook.

Praeger
An Imprint of ABC-CLIO, LLC

ABC-CLIO, LLC
130 Cremona Drive, P.O. Box 1911
Santa Barbara, California 93116-1911
www.abc-clio.com

This book is printed on acid-free paper ∞

Manufactured in the United States of America

Contents

Foreword by John Weeks   vii

Chapter 1   Introduction to Chiropractic Health Care
and Chiropractic Education   1
Carl S. Cleveland III

Chapter 2   Selecting a Chiropractic College   11
Brad Hough and Cheryl Hawk

Chapter 3   Applying to a Chiropractic College   39
Stacey Till and David Anderson

Chapter 4   Chiropractic Academic Education   51
*Stefanie Krupp, Ruth Sandefur, and
Rachael Pandzik*

Chapter 5   Chiropractic Clinical Education   75
*Stefanie Krupp, Ruth Sandefur, and
Rachael Pandzik*

Chapter 6   A Global Perspective on Chiropractic
Education   83
Phillip Ebrall

Chapter 7   Opportunities for Additional Training and
Experience   105
*Clinton Daniels, Stefanie Krupp, and
Shawn Hatch*

Chapter 8   Starting a Chiropractic Practice   137
Ronald J. Farabaugh

Chapter 9   Typical Chiropractic Practice   179
                  Marion W. Evans Jr., Cathryn S. Evans,
                  Lyndon Amorin-Woods, Christina Cunliffe,
                  and Jesse Politowski

Chapter 10   Chiropractic Specialization Career Paths   205
                  Stefanie Krupp and Clinton Daniels

Chapter 11   Academic Careers in Chiropractic   231
                  Phillip Ebrall

Chapter 12   Opportunities for Multidisciplinary
                  Practice   259
                  Jordan A. Gliedt and Cheryl Hawk

Chapter 13   Sports Chiropractic   275
                  Russ Ebbets

Chapter 14   Future Directions for the Chiropractic
                  Profession and Chiropractic Education   301
                  Carl S. Cleveland III and Michael R. Wiles

Index   311

About the Editor and Contributors   327

Foreword

Chiropractic at a Turning Point as the U.S. Medical Industry Turns toward Health

The policy and organizational campaigns to shift the medical industry in the United States toward a value-based system of health care have created challenges and opportunities for the chiropractic profession. Thanks to forward-acting members, the profession is increasingly well positioned to benefit from the mounting changes.

Moving Beyond the Era of Fee for Service

In the still-dominant fee-for-service environment, production-focused business models thrive. Manufacturers of high-end devices and providers of high-cost procedures benefit. Like other practitioners whose income is linked to repetitive delivery of procedures, many chiropractors also benefit by moving high volumes of patients through their practices.

However, the fee-for-service era has hit major problems related to both cost and quality. Widely accepted estimates suggest that a third of all health care delivery is wasted. The production orientation is associated with shockingly high levels of morbidity and mortality. Reformers responded by creating policy, payment, and delivery strategies through which those providing care would be accountable for outcomes.

These values have been promoted as the Triple Aim: enhancing the experience of patients, bettering population health, and lowering per capita costs. A chief tool for achieving these aims is a renewed interest in *evidence-informed care*. Another strategy is to catapult providers out of their separate silos and into collaboration and team care. *An era of interprofessionalism is emerging.*

Chiropractic in the Era of Value-Based Health Care

In recent years, many leaders of the chiropractic profession have been supporting developments that will help us thrive in the emerging era of value-based medicine. Researchers at multiple chiropractic colleges and universities and in appointments at academic medical centers have created an increasingly compelling case for cost savings. These go along with the patient satisfaction that has been a cornerstone of chiropractic practice. Chiropractors were successfully included in a federal program to support use of the electronic health records that are key to communication, outcomes, and continuity of care in the new system. After years of tilling the soil, a major chiropractic initiative began at the Veteran's Administration (VA). Opportunities for VA residencies now exist. Individual chiropractors can have their clinics certified through a process recognized by the National Committee for Quality Assurance as partners in new medical homes. Individual chiropractors can bolster their practice value via the chiropractor-led, multidisciplinary initiative Spine IQ, a federally recognized data registry to gather quality-of-care data.

This ground-tilling work for successful chiropractic practice in the new era does not end there. Multiple chiropractic educators serve—and have served—as leaders in efforts to foster interprofessionalism and inclusion through the Academic Collaborative for Integrative Health. Through that organization, they have created and joined teams of integrative practitioners and fostered a national dialogue through the National Academies of Sciences and local engagements with academic health centers. Aware that good works can fall in the forest with no one to hear them, thousands of individual practitioners and leaders of scores of chiropractic organizations and businesses unified the profession behind the Foundation for Chiropractic Progress in a stellar, multiyear, ongoing marketing effort.

What may be—for the patient—the cream on all of this transformational work is an emerging shift in clinical thinking and practice that goes to the heart of chiropractic philosophy *and* marketing. Numerous national and organizational guidelines have declared that, when it comes to the treatment of pain, nonpharmacological, complementary, and integrative approaches should come first. This echoes chiropractic's historic call for conservative treatment.

A special opportunity for chiropractic physicians is emerging here. The field is the most powerful and well organized of the licensed integrative health and medicine professions. Might chiropractic take the lead in fostering system investment in an ever-expanding and innovative practice of *conservative care first* to bring the necessary transformation? Some chiropractic leaders are already recognizing this historic opportunity. Such a change in care delivery will not only enhance patient care but also drive business success in individual chiropractic practices in the emerging era.

Might the field step into such leadership, not just for chiropractic but for the patients and professionals from all fields who recognize the centrality of this value in "value-based" health care? The potential in the emerging era is for chiropractic leaders to not merely lead chiropractic but also this move toward health care. This is an exciting future indeed!

John Weeks
Publisher-Editor, *The Integrator Blog News & Reports*
Editor-in-Chief, *Journal of Alternative and Comple'mentary Medicine*

CHAPTER ONE

Introduction to Chiropractic Health Care and Chiropractic Education[*]

Carl S. Cleveland III, DC

Chiropractic: Healing with a Human Touch

A CareerCast survey ranked "chiropractor" as the 11th-best job in 2013—higher than medical doctors and surgeons. The survey ranked 200 jobs from best to worst based on physical demands, work environment, income, stress, and hiring outlook.[1]

This ranking did not surprise doctors of chiropractic (DCs), the health care professionals concerned with the diagnosis, treatment, and prevention of disorders of the spine and other parts of the musculoskeletal system. These disorders plague 44.6 million Americans at an annual cost to society estimated at $267.2 billion.[2] Certainly this represents an opportunity to meet a health care need, considering the impact of extended sitting, violent sports, and car accidents prevalent in modern society.

---

[*] This chapter has been reprinted from Carl S. Cleveland III, DC. Chiropractic: Healing with a Human Touch. *The Advisor: The Journal of the National Association of Advisors for the Health Profession*, Vol. 34, No. 4, December 2014, pp. 19–35. Reprinted with permission from the editor.

A study by the Decade of Bone and Joint Disorders in *The Spine Journal* reported on the epidemic nature of back pain. It estimated the daily prevalence of chronic low back pain in the general adult population as 37 percent, the one-year prevalence as 76 percent, and the lifetime prevalence as 85 percent. Approximately 20 percent of sufferers described their pain as severe or disabling.[3] Back pain is also the leading cause of work-related disability and absenteeism and is associated with reduced mobility, quality of life, and longevity, along with increased rates of other health problems.

Today, nearly 120 years after its founding, chiropractic (from the Greek, meaning "done by hand") is taught and practiced throughout the world. The profession has earned broad acceptance from the public and in national health care systems. The chiropractic profession is the third-largest physician-level independent health profession in the Western world, after medicine and dentistry.

Satisfaction with the chiropractic approach to spine care also ranks in the 90th percentile in public, Medicare, and TRICARE patient polls. Indeed, satisfied patients have always been the mainstay of chiropractic care throughout its history. In a Congress-mandated pilot project conducted from April 2005 to March 2007, testing the feasibility of expanding chiropractic services in the Medicare program, 87 percent of patients in the study gave their chiropractor a satisfaction level of 8 or higher with 56 percent of respondents rating their chiropractor as a perfect 10.[4]

The U.S. Bureau of Labor Statistics projects employment of chiropractors to increase faster than the average for all occupations from 2014 to 2024, reporting that the increase cuts across all age groups. They attribute this in part to the nondrug and nonsurgical approach to patient treatment. Further, the Department of Labor Handbook states, "The aging of the large baby-boom generation will lead to new opportunities for chiropractors. Older adults are more likely to have neuromusculoskeletal and joint problems and they are seeking treatment for these conditions more often as they lead longer, more active lives."[5]

Conservative Care First

Today the DC is filling the role of the conservative spine and joint care practitioner, placing emphasis on manual techniques, including joint adjustment/manipulation, addressing both pain relief and restoring function.

The paradigm shift in spine care began with the ground-breaking 1994 report of the U.S. Public Health Service Agency for Health Care Policy and Research (AHCPR), Guideline 14, which concluded that only one in

100 cases of low back pain required surgery. It recommended spinal manipulation as a "proven treatment" to be used before medical methods.[6] In the following years, abundant research has followed that supports the effectiveness of spinal manipulation.[7]

The Chiropractic Perspective and Practice

The relationship between *structure*, primarily the spine and musculoskeletal system, and *function*, as coordinated by the nervous system, is central to the profession's approach to patient treatment, health, and well-being. Most patients consult chiropractors for back pain and other musculoskeletal pain of the spine or extremities, as well as headaches. Less frequently, patients present with other conditions, either caused, aggravated, or mimicked by neuromusculoskeletal disorders.[8]

The chiropractic perspective views health as a natural state of the individual and that any departure from that state represents a failure of the individual's inherent ability to adapt to changes in the internal and external environment, or is a result of adverse adaptation. Further, the chiropractic paradigm considers health as an expression of biological, psychological, social, and spiritual factors. The profession's principles value the intrinsic biologic ability or innate tendency of the body to self-regulate and to restore and maintain health through compensating homeostatic mechanisms, reparative processes, and adaptive responses to environmental challenges.

Further, the profession acknowledges the role of the nervous system in the control, coordination, and regulation of the body, and that spinal joint dysfunction, termed "subluxation" or "subluxation complex," can affect nerve function and interfere with the body's ability to regulate and maintain health. The core purpose of the chiropractic procedure is to relieve interference caused by disturbed spinal biomechanics through skilled manual assessment and correction, termed "spinal adjustment or manipulation."

This perspective represents a holistic biopsychosocial philosophy of health rather than a biomedical one and embraces a belief in optimizing health through good nutrition, constructive exercise, stress management, and a focus on the importance of good posture, as well as spinal and extremity joint biomechanics. The profession promotes a drug-free approach. However, DCs refer patients requiring medications or surgical interventions for appropriate medical care.

Chiropractic patient management includes manual techniques with particular competency in joint adjustment/manipulation, rehabilitation exercises, patient education in lifestyle and nutritional modification, and the use of adjunctive physical therapy modalities, orthotics, and other supports. Current accreditation and state licensing standards in the United States require DCs, as primary care, portal-of-entry providers, to establish a diagnosis, determine indications for providing chiropractic care, and consult with or refer to other health care practitioners when appropriate. *Chapter 9 details the components of typical chiropractic practice.*

Licensure and Legal Recognition

In the United States, all 50 states, the District of Columbia, Puerto Rico, and the U.S. Virgin Islands have statutes recognizing and regulating the practice of chiropractic as an independent portal-of-entry health provider. Although specific requirements vary by state, all jurisdictions require the completion of an accredited doctor of chiropractic (DC) program. Requirements for licensure include passing the examinations conducted by the National Board of Chiropractic Examiners, which includes the basic and clinical science subjects, clinical case studies, and a practical exam. Certain jurisdictions may require applicants to be examined over the law governing the practice of chiropractic in that state. Requirements for continuing education for license renewal vary with each state.

Chiropractic services are recognized and reimbursed through Medicare, and most state Medicaid Acts include doctors of chiropractic as primary health providers. Chiropractic services are covered by a substantial majority of health insurance policies. The U.S. Department of Labor, Office of Workers' Compensation Programs, Division of Federal Employees' Compensation, recognizes chiropractors as physicians for treatment of manual manipulation of the spine.

In 2000, President Clinton signed Public Law 106-398, mandating that chiropractic care be made available to all active-duty military personnel. In 2002, President Bush signed the Department of Veterans Affairs Health Care Programs Enhancement Act of 2001. This bill included a mandate to establish a permanent chiropractic benefit within the Department of Veterans Affairs (VA) health care system. *Chapter 12 gives an insider's view of chiropractic in the VA with interviews with DCs working in the VA.*

Including the United States, the practice of chiropractic is recognized and regulated by law in 48 countries. Common features of legislation and practice include a role as a primary care provider, allowing direct contact with patients, and the right and duty to diagnose, including taking and/or ordering skeletal imaging. *Chapter 2 lists accredited world chiropractic colleges.*

Admissions and the Doctor of Chiropractic Educational Program

The Council on Chiropractic Education USA (CCE-USA), recognized by the U.S. Office of Education since 1974, is the national accrediting body for the 16 chiropractic degree programs and solitary purpose chiropractic institutions in the United States. The council establishes minimum standards for chiropractic education; individual member chiropractic programs may establish additional requirements for admissions, curricular course content, and in the areas of clinical competency.

The accreditation standards of the CCE-USA require applicants seeking admission to the doctor of chiropractic program to have completed the equivalent of three academic years of undergraduate study (90 semester hours) at an institution accredited by an agency recognized by the U.S. Department of Education or an equivalent foreign agency. A grade point average of not less than 3.0 on a 4.0 scale is required for these 90 hours. A minimum of 24 semester hours in life and physical science courses, with at least half of these courses to include a laboratory component, is to be included within the 90 hours.

Further, the student's undergraduate preparation must include a well-rounded general education program in the humanities and social sciences and other coursework deemed relevant for successful completion of the doctor of chiropractic curriculum. *Chapter 3 details the requirements for entering chiropractic college.*

The educational program for the doctor of chiropractic degree in the United States typically represents a four-year academic program with a minimum of 4,200 instructional hours. The CCE-USA educational standards identify the following subject categories and courses:

- Foundations in Chiropractic: principles, practices, philosophy, and history of chiropractic
- Basic Sciences: anatomy, physiology, biochemistry, microbiology, and pathology
- Clinical Sciences: physical, clinical, and laboratory diagnosis; diagnostic imaging; spinal analysis; orthopedics; biomechanics; neurology; spinal adjustment/manipulation; extremities manipulation; rehabilitation and therapeutic modalities/procedures (active and passive care); toxicology; patient management; nutrition; organ systems; special populations; first aid and emergency procedures; wellness and public health; and clinical decision making
- Professional Practice: ethics and integrity, jurisprudence, business and practice management, and professional communications

- Information Literacy and Research Methodology: ability to access and understand information and critically analyze outcomes associated with research and scholarly activities.

The CCE-USA educational standards identify mandatory meta-competencies, outlining the skills, attitudes, and knowledge to prepare graduates to serve as primary care chiropractic physicians. These competencies require the chiropractic graduate to demonstrate ability to

- perform an initial assessment and diagnosis;
- create and execute an appropriate case management/treatment/intervention plan;
- promote health, wellness, safety, and disease prevention;
- communicate effectively with patients, doctors of chiropractic, and other health care professionals, regulatory agencies, third-party payers, and others as appropriate;
- produce and maintain accurate patient records and documentation;
- be proficient in neuromusculoskeletal evaluation, treatment, and management;
- access and use health-related information;
- demonstrate critical thinking and decision-making skills and sound clinical reasoning and judgment;
- understand and practice the ethical conduct and legal responsibilities of a health care provider;
- critically appraise and apply scientific literature and other information resources to provide effective patient care;
- understand the basic, clinical, and social sciences and seek new knowledge in a manner that promotes intellectual and professional development.

Outside of the United States, common international standards of education are being achieved through a network of accrediting agencies represented by the Councils on Chiropractic Education International (CCEI), an organization committed to quality assurance and defining chiropractic educational standards, ensuring their adoption and maintenance by accrediting agencies worldwide. *Chapters 4 through 6 discuss chiropractic academics, both in the United States and internationally.*

Being Part of Interdisciplinary Care

While most community-based chiropractic services are situated in private offices, *interdisciplinary practices* are now common, with chiropractic doctors, medical doctors, physical therapists, and others working as partners in private practices, occupational health and rehabilitation centers, and national sports medicine teams. As of the date of this publication, doctors of chiropractic provide services to active-duty military personnel in 66 interdisciplinary military treatment facilities worldwide (63 in the United States, others in Japan and Germany).[9]

Since 2002, chiropractic services have been included in the standard medical benefits package available to all enrolled veterans through the U.S. Department of Veterans' Affairs, and today chiropractic practitioners are employed in as many as 48 Veterans' Administration (VA) hospitals throughout the country. The VA treatment facilities are typically affiliated with medical schools, and as of July 2014, chiropractic graduates are eligible to participate in VA resident training hospitals side by side with medical students receiving clinical training in these facilities.[9]

It is estimated that 20 percent of disabled veterans and 30 percent of hospitalizations stem from low back pain, the largest disabling condition among active forces, resulting in more soldiers missing time from work than any other health condition.[10] A 2009 Johns Hopkins study, "Back Pain Permanently Sidelines Soldiers at War," found that the top reasons for medical evacuation from Iraq and Afghanistan were musculoskeletal disorders—24 percent compared to 14 percent who had suffered combat injuries.[11]

Interdisciplinary management of sports injuries and athletic performance management in professional, collegiate, high school, and recreational athletes are well represented by the profession nationally and across the globe. All NFL teams and most pro-sport teams have DCs as part of the medical staff. Bill Moreau, DC, serves as managing director of sports medicine at the United States Olympic Committee (USOC) in Colorado Springs, Colorado, where he directs the USOC Clinics, Games and the USOC National Medical Network. He has served as medical director for the U.S. medical team at the Sochi Olympics.

Twenty-eight chiropractors, including nine from the United States, treated athletes during the London 2012 Summer Olympics. Clinicians often report that elite athletes, often more than any other patients, insist upon chiropractic for its effectiveness in preventing and managing injury and enhancing and optimizing function and performance. *Chapters 12 and 13 provide more details of opportunities in interdisciplinary practice and sports chiropractic.*

A Rewarding Health Care Career

Within the present health care landscape, including the Affordable Health Care Act and the VA Reform Act, the cry heard loud and clear is to reduce costs and improve outcomes.

Considering that back pain and musculoskeletal disorders are now the number-one disabling conditions in the nation, including in the military, the need for nondrug, nonsurgical, and effective spine care is paramount for health care reform. Rising to address this need, the chiropractic profession is widely regarded as a leading example of a complementary health care discipline reaching maturity and extending its role within mainstream health care. Chiropractors today appear steadfast in their role as America's primary spine care provider in this epidemic of chronic pain.

Across this nation and internationally, responsible economists and policy makers are seeking the best outcomes in health care delivery, looking for cost containment with a move away from excessive and high-risk interventions, yet focused on achieving higher patient satisfaction through better results.

Strengthened with the evidence gained through research and outcome-effectiveness studies, doctors of chiropractic are attuned to consumers' increasing interest in a conservative, effective, and noninvasive approach to maintain health, and one less reliant on addictive opioid painkillers.

With mounting public interest in diet, nutrition, and exercise, and considering that aging boomers are seeking vitality and to remain active as they move through their golden years, the doctor of chiropractic is well positioned by education and clinical training to lead in conservative primary spine care and in the management of musculoskeletal disorders.

Being a doctor of chiropractic offers the opportunity to become a self-employed small business owner, earning respect as a health care provider within the community. Yet most important of all, being a doctor of chiropractic is about the priceless reward from the heartfelt gratitude expressed by the men, women, and children whose lives are changed through chiropractic care.

References

1. Jobs rated 2013: Ranking 200 jobs from best to worst. CareerCast Web site. http://www.careercast.com/jobs-rated/best-worst-jobs-2013. Accessed August 14, 2016.

2. U.S. Bone and Joint Decade. *The Burden of Musculoskeletal Disease in the U.S.* Rosemont, IL: American Academy of Orthopaedic Surgeons; 2008.

3. Haldeman S, Dagenais S. A supermarket approach to the evidence-informed management of chronic low back pain. *Spine.* 2009;8(1):1–7.

4. Stason W, Ritter G, Shepard DS, et al. *Report to Congress on the Evaluation of the Demonstration of Coverage of Chiropractic Services Under Medicare.* Washington,

DC: Centers for Medicare & Medicaid Services' Office of Research, Development, and Information; 2009.

5. Bureau of Labor Statistics. *Occupational Outlook Handbook*. Washington, DC: U.S. Department of Labor; January 2016–2017.

6. Bigos S, Bowyer O, Brown K, et al. U.S. Dept. of Health and Human Services, Public Health Service, Agency for Health Care Policy and Research, Clinical Practice Guideline, Number 14: Acute Low Back Problems in Adults AHCPR Publication No. 95-0642, December 1994.

7. Clar C, Tsertsvadze A, Court R, Hundt GL, Clarke A, Sutcliffe P. Clinical effectiveness of manual therapy for the management of musculoskeletal and non-musculoskeletal conditions: systematic review and update of U.K. evidence report. *Chiropr Man Therap*. 2014;22(1):12.

8. National Board of Chiropractic Examiners. *Practice Analysis of Chiropractic 2015*. Greeley, CO: National Board of Chiropractic Examiners; 2015.

9. Lisi AJ, Brandt CA. Trends in the use and characteristics of chiropractic services in the Department of Veterans Affairs. *J Manipulative Physiol Ther*. 2016 Jun;39(5):381–386.

10. Cohen SP, Nguyen C, Kapoor SG, et al. Back pain during war: an analysis of factors affecting outcome. *Arch Intern Med*. 2009;169(20):1916–1923.

11. Johns Hopkins Medicine. Back pain permanently sidelines soldiers at war. News and Publications, November 9, 2009. http://www.hopkinsmedicine.org/news/media/releases/Back_Pain_Permanently_Sidelines_Soldiers_At_War. Accessed November 20, 2016.

CHAPTER TWO

Selecting a Chiropractic College

Brad Hough, PhD; and Cheryl Hawk, DC, PhD, CHES

Students who have decided that a career in chiropractic is right for them will next need to select which chiropractic colleges to apply to. This chapter will describe the factors that should be taken into consideration in order to identify the best institution for the student's individual needs and preferences. It will also provide brief descriptions of currently accredited chiropractic colleges around the world.

The first consideration in selecting a chiropractic college is that the institution is accredited and that graduates are equipped to meet all the requirements to obtain licensure in their state and country. This is also essential in terms of obtaining federal student loans. Accrediting bodies exist for most international regions to ensure that colleges meet established standards. The Council on Chiropractic Education International is the umbrella organization for these regional accreditation agencies.[1] The World Health Organization's Traditional Medicine Department of Technical Cooperation for Essential Drugs and Traditional Medicine published a document addressing international educational standards for chiropractic.[2] This is important because of the need for standardization in countries where chiropractic practice is not yet as highly regulated as it is in countries where it has been well established.[2] The *WHO Guidelines on Basic Training and Safety in Chiropractic* addresses "two levels and four different settings for chiropractic education, each preparing health care practitioners to practice in the health care system as a chiropractor. These options are available to countries to meet their individual needs."[2]

The WHO guidelines list two categories:

1. Full chiropractic training programs for (a) students who have not previously been educated or had experience in any health care profession or (b) health professionals who desire training in chiropractic.

2. Limited chiropractic training programs meant to serve as an interim measure until the full program can be instituted, again for (a) students without previous health care training or (b) health professionals who desire chiropractic training. This second category is meant to operate in countries in which chiropractic is not yet regulated in order to establish that people already practicing chiropractic there meet minimal levels of competency.[2]

There are a number of additional considerations when choosing a school of chiropractic. It is important to explore these considerations to be sure that the program selected will meet one's individual needs and preferences. Potential chiropractic students should investigate these issues:

1. **How long does it take to complete the program?** Most chiropractic programs can be completed in 10 trimesters, or the equivalent in quarters or semesters. However, there are variations in how quickly these can be completed and whether there is flexibility in taking the program over a longer or shorter period.

2. **How strong is the program academically?** All colleges in the United States are required by their accrediting body, the Council on Chiropractic Education, to post information about the pass rates of their students on national board exams. This can give an indication of how well the students are academically prepared at that institution.

3. **Does the college provide some business skills training to assist graduates in managing their practice successfully and ethically?** Historically, chiropractors usually practiced as solo practitioners or with one or two other doctors of chiropractic (DCs). This trend still predominates. The 2015 *Practice Analysis* of chiropractic, the survey conducted every five years by the National Board of Chiropractic Examiners (NBCE), found that 75 percent of DCs are sole proprietors.[3] Even DCs working in multidisciplinary and other nontraditional settings are likely to be independent contractors or business owners rather than salaried employees. Therefore, it is important that chiropractic colleges provide substantial and ethical business training as part of the curriculum.

4. **Are clinical experiences introduced early in the curriculum to maximize students' experience with patient care?** The trend in medical education in general has been to integrate clinical experience into the curriculum as early as possible, even in the very first term of study. This model replaces the older one in which as much as the first half of health care professional

training was focused on basic science, with clinical experience reserved for the latter part of students' education. Gradually, chiropractic education is following the lead of medicine, as it has done in other aspects of training, and is moving clinical experience into the earliest part of the curriculum so that basic science study is grounded in the perspective of how it relates to clinical care of real patients.

5. *Are multiple chiropractic techniques as well as other procedures (such as exercise and rehabilitation, physical therapy modalities, and soft tissue techniques) part of the curriculum?* Since most chiropractors use a number of different procedures in order to achieve the best patient outcomes, it is important that there be opportunities to learn these during chiropractic college training rather than having to seek them out in postgraduate seminars.

6. *How many, and how diverse, are the clinical training opportunities available?* Chiropractic teaching clinics located only on the campus may not provide students with as broad an experience with patients of diverse demographics and conditions. Interested students should check the teaching clinics listed on the institution's website. Ideally, these will be in a variety of locations and venues, such as inner city, Veterans Administration, or in different types of health care settings. *Chapter 12 on multidisciplinary opportunities gives examples of a number of these types of experiences.* Since multidisciplinary practices are becoming increasingly prevalent internationally, institutions offering such experiences during chiropractic training will give students a head start when they graduate. Students should keep in mind that the types of teaching clinic experiences can vary a good deal among chiropractic colleges, largely due to variations in the types of settings locally available and/or the institution's capacity to establish collaborative arrangements.

7. *Does the chiropractic college have additional degree programs or affiliations with other institutions that do?* Many chiropractic colleges in the United States and other countries are now universities, offering several different degree programs. These are usually, but not always, health related, such as master's programs in health promotion, nutrition, radiology, rehabilitation, or sports and human performance. A smaller but growing number of chiropractic universities offer training in other independent health professions, such as acupuncture/Oriental medicine, massage therapy, naturopathic medicine, physician's assistant, and occupational therapy assistant.

Some of the degree programs can be taken concurrently, minimizing the amount of time required to receive an MS degree after earning the DC. Many MS programs are online or hybrid programs (partially online and partially on-site). It is wise for students to match their interests with the availability of relevant degree programs. Many students feel that earning an additional academic or professional degree improves their chances for career success and provides them with more options for employment.

8. *Are the institution's information technology resources up to date?* Health care professionals need to be versed not only in electronic health records but all the new communication technology, and so chiropractic colleges need to be on the cutting edge. This topic has become so important that we have provided a detailed discussion of it in the section below.

9. *Does the institution include preparation for licensure in multiple states and countries or offer assistance in obtaining it?* Students who are interested in practice mobility should consider whether their prospective colleges will prepare them to be licensed in different states and/or countries. U.S. chiropractic colleges routinely maintain licensure requirements for all U.S. states but may not necessarily do so for other countries. Contact admissions personnel for details on this.

Another factor to consider when selecting a chiropractic program is the institution's philosophy. One accepted way of classifying philosophical differences among chiropractors and chiropractic colleges is to locate them on a spectrum ranging from "broad scope" to "focused scope."[4] In this model, "broad scope" refers to chiropractors who use a number of different procedures within their scope of practice and do not restrict their practice to correcting subluxations (joint dysfunction) in the spine. "Focused scope" DCs would be those who practice primarily to remove

Table 2.1   U.S. Chiropractic Colleges' Position on the Spectrum from Broad to Focused Scope*

Broad Scope	Middle Scope	Focused Scope
National University of Health Sciences	Cleveland University	Life University
Southern California University of Health Sciences	Logan University	Life Chiropractic College West
Texas Chiropractic College	New York Chiropractic College	Sherman College of Chiropractic
University of Bridgeport	Northwestern Health Sciences University	
University of Western States	Palmer College of Chiropractic	
	Parker University	

*Only chiropractic colleges established before 2005 are included.

subluxations from the spine and usually do not use additional procedures. The majority of chiropractors, and now chiropractic colleges, in the United States (and to varying extents in other countries) tend to fall in between these two and are considered "middle scope."[4–6]

In terms of coursework, however, accreditation standards require that all colleges meet certain criteria. Other chapters will address coursework, standards, and licensure requirements in detail. Delivery methods of coursework and the type of clinical experiences provided may vary considerably among chiropractic colleges.

Table 2.1 shows the location of U.S. chiropractic colleges on the spectrum of broad to focused scope. These determinations were made through interviews with key personnel at the chiropractic colleges and were described in a report from the Institute for Alternative Futures.[5,6]

Technology Considerations

When selecting a chiropractic college for professional education, it is important to look at the technology in use at the institution and how it is being employed. A high-quality chiropractic program will use technology strategically to facilitate learning, support the overall student experience, and model best practices to prepare the graduate for a life of professional practice. When applied wisely, technology can make the chiropractic training experience more productive and enjoyable while setting the student up for success in future practice.

Technology for Teaching and Learning

There are a number of technologies that support learning. Anything from flashcard apps to video recordings of patient encounters can be used to improve a student's educational experience. The most foundational of all of these technologies is the Learning Management System (LMS). A good LMS provides an organized Web-based repository of all the requirements and content for a course, facilitates communication and collaboration, supports integration with textbooks and third-party applications, and tracks participation and assessments of learning. Blackboard, Canvas, Desire2Learn, and Moodle are examples of popular LMSs. An LMS will provide a pathway through the content of a course and help students stay organized and know what is required. At institutions without an LMS, students must develop and implement their own learning strategies and tracking mechanisms, while institutions who use an LMS effectively have students and faculty share the responsibility and the benefits.

As a complement to an LMS, many institutions also make use of a Web portal to provide students with self-service access to the college's student-facing business operations. For example, in many portals, students can register for classes, see their final grades, review the course catalog, pay their bill, and review and accept financial aid. A good portal system enables students to make efficient use of their time by conducting much of their college business after regular hours of operation.

In addition to online technology, the technology in the classroom itself plays an important role in the teaching and learning experience. At any modern chiropractic institution, classrooms will have a standard suite of presentation equipment (computer, projector, microphone, document camera, DVD player, etc.) to support the instructor and help the students follow the presentation of content. At some institutions, these standard tools are being supplanted by newer technology that replaces static document cameras with technology that enables real-time streaming from smartphones and tablets to high-definition screens in the classroom. The technology can certainly be used to display static images, but in technique classes where students are learning positioning and placement skills, this streaming technology is especially helpful because it allows the instructor to travel the classroom and project real-time video to illustrate the critical points from the lesson for the entire class to see, engaging the students and bringing the lecture to life.

Similar to streaming technology that is entering the chiropractic technique classes, anatomy and physiology classes are also making extensive use of technology to lead students through the body's systems in detail. To accomplish this, chiropractic institutions invest in specialized audiovisual theater technology that combines exceptional surgical lighting with high-quality cameras and remote control systems that are able to zoom from wide-angle displays to microscopic levels. Students benefit from the guided instruction of an expert and the exceptional image quality, helping them to visualize the body's systems and better preparing them for their own hands-on experience.

Another visual technology that helps better prepare chiropractors is an assessment center with the ability to record simulated patient encounters. In an assessment center, chiropractic students engage in scripted encounters with "patients" who have been trained to represent the symptoms of a variety of diseases and health issues. These practice encounters provide students with experiences that closely mimic the real-life presentation of the disease. Recordings allow students to review their performance in diagnostic interviews until they have mastered the process, are comfortable with the interview, and have developed the skills to interact well with patients. The technology supports multiple exam rooms and allows each one to house a different case presentation. All rooms can be simultaneously launched, monitored, recorded, and reviewed. Instructors can also review the sessions, enabling them to interact with all their students in a one-on-one format, enhancing the learning process.

Electronic testing is a relatively new technology that is being introduced at some chiropractic colleges. While paper-based testing is still quite common, electronic testing has become well established in many professional education programs (e.g., legal, health care). Forward-leaning institutions are adopting these testing systems and delivering exams on computers, laptops, or tablets. One of the chief benefits of this technology is that it allows students to receive more rapid feedback, often automatically and immediately grading the objective portions of an exam. It also provides faculty and administrators with much-needed deep insight into the learning that is or is not occurring both in an individual class and across the curriculum. The immediacy of electronic testing enables students to seek assistance before they fall behind and allows for just-in-time corrections in the classroom during the term, helping instructors know what needs to be covered in greater detail and ultimately helping students learn the material better.

Supporting Technology

In addition to using technology to support teaching and learning, leading chiropractic institutions have embraced today's mobile technology of laptops, tablets, and smartphones. Before mobile technology can be widely adopted, the institution must first implement a variety of supporting technologies that enable the effective use of these devices by their staff, faculty, and students in the classroom and around campus. The initial step in elevating mobile to be a first-class technology is a significant investment in a robust wireless network to provide high-speed access throughout the campus—all classrooms, study areas, work spaces, and public spaces. While spreading coverage widely across the campus is important, it is not enough. The network must also be built and tuned to handle the high-density usage patterns common in today's classrooms. With the proliferation of mobile technologies, students and faculty often carry three or more network devices (e.g., laptop, smartphone, and tablet), creating far greater demand on network resources in classrooms than in a one-person, one-device model. Because of the sheer number of devices seeking connections, and the amount of data being consumed in these environments, wireless networks built with older technology, or those not designed with the expectation that each user will have multiple devices, are easily overwhelmed. In today's mobile-centric world, colleges must have a robust network infrastructure to be able to leverage technology for chiropractic education.

In addition to the wireless network on campus, colleges need to invest in high-capacity Internet service. Increasingly, students, faculty, and staff at chiropractic colleges rely on resources from the Internet for teaching and learning, as well as online resources for communication and collaboration. In many cases, services that have previously been developed and maintained on the premises (e.g., email) are now located off-site in the cloud or in a vendor's data center and are accessed through the campus's Internet gateway. For proper performance, this new cloud-services model means that users must be able to both upload and download very large amounts of data through a network that is also highly responsive (low latency). Campuses without one or both of these capabilities have difficulty offering modern services that meet expectations—large files move slowly, processes that require many round trips to the cloud feel sluggish, time is wasted, and students and faculty grow frustrated. Campuses with both of these capabilities are better positioned to meet both current and future needs as the use of cloud systems grows.

A relatively new but growing expectation is for modern chiropractic colleges to have access to virtually unlimited online storage. Today's students and faculty regularly make use of multiple forms of media (e.g., text, photos, audio, videos, animations, presentations, etc.) throughout the teaching and learning experience. As instructional media becomes more sophisticated, storage requirements grow exponentially. A mobile-friendly college recognizes this need and provides its students and faculty with large online storage capabilities to ensure that the resources supporting learning are available from any kind of device, anywhere the student or faculty member may be. While once a costly option that few colleges offered, online storage is now a commodity service that is very inexpensive or even free to supply.

With the ascendancy of the Web, access to information has become a hallmark of the modern college, but it requires deliberate attention to ensure that Web-based information is easily accessible from the myriad of computing devices now in use. To address this challenge, colleges have adopted responsive design, a mobile-friendly technology designed to deliver Web pages in a variety of formats in real time. Websites that use these responsive-design techniques dynamically reformat the presentation of the information to fit the capabilities of the device requesting it, whether it's a smartphone, tablet, or computer. When a student or faculty or staff member accesses information with this next generation of the Web, pages are rearranged, data collection is modified, screen elements are prioritized, and the user experience is enhanced for each individual. Colleges that have truly adopted mobile devices and a "bring your own device" (BYOD) philosophy have undoubtedly already moved to a responsive design approach for their website and key communication systems.

Printing is an important but often overlooked technology that is directly impacted by a mobile BYOD philosophy. When chiropractic colleges fully embrace technology, they must wrestle with how to allow students, faculty, and staff to print from their personal mobile devices over the institution's wireless network—something that would not have been allowed just a few years ago. Solving this dilemma involves rethinking the traditional view of concentrating shared resources and instead adopting a policy of distributing printing devices to places where students, faculty, and staff work. It also requires implementing a different security model that segments the network into zones of variable security rather than maintaining a uniform high-security posture. The result is a network that simultaneously supports users working with sensitive data (high security) and users printing homework assignments from their personal devices (low security) without compromising the institution's overall security posture.

Even in an age of nearly ubiquitous mobile devices, sometimes students need a computer. Today's chiropractic colleges maintain computer labs to provide access to specialized educational resources and as a place for general computing services (word processing, email, Internet, creating/viewing presentations, printing, etc.). Well-equipped lab environments offer a more productive computing experience than is available with mobile technology, employing much larger monitors, faster computers, and a rich collection of software. Students at modern chiropractic colleges supplement their tablets and smartphones with full-size computers when they have a significant amount of creative work to produce (e.g., writing a paper or creating a presentation) or when they need to access educational resources that require a computer (e.g., DVDs or software). Lab computers continue to be an essential part of the overall campus technology environment, providing extra power and ease of use when needed.

A final supporting technology isn't really a technology; it is technology support. Whether through email, telephone, the Web, or face to face, the support resources for technology at a chiropractic college can make or break technology use. While it is common for the face-to-face staff to be available during reasonable windows of time in the work week, critical applications should offer extended support hours (often by text, email, or phone). Troubleshooting is the most commonly relied-upon service, with many colleges now supplementing their staff with short on-demand videos that demonstrate how to resolve the most common issues. These online resources often offer the most direct route to resolving simple issues and are available 24/7, 365 days a year. Consider the availability of all the support resources when evaluating the college's technology.

Technology's Role in Modeling Professional Practice

Upon graduation, chiropractic students will enter a rapidly changing health care environment where technology is being increasingly incorporated into the entire experience—patient intake, diagnosis, treatment planning, patient education, record keeping, billing, communication, and more. Expectations for the use of technology to improve health care are coming from state and federal agencies, professional organizations, vendors, other health care providers, third-party services (e.g., billing services), but most especially from patients. As technology has become embedded in daily life, the expectation to find it in chiropractic care is a natural outcome. The most forward-thinking chiropractic programs recognize these developments and prepare their students to excel in the new professional practice setting.

As with so many of the developments in chiropractic education, the process of building fluency with technology begins with college faculty. When faculty are comfortable with a variety of communications and learning technologies and use them regularly in their teaching, they set a standard for students and illustrate how technology adds value to a process. As students move through the curriculum, more technologies are introduced to enhance their learning (e.g., video recordings of structured patient encounters), while other experiences prepare them for their upcoming clinic practice (e.g., electronic health records, digital X-rays). Students also begin to develop fluency when they use technology they will later find in professional practice (e.g., tablets) for personal productivity and to support their learning. All of this experience with technology comes together in real practice when students engage patients in the clinical experience portion of their professional preparation and use various technologies to find, enroll, diagnose, educate, and treat real patients.

The way members of an institution use technology reveals much about what they believe the future of chiropractic will be like and what the preparation for professional practice will be like at that institution. Technology does not replace the knowledge and experience of a chiropractor; it enhances the doctor's ability to serve patients. When technology is properly integrated into the curriculum, by the time students complete their chiropractic training, they will be skilled with digital communications, knowledgeable users of state-of-the-art diagnostic tools, experienced with new forms of record keeping and managing patient data, and confident in their ability to use technology in professional practice. In short, they will be prepared to participate in the new models of health care.

Geographic Location

After these considerations, a student's final choice of a college may come down to geographic location. Proximity to the family, employment considerations for spouse or significant other, and preferred part of the country—or choice of country—are often deciding factors for many students. However, it is unwise to select the college based on proximity to where you intend to practice. Because many students tend to stay close to their alma mater, the density of chiropractors near most chiropractic colleges is greater than in other areas and may make starting a practice more difficult.

The number of chiropractic colleges outside of North America is growing rapidly, although the growth in North America has slowed almost to a stop. World chiropractic colleges providing training to the 88 member countries of the World Federation of Chiropractic are listed below, including their addresses and website URLs. Chiropractic colleges are located in 16 countries; all but three countries have one or two colleges. Australia and the U.K. each have three, and the United States has the greatest number of colleges, with 17 located in 13 states. Several of the colleges are separate campuses of a single chiropractic institution—Palmer College of Chiropractic has campuses in Iowa, California, and Florida; Life University has campuses in Georgia and California. National University of Health Sciences has one campus located in Illinois and a second site in Florida, but they are not considered distinct colleges. These institutions are listed separately because geographic location is an important part of the decision-making process when selecting an institution. Included in each listing are additional programs offered, either academic (such as master's programs) or in other health professions. Generally, colleges that are part of a university will offer additional programs, while most single-purpose chiropractic colleges will not. Many single-purpose chiropractic colleges in the United States, as well as U.S. chiropractic colleges in university systems, have chiropractic assistant/technician programs as well. Chiropractic assistant (CA) or chiropractic technician (CT) is an allied health profession working in chiropractic offices. Some chiropractic students' spouses train as CAs/CTs while their spouse pursues a DC degree.

Following is a list of chiropractic institutions along with additional programs offered. All the institutions were contacted for additional information. This information is included for those institutions that responded, with their permission.

United States

California

Life Chiropractic College West. Hayward, CA; website: www.lifewest .edu

Life West offers a chiropractic program only.

Life Chiropractic College West is located in the heart of the San Francisco Bay area. Life West specializes in chiropractic education and offers an outstanding doctor of chiropractic degree. The curriculum at Life West features an integrated emphasis on chiropractic philosophy and technique that draws passionate students from around the world.

Life Chiropractic College West was founded in 1976 (originally Pacific States Chiropractic College) and provides solid academic and clinical experience. The Life West learning community is known for its diversity, integrity, and cooperative spirit.

The San Francisco Bay area gives Life West students an unparalleled experience in lifestyle as well as access to a wide variety of mentorship and career opportunities.

Life West's mission is "Creating a Brighter Future for Humanity." Life West provides a well-balanced approach to education, integrating the fundamental elements of practitioner success: science, technique, philosophy, and business skills. It is committed to producing academic and clinical research, adding to the body of knowledge available to and for the chiropractic profession.

Palmer College of Chiropractic West. San Jose, CA; website: www.palmer .edu

Palmer College of Chiropractic West, part of the three-campus Palmer system, offers a chiropractic program only. *See "Palmer College of Chiropractic" under "Iowa" subhead for general information about Palmer campuses.*

Southern California University of Health Sciences. Whittier, CA; website: www.scuhs.edu

In addition to the DC program, SCUHS offers both a master's of acupuncture and Oriental medicine (MAOM) and a doctorate of acupuncture and Oriental medicine (DAOM). It offers certificate programs in Ayurveda and also in massage.

Los Angeles College of Chiropractic (LACC) has been a leader in chiropractic education since 1911. As LACC moves into its second 100 years, it is continuing to provide excellence in health care education, which leads to excellence in interprofessional health care.

LACC graduates are evidenced based while being tolerant of those who may have a different philosophy. They have a passion for continued learning in areas that would best benefit their patients. They view the chiropractic adjustment as their primary tool but are constantly looking to expand that toolbox to better improve their approach to patient care. They also graduate with business skills that give them the confidence to succeed in practice.

Information literacy is a hallmark of our graduates. They are able to answer clinical questions through analysis of the literature.

LACC is well known for providing excellent clinical education. This includes a philosophy that is based on evidence and outcomes and an education integrated with other forms of health care and within the education itself.

Connecticut

University of Bridgeport College of Chiropractic. Bridgeport, CT; website: www.bridgeport.edu/chiro

In addition to the DC program, UBCC students can earn a concurrent master's degree in human nutrition or acupuncture. The university offers degrees, as separate programs, for several other health professions as well.

Florida

Palmer College of Chiropractic, Florida Campus. Port Orange, FL; website: www.palmer.edu

Palmer College of Chiropractic Florida, part of the three-campus Palmer system, offers a chiropractic program only.

See "Palmer College of Chiropractic" under "Iowa" subhead for general information about Palmer campuses.

National University of Health Sciences, Florida Site. Pinellas Park, FL; website: www.nuhs.edu

This campus is part of the National University of Health Sciences system. *See description under "National University of Health Sciences" under "Illinois" subhead for general information about National University of Health Sciences campuses.*

Georgia

Life University. Marietta, GA; website: www.LIFE.edu
In addition to the DC program, Life U. has master's programs in sport health science (concentration in chiropractic sport science, exercise sport science, nutrition and sport health science, sport coaching, or sport injury management), positive psychology, athletic training, and clinical nutrition.

Illinois

National University of Health Sciences, Chiropractic Medicine Program. Lombard, IL; website: www.nuhs.edu
In addition to the program in chiropractic medicine, National University of Health Sciences (NUHS) offers a doctor of naturopathy (ND); a master's in acupuncture or Oriental medicine, a postprofessional master's in advanced clinical practice, and a certificate in massage therapy. NUHS has set the highest standards in training for careers in health care since its founding in 1906 as a chiropractic college. Since then, the Illinois institution has added graduate degrees in naturopathic medicine, acupuncture, and Oriental medicine, as well as undergraduate degrees in biomedical sciences and massage therapy. In 2009, the university further advanced its offerings by opening a second chiropractic degree program in Florida.

An historic leader in evidence-based health care, National University publishes three Medline-indexed scientific journals and has received over $5 million in federal and private research grants. National University also provides whole health patient-centered care in five integrative medical clinics. Professional degree students can choose to intern in numerous hospital rotations, including several at VA medical facilities or a Salvation Army center serving the medically underserved population.

National University trains its chiropractic and naturopathic medicine students as primary care doctors who view physicians and other health care providers as colleagues, not competitors. This dynamic immersion in integrative medicine enables students and faculty from differing medical specialties to work together as colleagues, not competitors, sharing their individual skills for better patient outcomes.

National University of Health Sciences continues to look forward to new ways to grow and advance the institution, such as the addition of online courses and additional degree offerings in the field of natural health care.

Iowa

Palmer College of Chiropractic, Davenport Campus. Davenport, IA; website: www.palmer.edu

In addition to the DC program, PCC offers a master's in clinical research.

Palmer College of Chiropractic, with campuses in Davenport, Iowa, San Jose, California, and Port Orange, Florida, is the founding and largest college of the chiropractic profession. D. D. Palmer, the discoverer of chiropractic, founded Palmer College in 1897, and it has become known as "*The* Trusted Leader in Chiropractic Education." Palmer's 26,000 alumni comprise more than one-third of all chiropractors in the United States.

The Palmer Center for Chiropractic Research is the largest institutional chiropractic research facility in the world and has received more than $35 million in federal funding since its inception. Palmer is the only chiropractic institution to receive three Developmental Center for Research on Complementary and Alternative Medicine grants from the National Institutes of Health, and it is the first chiropractic college to establish a master's degree program in clinical research.

Palmer's faculty is highly respected for teaching excellence and scholarship, and a number of faculty members have authored textbooks in use at most chiropractic colleges. Palmer College of Chiropractic also has the largest clinic system in chiropractic education, and the majority of its faculty clinicians have advanced training in specialties such as pediatrics, rehabilitation, radiology, sports chiropractic, and neurology.

Kansas

Cleveland University–Kansas City, College of Chiropractic. Overland Park, KS; website: www.cleveland.edu

In addition to the DC program, CCC offers a master's in health promotion.

Steeped in history, yet meeting the challenges of contemporary health care education, Cleveland University–Kansas City offers a personalized approach to education for a rewarding career in chiropractic and health sciences. Founded in 1922 by one of the first families of chiropractic, the university is best known for preparing doctors of chiropractic with a balanced approach to the philosophy, science, and art of chiropractic; however, today it has expanded its curriculum to include the master's in health promotion, the bachelor's of science in human biology, and associate of arts in biology degrees.

Students looking to enroll at Cleveland are often individuals pursuing or holding undergraduate degrees in biology, kinesiology, exercise, related health sciences, or other pre-health programs. They are most likely in the 18–30 age group and interested in promoting a holistic approach to health and wellness.

Students may enroll in the standard four-year doctor of chiropractic curriculum or apply for the accelerated 3 1/3–year program. Students in the concurrent BS/DC program graduate with the undergraduate human biology degree and doctor of chiropractic degree.

With an early introduction to hands-on learning, a supportive and welcoming community, and a passion to help shape the future of health care, students of Cleveland University–Kansas City leave with more than a degree. They're prepared to launch their careers and make a difference for their patients and for themselves.

Minnesota

Northwestern Health Sciences University. Bloomington, MN; website: www.nwhealth.edu

In addition to the DC program, NWHSU offers a master's degree in acupuncture (MAc) and Oriental medicine (MOm) and a certificate in massage therapy.

Missouri

Logan University. Chesterfield, MO; website: www.logan.edu

In addition to the DC program, Logan offers a master's in health informatics (online), master's in nutrition and human performance (online), master's in sports science and rehabilitation, and doctorate of health professions education (online).

As one of North America's top chiropractic universities, Logan University offers students a demanding science-based curriculum taught by highly qualified faculty in state-of-the-art educational and learning facilities. Through an innovative, outcome-based academic curriculum that emphasizes evidence-informed care, diverse clinical immersion opportunities, emerging technology, and proven practices, Logan University graduates are trained, confident, and better prepared for the future.

Innovative clinical education continues to be a hallmark of Logan with hands-on learning in real-world settings. At Logan University, students are provided with the knowledge, tools, and experiences to successfully transition from classroom to clinic. Logan's state-of-the-art assessment center offers monitored exam rooms for faculty observation, formative feedback, and sharing best practices for improved outcomes. Hands-on internship programs give Logan student interns exposure to a diverse patient population and complex clinical cases. Opportunities are available at organizations that allow students to step outside of the traditional classroom and into environments where interns can treat a variety of individuals, including veterans (Department of Veterans Affairs, Scott Air Force Base), the physically disabled (Paraquad), and underinsured at federally qualified health centers (Myrtle Hilliard Davis Comprehensive Health Centers).

New York

D'Youville College. Buffalo, NY; website: www.dyc.edu

New York Chiropractic College. Seneca Falls, NY; website: www.nycc .edu

Founded in 1919 as the Columbia Institute of Chiropractic, New York Chiropractic College (NYCC) has evolved to become a leading institution for the education of natural health care professionals and academicians. Doctor of chiropractic students have the option to supplement their education with additional degrees in acupuncture and Oriental medicine, clinical nutrition, or human anatomy and physiology instruction. Post-professional degree programs in diagnostic imaging and clinical anatomy are also available.

Located in Seneca Falls, New York, the beautiful 286-acre campus includes state-of-the-art classrooms, robust technology, and diverse learning resources to support the college's commitment to academic excellence, quality patient care, and professional success. Rigorous evidenced-based curricula, supplemented by strong academic support and career development programs, ensure that students are well prepared to excel in today's complex, collaborative, patient-centered health care environments.

Modern health centers in Buffalo, Long Island, Rochester, and Seneca Falls—along with clinical opportunities through academic affiliations with Veterans' Administration Centers, State University of New York campus health centers, and other sites—provide students with the finest clinical experiences available in chiropractic and acupuncture education.

Oregon

University of Western States. Portland, OR; website: www.uws.edu

Founded in 1904, University of Western States (UWS) is the second-oldest chiropractic physician program in the world. It has since evolved into a leading institution for an evidence-informed, science-based education, with a focus on health and wellness. UWS is institutionally accredited by the Northwest Commission on Colleges and Universities (NWCCU).

University of Western States has enduring commitment to educating health sciences practitioners with a passion for patient care. The university motto "For the good of the patient" guides every aspect of the institution and enables UWS to fulfill its mission of improving the health of society through conservative, patient-centered care.

Extending this pursuit beyond campus, UWS has cultivated several key community partnerships and is a founding member of the Oregon Collaborative for Integrative Medicine (OCIM). This collaborative provides students, faculty, and staff the opportunity be a part of interdisciplinary education, research, and advocacy for patients in support of integrated care.

In 2015, UWS launched the Northwest Center for Lifestyle and Functional Medicine (NWCLFM) to educate health professionals, support community outreach, and conduct research in the areas of lifestyle, sports and functional medicine, health promotion, and diet and nutrition.

UWS is located in Portland, Oregon, a beautiful city situated in the progressive Pacific Northwest. This area embraces innovative approaches to health and well-being, which is reflected in the whole-person health care education taught at University of Western States.

South Carolina

Sherman College of Chiropractic. Spartanburg, SC; website: www .sherman.edu

Texas

Parker University. Dallas, TX; website: www.parker.edu

Dallas-based Parker University, formerly known as Parker College of Chiropractic, is one of the world's leading educators of health care professionals. Founded in 1982, this private, nonprofit educational institution prepares men and women to become doctors of chiropractic and other leaders in health care–related professions. Parker University offers 12 different degree programs as well as continuing education specializations and certifications. Parker University also includes the Parker Research

Institute, which provides sound, scientific evidence supporting health and wellness; two chiropractic wellness clinics in the Dallas-Fort Worth Metroplex; Parker Seminars, the largest chiropractic seminar organization in the world, and Parker SHARE Products that provide innovative, high-quality products and current information on chiropractic wellness.

Texas Chiropractic College. Pasadena, TX; website: www.txchiro.edu

Australia

Macquarie University, Department of Chiropractic. Sydney, NSW: website: www.chiro.mq.edu.au

Macquarie's Department of Chiropractic has long enjoyed a reputation for excellence. Their chiropractic degrees are particularly popular with both domestic and international students, who learn in state-of-the-art facilities and benefit from hands-on experience in the university's three chiropractic clinics.

The university recently reaffirmed its commitment to offering outstanding chiropractic teaching and research programs. The bachelor of chiropractic science and master of chiropractic will be enhanced to include more opportunities to pursue chiropractic research, including through the master of research degree.

The master of chiropractic degree has alternate entry pathways available. Graduates with degrees in human health science with substantial studies in anatomy and physiology and a GPA of 2.5/4 are eligible to apply. For more information or to ask a question about the master of chiropractic programs see http://courses.mq.edu.au/postgraduate/master/master-of-chiropractic.

The bachelor of chiropractic science is Australia's most established and respected chiropractic school. For more information or to ask a question on the bachelor's program, see http://courses.mq.edu.au/undergraduate/degree/bachelor-of-chiropractic-science.

Murdoch University, School of Health Professions. Murdoch, W. Australia: website: www.chiropractic.murdoch.edu.au

RMIT University, Division of Chiropractic. Bundoora, Victoria; website: www.rmit.edu.au/chiropractic

The RMIT (Royal Melbourne Institute of Technology) chiropractic program is one of the first government-funded chiropractic training programs in the world. The evidence-based, double bachelor's degree is of five years' (10 semesters') duration and sees students engage in clinical training during semesters 7–10. Set within one of the largest institutions in the country, the program makes full use of the rich basic science resources a full university environment provides. Interprofessional learning with other health disciplines is a strong feature of chiropractic training as is work-integrated learning in local and international environments. The RMIT graduate is a primary contact, evidence-based health care practitioner with a passion for lifelong learning and critical inquiry.

Brazil

Centro Universitario Feevale, Faculdade de Quiropraxia. Novo Hamburgo, Brazil: website: www.feevale.br

Universidade Anhembi Morumbi, Faculdade de Quiropraxia. São Paulo, Brazil; website: www.anhembi.br

Canada

Canadian Memorial Chiropractic College. Toronto, Ontario; website: www.cmcc.ca

The Canadian Memorial Chiropractic College (CMCC), located in Toronto, Ontario, Canada, is an accredited private postsecondary academic institution established in 1945.

CMCC is one of the most innovative chiropractic institutions in North America and is recognized as a world leader in chiropractic education and research. Among its 12 teaching and research laboratories is North America's first simulation laboratory designed to enhance training in chiropractic technique through the use of Force Sensing Table Technology and human analog mannequins developed by researchers at CMCC.

CMCC offers a second-entry undergraduate professional degree and postgraduate and continuing education programs and works collaboratively with a number of local hospitals and health care centers for the purposes of clinical training and research. CMCC provides a vibrant educational community to its 750 students and 200 staff and faculty, many of whom are specialists and leaders in their field.

Students complete their final year of studies interning at one of the school's community-based clinics, providing supervised patient care to a wide variety of patient populations in these communities. CMCC's well-prepared graduates maintain excellent pass rates on both the Canadian and American board exams.

Université du Québec à Trois-Rivières, Département de chiropratique. Trois-Rivières, Québec; website: www.uqtr.ca

Chile

Universidad Central de Chile, Chiropractic Program, Faculty of Health Sciences. Santiago, Chile; website: www.ucentral.cl

Denmark

University of Southern Denmark, Institute of Sports Science and Clinical Biomechanics. Odense, Denmark; website: www.sdu.dk

The education in clinical biomechanics was launched as a Nordic chiropractic education in 1994. It is a five-year full-time university-based program consisting of a three-year BSc and a two-year MSc. A further one-year postgraduate internship is required to obtain a full license to practice in Denmark. The educational scope is broad and aims at producing specialists in the field of musculoskeletal disorders who are fully equipped to be active players within the Danish health care system.

The content of clinical biomechanics is evidence based and taught by active researchers, and 20 percent of the curriculum deals with research-related issues. To ensure the highest academic standards, almost the entire BSc curriculum is integrated with the medical education. The program is divided into three tracks—the biomedical, academic, and profession tracks—with the biomedical subjects accounting for four-sixths of the curriculum. Teachings at the BSc level are focused on the biopsychosocial model of health and disease. The MSc program is the clinical part of the education, focusing on differential diagnosis, diagnostic imaging, clinical skills, patient management, and internships. The main one-year internship is located at a rheumatology outpatient department where the interns are part of several multidisciplinary teams.

France

Institut Franco-Européen de Chiropratique. Ivry-Sur-Seine, France; website: www.ifec.net

The Institut Franco-Européen de Chiropraxie (IFEC) was established in 1984. Chiropractic practice became legal in France in 2011 and was recognized by the government. IFEC was accredited by France's Ministry of Health in 2013.

Japan

Tokyo College of Chiropractic. Tokyo, Japan; website: www.chiro.jp

The first chiropractic education of international standard started in 1995 as RMIT University Chiropractic Unit Japan in collaboration with RMIT University, Australia. All courses were taught in the Japanese language and by Japanese educational staff. This was the first chiropractic program of high standard in Asia, and it was accredited by ACCE (Australasian Council on Chiropractic Education) in 2005.

The Tokyo College of Chiropractic (TCC) is formerly known as RMIT University Chiropractic Unit Japan and succeeded its precursor as independent yet with the same management. The TCC has more than a decade of experience in teaching and producing a high standard of graduates.

The aim of the chiropractic program is to produce chiropractors most suited for practicing in Japan. TCC graduates are accepted as full members by the Japanese Association of Chiropractors (JAC), the representing organization from Japan to the World Federation of Chiropractic (WFC).

The program is four years, full time, with more than 4,200 hours in the class and the clinic and is accredited by CCEA (Council on Chiropractic Education Australasia). Graduates receive the doctor of chiropractic (DC) degree.

There are many qualified chiropractors, medical doctors, and PhDs teaching at Tokyo College of Chiropractic. Other part-time lecturers also teach at medical or dental schools.

TCC is located at Shimbashi, a major business district adjoining to the world-famous international area, Ginza, in central Tokyo. In addition to the main campus, which includes the outpatient teaching clinic, TCC teaches in physiology and biochemistry labs at the Omori campus of Toho University and in the anatomy lab, technique lab, and classrooms at the Tokyo University of Medicine.

Classes commence annually after graduation in March, and selection requires an interview and a passing grade on a pre-chiropractic studies examination.

Korea (Republic of Korea)

Hanseo University, Department of Chiropractic. Seosan City, Korea; website: www.hanseo.ac.kr

Hanseo University was founded in 1991 by the founder and current president, Dr. KeeSun Ham. The Department of Chiropractic (HUDC) was established in 1997 under the leadership of Dr. SeunHae Han. Known as "the Cradle of Chiropractic Education in Asia," this was the first official chiropractic program to adopt the World Health Organization guidelines on basic education and safety in chiropractic in Korea. This is also the first chiropractic program officially approved by the Ministry of Education and Human Resources Development of Korea. HUDC initially collaborated with the Royal Melbourne Institute of Technology in Australia. Currently, it works in partnership with the University of Bridgeport College of Chiropractic in the United States with its foundation provided through the Department of Health Management (pre-chiropractic program) since 2002. As the first independent chiropractic program in Asia, HUDC received accreditation from the Council on Chiropractic Education Australasia Inc. in November 2010. HUDC also serves as the only official test site for the National Board of Chiropractic Examiners in Asia.

Malaysia

International Medical University. Kuala Lumpur, Malaysia; website: www.imu.edu.my

Mexico

Universidad Estatal del Valle de Ecatepec, Chiropractic Program. Estado de Mexico, Mexico; website: www.uneve.edu.mx

Universidad Veracruzana started developing a chiropractic college in 2011 with the collaboration of Colegio de Profesionistas Cienctificos Quiropracticos de Mexico A.C. in Veracruz, Mexico. This program is designed to meet national and international standards of education for chiropractic programs around the world and in keeping with the guidelines of the World Health Organization.

This chiropractic program developed within the Faculty of Medicine of Veracruz. This was the first time in Latino America that a chiropractic college was located within a public medical college. Its purpose is to provide chiropractic students with a strong basic science education taught by the medical faculty and a strong chiropractic sciences education taught by experienced doctors of chiropractic trained in the United States, France, and Mexico.

The program started in August 2013 with 15 students enrolled in the chiropractic program. In 2015, the program had 70 chiropractic students enrolled and the demand is growing. The Universidad Veracruzana is making formal arrangements with local hospitals to allow students to do clinical rotations inside the hospitals. Additionally, in 2015, the Universidad Veracruzana contracted with the naval hospital to allow chiropractic interns to provide care for the Mexican marines. A key feature of this program is that chiropractic and medical students share the same facilities and basic science.

Universidad Veracruzana is ranked ninth among all private and public universities in Mexico and number 55 in all of Latin America. The Universidad Veracruzana has five campuses with a total of 79,180 students.

Universidad Estatal del Valle de Toluca. Ocoyoacac, Mexico; email: unevt@live.com.mx

New Zealand

New Zealand College of Chiropractic. Auckland, New Zealand; website: www.chiropractic.ac.nz

South Africa

University of Johannesburg, Department of Chiropractic. Johannesburg, South Africa; website: www.uj.ac.za

The University of Johannesburg is currently within the top 4 percent of universities globally and is a member of the prestigious U21. The Department of Chiropractic is housed within the Faculty of Health Sciences, along with programs of radiography, nursing, emergency medical care, optometry, homeopathy, podiatry, human anatomy and physiology, biomedical technology, somatology, and sport and movement studies.

The course is a structured five-year full-time program, with a final exit level of a master's degree in chiropractic, this being the required level of qualification for registration with the Allied Health Professions Council of South Africa (the statutory regulation authority for the profession).

The program is designed within the context of South Africa to allow graduates to practice within a multidisciplinary environment, with the basis of the course being focused on the biopsychosocial model and evidence-based practice within the musculoskeletal environment. The program is accredited by the European Council on Chiropractic Education.

Durban University of Technology, Department of Chiropractic. Durban, South Africa; website: www.dit.ac.za

Spain

Barcelona College of Chiropractic. Barcelona, Spain; website: www. bcchiropractic.es

The Barcelona College of Chiropractic (BCC) is the first college of chiropractic in the Mediterranean region, having opened its doors in October 2009 and running a five-year full-time program of study. The legal entity representing the BCC is the Fundació Privada Quiropràctica (FPQ), a nonprofit foundation compliant with Spanish law and registered as a foundation with the Generalitat de Catalunya. It is the world's first bilingual college of chiropractic, having two official languages—English and Spanish. It is a private college, holding collaborative agreements with two of Spain's best public universities—Universitat Pompeu Fabra (UPF) and Universitat Autònoma de Barcelona (UAB). The BCC delivers many of its classes on the UPF's city-center campus. Additionally, the UPF is involved in the teaching of the program and students receive a master's in chiropractic from the UPF upon graduation. The other agreement, with the UAB, relates to the BCC's use of the anatomical dissection facilities and staff. The BCC is not presently accredited but will apply for full accreditation with the European Council on Chiropractic Education during 2016. The college presently has 130 students who come from more than 20 different countries.

Madrid College of Chiropractic-RCU. Madrid, Spain; website: www .rcumariacristina.com

The Real Centro Universitario Escorial Maria Cristina (RCU) was founded by the Regent Queen Maria Christina of Austria in 1892. It is a private university center affiliated with a major public university for degree-awarding purposes. In 2007, the RCU established the chiropractic program (aka Madrid College of Chiropractic), the first one in Spain. Chiropractic education is offered in a combined program of four years followed by a one-year master's in chiropractic (MChiro), accredited by the European Council on Chiropractic Education since December 2012.

The program is delivered in Spanish and English, with opportunities for international exchange programs in universities and colleges abroad. To this date, chiropractic remains unregulated in Spain and there is no protection of the title and the scope of practice.

Switzerland

University of Zurich. Zürich, Switzerland; website: www.uzh.ch

This is a six-year program composed of a three-year bachelor of medicine and three-year chiropractic medicine. The school is open only to Swiss students who have been accepted into the medical school to study chiropractic.

Turkey

Bahçeşehir Üniversity, Chiropractic Program. Beşiktaş/İstanbul, Turkey; website: http://www.bahcesehir.edu.tr/icerik/9570-kayropraktik-yuksek-lisans-programi
-program-tanimi

The chiropractic program was launched in September 2015.

United Kingdom

Anglo-European College of Chiropractic. Bournemouth, Dorset, England; website: www.aecc.ac.uk

The AECC is the oldest educational institution for chiropractors in Europe and offers a full-time university-validated and professionally accredited master's degree program in chiropractic. It is a not-for-profit and independent higher education institution, located on the south coast of England in Bournemouth. The AECC's state-of-the-art teaching clinic contains advanced diagnostic imaging equipment, such as quantitative fluoroscopy for spinal motion analysis and an open and upright MRI scanner. Clinical training includes hospital and general practitioner placements.

Alongside chiropractic education and training, the AECC co-delivers a BSc degree in clinical exercise science and offers a number of postgraduate MSc programs for qualified chiropractors and other health care professionals. In particular, the college has built a reputation in postgraduate musculoskeletal diagnostic ultrasound education and training and is now a leading provider in the U.K. as well as delivering the program in other countries.

An essential part of the academic character of the AECC lies in its commitment to research and in recognizing the value of research activity in informing the taught knowledge base; as such, the college has a strong tradition of supporting PhD students.

The AECC is committed to providing students with an environment that fosters the acquisition of understanding and skills at the forefront of knowledge, the attitudes to continue to learn throughout professional life, and quality learning opportunities and experiences to equip them to practice to the highest professional standards in their chosen careers.

McTimoney College of Chiropractic. Abingdon, Oxfordshire, England; website: www.mctimoney-college.ac.uk

Established over 40 years ago, the McTimoney College of Chiropractic (MCC) is located just south of Oxford in the heart of England, with a second campus located in central Manchester in the north of the country. MCC is one of only three U.K. institutions accredited by the General

Chiropractic Council (GCC), and all programs are validated by BPP University, one of the largest private universities in the U.K.

Known for its friendly and supportive learning environment, the integrated master's in chiropractic degree (MChiro) is the key route for registration with the GCC and a career in chiropractic. The college offers a standard four-year full-time and a unique five-year full-time extended delivery option that allows students to continue to work while studying. The college also offers a Foundation Pathway program for those who don't have the entry-level requirements. There is a very good ratio of tutors to students, especially in the practical and clinical training modules, and the college has a strong track record of publishing student research projects.

University of Glamorgan, Welsh Institute of Chiropractic. Pontypridd, Wales; website: www.southwales.ac.uk/chiro

The Welsh Institute of Chiropractic (WIOC) has been an integral component of the School of Health, Sport and Professional Practice in the Faculty of Life Sciences and Education at the University of South Wales (USW) since 1997. The chiropractic degree is the only program in the U.K. that is fully integrated into the university infrastructure, offering students a wide educational experience. The WIOC offers a full-time five-year (1 + 4) undergraduate integrated master's degree (master of chiropractic [MChiro]), with two points of entry depending on the level of pre-chiropractic education. The funded pre-chiropractic foundation year for students prepares students lacking science subjects to pursue a health professional career. The MChiro is accredited by both the General Chiropractic Council (GCC) in the U.K. and the European Council on Chiropractic Education (ECCE). Graduates of the MChiro can directly register with the GCC and practice legally in the U.K. or return to practice in various home states within the European Union. ECCE accreditation facilitates applications for registration to practice in other countries around the world. The course aims to produce caring and competent chiropractors who are capable of practicing independently and safely. In addition to designated specialist teaching facilities, clinical training is conducted on site within the fully equipped WIOC outpatient clinic to facilitate student educational experience.

References

1. Ebrall P, Draper B, Repka A. Towards a 21 century paradigm of chiropractic: stage 1, redesigning clinical learning. *J Chiropr Educ.* 2008;22(2):152–160.

2. World Health Organization. WHO guidelines on basic training and safety in chiropractic. Geneva: World Health Organization; 2005.

3. Examiners NBoC. *Practice Analysis of Chiropractic.* Greeley, CO: NBCE; 2015.

4. McDonald W, Durkin KF, Pfefer M. How chiropractors think and practice: the survey of North American chiropractors. *Seminars in Integrative Medicine.* 2004;2(3):92–98.

5. Institute for Alternative Futures. *The Future of Chiropractic Revisited: 2005–2015.* Alexandria, VA: Institute for Alternative Futures; 2005.

6. Institute for Alternative Futures. *Chiropractic 2025: Divergent Futures.* Alexandria, VA: Insitutute for Alternative Futures; 2013.

CHAPTER THREE

Applying to a Chiropractic College

Stacey Till, MSEd; and David Anderson, DC, MS-HSA

In exploring the options that a career in chiropractic can provide, students should consider multiple areas. First, potential students should explore their level of interest and desire to pursue the profession. Then, they should review the educational requirements to determine potential gaps in their past education. Additionally, they should check out individual chiropractic college campuses. Once students find a campus or two that meets their needs, they should begin the application process. Finally, they should explore ways to pay for educational expenses.

Choosing Chiropractic

For many years, people were mainly drawn to a career as a doctor of chiropractic (DC) due to a positive personal experience with the profession. Often, either the student, a relative, or a close friend had had a life-changing experience that greatly improved health and function, which caused the prospective student to investigate the profession. A large number of students report a desire to help others with a goal of providing a similar positive experience.

Today, while many students enter the profession for the above reason, more students are choosing chiropractic as a career without firsthand knowledge. Students today note positive information in sources like the government's occupational outlook. Also, as more athletic teams from high school to the professional level employ DCs, students sometimes learn about the profession in relation to their favorite athlete or team.

No matter their path, students typically note several facets of chiropractic that draw them to the profession, including chiropractic's less-invasive approach to health concerns and the relational aspect of the chiropractic profession wherein chiropractors can build a close doctor-patient relationship. Through the hands-on nature of the treatments provided, students expect a stronger bond with patients. Finally, students often note the ability to be entrepreneurial and run a small business as an attractive feature of the profession.

Once students choose to pursue chiropractic as a career, they should expect a rigorous course of study. Students interested in pursuing the profession should possess an aptitude for science. The chiropractic curriculum devotes significant time to the areas of human anatomy and physiology, biochemistry, microbiology, pathology, radiology, and chiropractic technique. The curriculum is challenging, and most of the material presented will be new. Students will be evaluated on their demonstration of empathy and communication skills in the areas of patient care and interprofessional communications. Typical chiropractic curricula expect at least 25 hours per week in class and in laboratory work. This is twice the expectation of a standard undergraduate curriculum. Students entering chiropractic college should expect to dedicate more than 60 hours a week to the study of chiropractic.

Enrollment Standards (Prerequisites to Enrolling in Chiropractic Colleges in the United States)

The Council on Chiropractic Education (CCE) provides accreditation, oversight, and guidance to the programs in the United States. It is also the responsibility of the CCE to outline the minimum educational requirements for acceptance to these programs. Until recently, the standards prescribed by the accrediting body were specific and rigid, including a full academic year of life and physical science: biology, general chemistry, organic chemistry, and physics, each with corresponding laboratory components. Although these standards existed for many years, there was no formal work done by the CCE or the chiropractic colleges themselves to evaluate if those requirements provided the best preparation for incoming students or if they were necessary at all for the successful completion of the degree.

In an effort to allow chiropractic colleges additional flexibility in reviewing candidates for admission, the standards were rewritten in 2013. The current minimum standards include no less than 90 semester hours of college-level coursework, including no less than 24 hours of life and physical science credits. Half of these courses must have a corresponding laboratory component. Additionally, students must have achieved no less than a 3.0 grade point average on a 4.0 scale for the required 90 hours. These are minimum standards; individual chiropractic colleges are able to publish standards that set the entrance bar higher than those listed above.

Historically, this type of admission standard has been met through the student completing coursework at a two- or four-year institution. Traditionally, majors or courses of study for students entering chiropractic programs follow those of other health professions: biology, chemistry, or premedical. However, with the increased flexibility in standards, chiropractic colleges are now attracting more students with majors in the movement sciences, such as kinesiology and athletic training. These students have typically not completed full academic years of study in the four science areas listed above but do meet the 24-hour science requirement that is a part of current standards. Further, the hands-on nature of these types of degree programs prepare students well for a degree in chiropractic.

While these standards seem fairly rigid, individual chiropractic colleges are able to evaluate candidates in comparison to the rigorousness of the corresponding program of study. They have some flexibility in reviewing candidates who fall outside of the standards listed above, who have grade point averages below the 3.0 minimum, or who have less than the required 24 hours of science. This change in admissions standards has allowed students with unconventional backgrounds to enter chiropractic college without the burden of additional undergraduate coursework. When reviewing candidates with nontraditional backgrounds, the CCE provides this guidance to colleges: "The admissions policies and practices are documented and designed to ensure that admitted students possess the academic and personal attributes for success in developing the skills, knowledge sets, attitudes and behavior that are necessary to succeed in the rigors of the academic program and pass the exams necessary to obtain a license to practice, and to perform as a knowledgeable, skillful, caring, and ethical Doctor of Chiropractic capable of best serving the public and the chiropractic profession" (Council on Chiropractic Education 2013). Students with majors in music, philosophy, business, or other nonscience-based degrees have been successfully admitted to chiropractic college using the more flexible standards.

Because of each chiropractic institution's interpretation of these standards, as well as the variations in the rigor of the individual programs, prospective students may find when applying to several programs that an offer of admission is provided by one institution, whereas another institution may require that the student complete additional preparatory coursework to be accepted.

Completing the Prerequisites

Students have many options for completing the coursework to prepare for chiropractic college. Students completing prerequisite coursework at community colleges may be able to complete a bachelor's degree concurrently with the chiropractic degree. This option allows students to complete 90 semester hours of specific coursework at the community-college level before enrolling in the chiropractic program. Students should investigate this option when starting community college, coordinating with potential chiropractic programs to ensure accurate degree planning.

In addition to the bachelor's degree completion program mentioned above, four-year undergraduate institutions have entered into partnerships with various chiropractic colleges. These partnerships allow students to complete three years of coursework at the undergraduate institution and spend their fourth undergraduate year completing the first year in the chiropractic program. This fourth year then transfers back to the undergraduate institution, and the student earns a bachelor's degree from the undergraduate institution. This popular option allows students to receive a bachelor's degree from a "home" institution as well as to complete the doctor of chiropractic program. These programs are often labeled "3+1" or "3+3" programs. Students interested in this option should contact the chiropractic college prior to the freshman year of undergraduate education to verify the participating institutions and the appropriate degree program at that institution.

Students should also coordinate any prerequisite courses needed with the chiropractic college of their choice. Often, undergraduate preparatory coursework is offered through the chiropractic institution or a partner school. The curriculum of these courses is designed to prepare students for the rigors of a chiropractic program. Chiropractic institutions around the country offer options in this area in accelerated, on-campus, and even online formats.

Application Criteria

Unlike other health professions, chiropractic does not use a common application or an application service to evaluate candidates. Students must complete an application for each individual college. Each institution will detail items required for the application in addition to all postsecondary academic transcripts, letters of recommendation, personal essay or statement of intent, and a personal interview. Students should contact the admissions office of institutions they are interested in to receive the full details of the application.

The chiropractic colleges' decision to not use a common application has both benefits and drawbacks to prospective students. On the positive side, students are able to form close relationships with admissions professionals at their chosen schools. This can help if students need to explain anomalies in their background or experience that may not be properly conveyed through the common application system. However, on the negative side, because of the lack of a centralized repository for application information, there are no data available to definitively outline the backgrounds of students entering the chiropractic profession. Chiropractic institutions are not required to provide details on applicants or admitted students' academic backgrounds. Therefore, we do not have true data on numbers of applications or admitted students across the profession.

Making an Informed Decision

The lack of entrance data on acceptance rates can leave students feeling uninformed about how to approach their desired campuses. However, this does not mean the process of assessing campuses is more difficult for prospective students. Prospective students can access a wealth of information about chiropractic programs on the individual colleges' websites, including the schools' approach to the teaching of chiropractic as well as the profession overall. Websites include videos and pictures, so prospective students can see how the campus looks, its overall size, and the metropolitan area in which it is located.

To further assist prospective students in making an informed decision about a chiropractic college, most campuses provide a formal visit program on weekdays and extended weekend visits throughout the year. Typically, these programs allow prospective students to interact with admissions staff, have their questions answered, and spend time with current students and faculty.

Many chiropractic colleges connect prospective students with practicing alumni in their area, allowing aspiring students to shadow local doctors and get answers to questions about the profession firsthand.

Financing a Chiropractic Education

Tuition at chiropractic colleges ranges from $20,000 to $25,000 per academic year, with the total tuition cost of the degree ranging from $100,000 to $130,000. Additionally, students are expected to purchase textbooks, supplies, and basic diagnostic instruments. This cost can range from $700 to $2,000 in some terms, depending on the books and equipment required. Finally, living expenses can be an important factor in determining the overall cost. As most chiropractic colleges do not offer dormitory-style housing, students will typically seek housing in apartments near campus (either by themselves or shared with other students) and be responsible for food expenses and travel to and from campus. The total cost to attend a college will be significantly impacted by the student's living expenses.

Chiropractic colleges in the United States are able to offer federal financial aid to eligible students. Because chiropractic college is considered a graduate-level program, students applying for aid are considered independent students, regardless of how they are claimed on their parents' taxes.

The process begins with completion of the Free Application for Student Aid (FAFSA), which is the first step for any student to determine eligibility for federal financial aid. The FAFSA is completed annually while the student is in school to determine initial and continued eligibility.

Current limits allow a student to borrow $33,000 per academic year in direct unsubsidized Stafford loans. This limit will be divided over semesters, trimesters, or quarters, depending on the academic calendar of the college. Typically, federal student aid is applied first toward any charges incurred at the college or university. Any excess funds are returned to the student in the form of a refund; this refund amount can then be used to pay for living expenses.

Students are able to borrow an aggregate maximum of $224,000 in Stafford student loans. This aggregate amount takes into consideration Stafford loans, both subsidized and unsubsidized, that have been previously borrowed at undergraduate and graduate levels. Subsidized Stafford loans are only available to undergraduate students, and the government pays the interest on these loans for the student in certain scenarios. Direct unsubsidized loans begin accruing interest from the time the loan is disbursed; many students choose to defer the interest and not pay it while they are in school.

If the cost of tuition is close to or exceeds the allowable limit for direct unsubsidized Stafford loans, additional financial aid dollars can be sought in the form of credit-based loans. There are several options for this type of funding. In addition to the credit evaluation, a cosigner may be required. Interest rates charged for these types of loans tend to be higher, so students are strongly encouraged to carefully evaluate whether they can pay for school and living expenses without using credit-based loans.

Applying for federal financial aid (completion of the FAFSA) can also give students the opportunity to pursue federal work-study employment. These opportunities are managed by the chiropractic college, and hourly rates of pay are determined by the type of work being performed.

Scholarships for chiropractic students are typically specific to the institution. As the scholarships are often funded by donors, eligibility requirements can vary greatly. Scholarship criteria will usually focus on the student's financial need and academic ability. Additionally, scholarships can also be awarded for students from a particular region of the country or with a particular path to the chiropractic profession (second-career students or single parents, for example). Financial aid offices often report that they have few scholarship applications to review, probably due to the busy nature of the curriculum. So students are always encouraged to apply for any and all scholarships they're eligible for as a great way to offset the overall cost of the education.

Chiropractic Students' Perceptions of Chiropractic College

Five students from four countries (Australia, Canada, the United Kingdom, and the United States) shared their journeys to chiropractic college and their experiences there. Yoshi is a student at RMIT in Australia; Melissa is a student at Canadian Memorial Chiropractic College in Toronto, Canada; Julie, James, and Sharee are students at BPP University in the U.K.; and Raven is a student at Texas Chiropractic College in the United States.

When asked, "How did you decide to become a chiropractor?" students identified factors such as personal experience of the powerful effects of chiropractic and an interest in helping people, especially through natural methods.

> In my early adolescence, I suffered from a TMJ [temporomandibular joint] issue, which was highly debilitating and stressful. After a couple of visits

to a chiropractic clinic, I was pain free and felt more confident and present within myself. It was quite amazing how gentle the technique was and how quickly the results ensued. As I came toward the end of my final high school years, I decided that I would become a chiropractor. (*Yoshi, Australia*)

During my master's degree, I realized that I wanted to pursue the health care field but needed to figure out which avenue to take. I had seen a chiropractor due to chronic and debilitating back pain during my varsity soccer career and was pain free as a result. In addition, I had taken a health and injury biomechanics course that was taught by a chiropractor and researcher. Both of these experiences, as well as the content of the course I took, made me pursue chiropractic. (*Melissa, Canada*)

I was having some health issues and a colleague suggested I visit a chiropractor. His belief and knowledge of chiropractic was powerful. I underwent an intensive course of care, which helped me greatly. Then I was fortunate to have the opportunity to work with him in his office as a clinic assistant, where I saw the powerful healing that clients were going through. I realized that I would have to become a practitioner and be able to help serve people myself. (*Julie, U.K.*)

Having worked in human resources for over 20 years, I regularly came into contact with people who were not happy in their job but didn't know what they wanted to do. During a period of reflection in 2005 after our son passed away, it suddenly came to me that I wanted to work in a job where I could help others whilst doing something that I believed in. I am now in my 40s, and experience has shown me how fragile life can be and how precious good health is. Now in my final year and about to graduate in a few months, I feel privileged and proud to think that I will soon be able to call myself a chiropractor! I can't wait! (*Sharee, U.K.*)

I first found out about chiropractic after having survived a serious illness in hospital. I was initially very skeptical but went to the chiropractor aiming to fix my residual low back pain. I realized soon after that my skepticism was misplaced and chiropractic could do so much more than I had initially given it credit for. I felt amazing after just one session. As a result of feeling so wonderfully different, I wanted to know more about why it worked and how it seemed to affect more than just my low back pain! (*James, U.K.*)

When working in a pharmacy, I saw how many patients were on multiple medications. Although some medications are needed, many can be avoided through proper diet and healthy living. As a health screener at the pharmacy, I met many patients who had constant pain. Also, I met a few patients who were addicted to their medications. To help, I began looking up alternate ways, other than medicine, to help them cope with the pain and I stumbled upon chiropractic. I did my research and before I knew it I had applied to Texas Chiropractic College. *(Raven, United States)*

Students found some unexpected—and some expected—benefits and challenges after entering their chiropractic training.

Chiropractic college was significantly more intense that I initially envisioned. The heavy emphasis on neurology, anatomy, and physiology is something that is hugely overwhelming. Exam times were always stressful as there were always more than seven or eight exams, both regular exams and practical exams. *(Yoshi, Australia)*

Chiropractic was essentially what I expected it to be academically. Socially, there were definitely some surprises due to the long hours spent with the same people. I was surprised at the amount of "drama"! *(Melissa, Canada)*

Was delighted to find such wonderful teachers who are all so dedicated to chiropractic. *(Julie, U.K.)*

I had never been to college or university before, so I was very apprehensive to start. I was worried about the level of academia, time commitments, and I was also nervous about whether I would "fit in." The course structure, level of academia, and time commitment required were pretty much what I expected, but I did not expect to establish the friendships that I have with my peers. We are such a diverse group but have all bonded and supported each other all the way. I am going to miss them all. *(Sharee, U.K.)*

I was constantly surprised at chiropractic college. A huge part of why I was surprised was because I kept realizing just how much our general perceptions of health and healing in society are not always correct. *(James, U.K.)*

School is tough. That is the only way to describe it, but I know it will pay off when I see improvement in my future patients' health. This is exactly what I expected. *(Raven, United States)*

When asked, "How did your experience in chiropractic college change you?" all the students found chiropractic college fostered deep personal growth.

The last five years at chiropractic college have been full of ups and downs and a lot of self-reflection and realization. There have been times when I've wanted to leave the program due to its intense nature, have questioned whether chiropractic even works and whether I even want to become a chiropractor. With the friends I've made within the program as well as opportunities externally, I've been fortunate enough to make connections with students and practitioners all over the world. As such, this has given me a greater perspective of what chiropractic is globally and through different generations. *(Yoshi, Australia)*

My experience in chiropractic college has had a profound effect on me as a person. I find that I am more self-aware and so am constantly trying to present myself in a positive, open, and friendly manner. I am also more patient, a better listener, and am better at thinking on my feet. My confidence has grown significantly as a result of this program as well as interacting with patients throughout my clinical term. *(Melissa, Canada)*

It has been a roller coaster of emotions and challenges. Have bonded with some lovely people. I have learnt a lot about myself, what I'm capable of. *(Julie, U.K.)*

My experience in college has changed me in so many ways, and I am not the same person that I was four years ago! I am much more open and keen to learn new things—I don't think I will ever stop learning! My perception of "good health" is totally different now too. It's not simply the absence of disease that I aspire to for good health. *(Sharee, U.K.)*

My experience in chiropractic college changed everything about me. Before I joined the college, I trained as a lawyer and had developed all the traits that lawyers tend to. I found not only my knowledge of chiropractic developed but also I unwound, grew as a person, and developed a completely different level of confidence in all that I do. *(James, U.K.)*

First and most importantly, I am extremely disciplined. I learned the word "no," meaning I had to tell myself what was not important and limit those distractors. *(Raven, United States)*

The students were excited about the future for which their training has prepared them expressed many plans and goals, such as:

• to travel the world for a couple of months before beginning work as a chiropractor. Next semester we commence fieldwork with practitioners out in the field, a clinical internship, for eight weeks. Based on the different clinics and chiropractors I work with, I will decide whether or not to work in Australia. I'm looking to work in rural areas away from the cities as they seem to be saturated with chiropractors here. I would love to work internationally whilst I build up my clinical experience and confidence. Eventually, I'd love to open a multidisciplinary practice with holistic medical physicians, naturopaths, Chinese medicine practitioners, physiotherapists, and dieticians. *(Yoshi, Australia)*

- to make a difference in the way athletic development is perceived or how children are trained early on in their athletic career. Part of this dream is becoming a sports fellow, and I will begin the process this fall as a sports science resident at CMCC. *(Melissa, Canada)*

- to be the best chiropractor I possibly can, keep improving my skills, and help to educate people about the gift and importance of regular chiropractic care. *(Julie, U.K.)*

- to come home at the end of each day and feel I have helped my clients—not just in relieving pain but in achieving good health. Longer term, I would love to inspire the next generation of chiropractors. *(Sharee, U.K.)*

- to provide chiropractic care to a wider range of people and be able to raise awareness and support chiropractic in improving the health and well-being of the nation. If chiropractic has changed my life so much for the better, it will and can for others. *(James, U.K.)*

- to work in the VA [Veterans Administration] as a chiropractor. Eventually, I would like to open an evenings and weekends practice that would focus on sports (because of my interest in kinesiology and sports studies). *(Raven, United States)*

Finally, they each gave advice to students who are considering a career in chiropractic.

The friendships and opportunities that have come about as a result of studying chiropractic are immeasurable. Five years initially seemed like a long time, but it has flown by very quickly. Speaking to friends who study in other institutions, it really is noticeable how supportive our cohort is. *(Yoshi, Australia)*

Make sure you are passionate. If you love what you are learning, you will learn more and you will be better. This profession is one where you are constantly learning and growing; be open to that change, growth, and development. Be ready to work hard, but know that it is all worth it in the end because chiropractic is a profession of passion, of growth, and of satisfaction. You will be amazed at what you can do with your hands. *(Melissa, Canada)*

I would encourage anyone, any age to consider a career in chiropractic. Although I took the full-time four-year pathway, to be able to study in the five-year program is just an extraordinary opportunity for the more mature applicant to be able to change their direction and have the chance to train for this great career. *(Julie, U.K.)*

I would say, "Go for it!" There is a choice of colleges and courses, so find the one that suits you. It is a career where you will work with people, help others, and you can set up your own business, or you can work as part of a team within a practice. It is also a career where you can specialize in different techniques, fields (e.g., pediatrics), and therapies. You never stop learning! *(Sharee, U.K.)*

Don't put it off! Joining the chiropractic profession was one of the best decisions I have ever made, and I most certainly do not look back at the old me. The best advice I'd give is to go to a chiropractor and experience it yourself. If you like what you see and feel and want to know more, apply! Speaking to your chiropractor can also help in gaining additional information and support as you are going through your training. The chiropractic profession is like a big family—if you need help or support all you need to do is ask! It is natural to worry about whether we will be able to cope with a new course or career, but the path to success and self-empowerment is most certainly by taking yourself out of your initial comfort zone and taking each step as it comes. I worried when I signed up (I didn't even know if I could learn any new information), but only a few short years later I gained a first-class degree, gained professional respect with both members of the public and my peers, and have just set up my own clinic. It's well worth signing up to! *(James, U.K.)*

Chiropractors focus on the well-being of their patient. They are interested in health and recovery, rather than hiding symptoms with prescriptions that would lead to other problems. If you truly want to help your patient, I believe chiropractic is the best way to go! *(Raven, United States)*

CHAPTER FOUR

Chiropractic Academic Education

Stefanie Krupp, DC, MS; Ruth Sandefur, DC, PhD; and Rachael Pandzik, DC

This chapter explores the core academic curriculum common across chiropractic institutions in the United States as well as what makes an academic program distinct. The evolution of chiropractic education provides context for historical influences and curriculum development occurring across institutions, which also generates a framework to understand the current trends in health science education. The chapter concludes with supplementary resources provided by chiropractic institutions that complement and support the academic content.

Accredited chiropractic programs in the United States lead to a doctor of chiropractic (DC) degree. These four-year professional programs may be structured in a semester, trimester, or quarter system depending on the institution, with new cohorts beginning in every, or almost every, term. Chiropractic programs are referred to as "lock-step," meaning every student takes the same courses at the same point in their curricular progression. Offering year-round courses, some programs appear accelerated but often can accommodate breaks or modified schedules, allowing students to customize their pace. Programs are full time with a vigorous course load. Because of the manner in which content builds and the hands-on clinical nature of chiropractic, successful mastery and integration of course content is essential. This may require substantial out-of-class study time and use of institutional resources such as the library, tutoring programs, and open lab hours.

The standard chiropractic curriculum covers the following topics:[1]

- anatomy
- cell and systems physiology
- histology
- embryology/developmental anatomy
- biochemistry
- microbiology
- neuroscience and clinical neurology
- pathology and pathophysiology
- physical, clinical, and laboratory procedures and diagnosis
- diagnostic imaging procedures, technology, and diagnosis; radiology report writing
- biomechanics, spinal and extremity analysis, including gait and posture
- orthopedic and neurological examination and diagnosis
- principles and practice of chiropractic
- chiropractic adjustive techniques
- physiotherapy (rehabilitation and adjunctive procedures)
- differential diagnosis and general diagnosis
- clinical decision making, documentation, and diagnostic coding
- treatment plans, patient outcomes, and prognosis
- information literacy, research methods, evidence-based practice principles
- special populations, including pediatrics, geriatrics, and women's health
- first-aid and emergency procedures
- public health
- dermatology
- psychology
- toxicology and pharmacology
- nutrition science, clinical nutrition, wellness and lifestyle counseling
- ethics, jurisprudence, and practice management, including billing and coding
- communication and patient education

At present, chiropractic college curricula across the United States are fairly similar, primarily due to the strong influence of accreditation standards and the national board examinations testing specific content knowledge and skill sets. Curricula can generally be organized into two main areas of study: basic sciences and clinical sciences. Clinical sciences include chiropractic practice (also referred to as chiropractic sciences or chiropractic technique) and associated clinical practice topics, such as practice management and public health; although often chiropractic practice and associated clinical practice topics may be considered separate and distinct from clinical science content. Embedded in these main content areas are evidenced-based (EBP) or evidence-informed (EIP) practice, interprofessional education (IPE) and integrative practice, professionalism, and communication. Clinical internships serve as capstone experiences of the professional degree (covered in Chapter 5). Often prior to entering various phases of the clinical environment, students may be required to pass written and practical examinations, called objective structured clinical examinations (OSCEs). OSCEs are designed to evaluate students to ensure they possess the clinical competency necessary to enter into patient care and/or to graduate.

For programs outside of the United States, information can be obtained through universities and institutions offering chiropractic education as well as through national licensing boards, chiropractic associations, and the International Board of Chiropractic Examiners (IBCE). Canada has its own series of board examinations offered through the Canadian Chiropractic Examining Board (CCEB), which are generally similar in content and format to the national board exams in the United States. Foreign countries may accept degrees and board certifications from the United States for licensure.

Historical Context of Chiropractic Education

The birth of chiropractic in the United States dates back to September 18, 1895, when the practice was founded by Daniel David (D. D.) Palmer. Early developers of the chiropractic profession were eager to share it with others. Thus, chiropractic schools began to spring up around the country in the early 1900s.[2] In the first half of the 20th century, chiropractic colleges primarily used instructional content developed by the respective college leaders and instructors. Because chiropractic was based on a new health care paradigm of a conservative and holistic model of care, some information contained in traditional medical texts was not suitable. In addition, this new profession had yet to publish chiropractic science textbooks. Presidents or founders often exerted influence upon their educational programs, instilling their own philosophy, beliefs, and techniques.

This led to differences among colleges and their curricula, often serving as the basis for minor rivalries.[3]

As the chiropractic colleges evolved, the basic science curriculum was largely taught from unaltered medical texts used in traditional medical programs. In the chiropractic and clinical sciences, even though a number of courses were still being taught from instructors' notes, many began incorporating medical texts. To remain viable, it was imperative that chiropractors be trained to recognize conditions requiring immediate medical intervention. These included conditions that were unlikely to respond to conservative care, or those simply considered "off-limits" for chiropractors to treat (such as cancer) and that require referral to an appropriate physician.

Starting in the early 1960s, the chiropractic college curriculum became a focus of the American Chiropractic Association (ACA).[4] The ACA, formed in 1963, is the largest professional organization representing chiropractors in the United States. The ACA proposed a curriculum that included more diagnosis- and medical-oriented subjects in order to lead the profession toward a more evidence-based and less philosophical stance.[4] However, opponents of the ACA claimed the emphasis on scientific approaches was delving too far into the medical arena. Chiropractors have long fought to be recognized as distinct from medical doctors, and the incorporation of similar curricula and texts was perceived to undermine those efforts.

The ACA attention and effort was instrumental in establishing a government-recognized accrediting agency charged with overseeing and ensuring the quality of chiropractic education. The Council on Chiropractic Education (CCE) was recognized by the U.S. Department of Education in 1974, and it became the professional accrediting agency for U.S. chiropractic educational programs. Currently, all U.S. chiropractic colleges are accredited by the CCE. The curriculum and most other functions of chiropractic colleges are monitored with cyclic review and reaccreditation periods by the CCE, in addition to the regional higher education accrediting associations in the United States.[5]

An early but adverse effect of gaining CCE accreditation was the limitation that colleges could no longer enroll students in night classes. This excluded many adult learners who desired a career change while still working full time. Preprofessional requirements for matriculation became more robust, further narrowing the field of prospective students. Additionally, CCE demanded significant upgrades to basic sciences courses as well as requiring instructors to hold advanced degrees in their subject area of instruction, such as a PhD, or at least a master's degree, with PhDs outnumbering master's degree faculty. Colleges had to employ basic scientists and compete with salaries offered by medical schools. Fortunately, students attending programs accredited by CCE were now eligible for government-supported student loans, making chiropractic programs more financially attainable for many students.

Another influence on the chiropractic college curriculum was the advent of the National Board of Chiropractic Examiners (NBCE), established in 1963. Prior to this, the practice of chiropractic was regulated on a state-by-state basis, each issuing licenses using separate criteria and testing practices. The NBCE aimed to provide testing that would allow students who passed a series of structured tests the opportunity to obtain a license in any state.[5] Acceptance by individual states was a gradual process, and as of today, all 50 states accept the NBCE exams as a criterion for licensure, although many states have separate jurisprudence or other exams as additional requirements.

Because all chiropractic graduates take the same national board exams and have the same professional accreditation body, the curriculum across U.S. chiropractic colleges is strikingly similar. This phenomenon is fairly standard across the spectrum of professional schools. Medical, dental, and law programs teach to their respective licensing exams. Student pass rates of licensing exams are used as a recruitment tool, and, in some instances, ongoing accreditation depends on these pass rates. Studies have compared the curriculum of chiropractic colleges with those of medical schools.[6] Considering the diverse paradigms of these two health care professions, the similarities in curricula are striking. This is primarily because the basic sciences (anatomy, physiology, histology, etc.) and clinical diagnosis are fundamental to all professional health care professions, and these subjects comprise a large portion of the curriculum.

Historically, the difference between the medical and chiropractic curricula has been considerable. When chiropractic was established as a profession, it was presented as an antithesis to the invasive medical procedures of the day. Chiropractic, based on the principles of the self-healing capabilities of the human body, stipulated that no foreign substances would be introduced into the body, including surgical instruments and pharmaceuticals. As summarized in *Job Analysis of Chiropractic*,[7] "Chiropractic also is based on the premise that the body is capable of achieving and maintaining health through its own natural recuperative powers, provided it receives the necessary health maintenance components, including proper food, water, adequate rest, exercise, clean air, adequate nutrition and a properly functioning nervous system."

The foundation of chiropractic sciences is the biomechanical, neurological, and philosophical understanding as it applies to the chiropractic adjustment. The hallmark chiropractic treatment method, termed an "adjustment" or "manipulation," proposes to manually remove interference with nerve flow to affected parts of the body in order to facilitate the body's natural healing process. Traditionally, chiropractic theories have posited that manipulation is intended to remove "subluxations" in the spine.[8] The term "subluxation" (also known as "the vertebral subluxation complex" [VSC], "joint fixation," or "restriction," among other terms) has been the single most vital, yet controversial, concept in the profession of chiropractic. Philosophy-oriented programs often choose the term "subluxation," whereas more moderate programs opt for "restriction" or "joint fixation." Many leaders in the profession recommend adopting standard terminology that would unite rather than divide the profession.[9]

Even after the changes to the chiropractic college curricula as a result of CCE and NBCE influences, a number of colleges continued to include, along with the science-based coursework, the original chiropractic paradigm presented by early educators. However, the opposition of philosophical to moderate viewpoints resulted in the formation of chiropractic "factions."[10] A universal agreement about the concept of subluxation still does not exist either within the chiropractic profession or the scientific community.[8] Nevertheless, in over 100 years of chiropractic's existence, millions of adjustments, many thousands of anecdotal success stories, and thousands upon thousands of satisfied patients have attested to the benefit of chiropractic treatment. The significance of the subluxation is apparent in all chiropractic curricula, however, since the chiropractic and clinical sciences fundamentally revolve around the detection and correction of subluxations. A recent study of practicing chiropractors in North America showed that a majority consider themselves to be occupying middle ground with respect to the opposing views of the traditional (philosophical) versus moderate chiropractic paradigm.[11]

Colleges choose which principles, techniques, and protocols to include in their curriculum. In the early days, college founders or presidents may have chosen techniques based on their particular bias or because the technique was their own discovery. Chiropractic techniques often came into being by the efforts of individual chiropractic practitioners. Practitioners who developed techniques did so by studying, often for years, the beneficial results of patients under their care. These practitioners shared their findings by teaching classes so other chiropractors could learn their methods. Techniques were sometimes named for the originator. Over the years, a large number of techniques were developed, and many of them have gathered large groups of dedicated supporters.[7] The popularity of a technique was often a factor in whether it was included in a college's curriculum. Colleges depended on practitioners to refer students to their institutions, and practitioners were more likely to refer students to a college that taught their preferred methods or techniques. A few colleges opted for more generic techniques not associated with a particular technique originator. Though it may appear that the number of hours devoted to teaching technique courses varies between institutions, the course names may not fully disclose the actual content.[12]

A discussion about the chiropractic college curriculum would not be complete without mentioning the role of teaching strategies and philosophy, termed "pedagogy" or "andragogy." In the early days of chiropractic education, instruction was provided by chiropractors whose desire was to pass their knowledge and skills on to others, helping to advance the profession. Those instructors most likely had not received training in teaching methods and may not have taken any college coursework other than the chiropractic curriculum. Improvements brought about by the CCE in the mid-1970s included requirements about the qualifications and credentials of instructors. Colleges were to give priority to DC faculty holding additional credentials and degrees. For example, specialty courses, such as radiology, were to be taught by credentialed DCs holding additional board certifications sanctioned by the ACA. The CCE also encouraged institutions to present faculty in-service programs similar to those offered to public institution educators, to support faculty attendance at higher education conferences, and to provide support for faculty wishing to advance their teaching careers by enrolling in advanced degree programs. These measures were designed to increase the ability of chiropractic instructors to effectively teach in the chiropractic program.

Chiropractic colleges monitor and update curriculum as necessary to keep in accordance with reaccreditation requirements and improve the student experience. Current trends in health science education are fostering the transition of programs to competency-based education. A competency-based approach is centered on the assessment of student knowledge and skillful performance, rather than solely achieving passing grades and gaining content exposure. Paired with timely feedback, the integration of knowledge across stages of training provides a link between assessments and practice that can further enhance student academic and professional development.[13] Course and learning objectives and corresponding assessments not only focus on the demonstration of knowledge but also prompt active and responsive learning. Excellent clinical reasoning and critical-thinking skills are essential for practicing doctors to quickly identify, respond to, and properly manage all types of patient conditions. Chiropractic education provides the foundation student doctors need to apply their knowledge and skills in a clinical setting, first in a mentored setting during clinical internship experiences and, ultimately, independently in clinical practice.

Core Chiropractic Academic Curriculum

Doctor of chiropractic programs prepare graduates for health care practice as portal-of-entry providers. Chiropractic programs have extensive lecture and laboratory hours for basic and clinical sciences and chiropractic technique, which account for the significant amount of in-class time for the chiropractic programs in the United States. As mentioned in the previous section, content in chiropractic colleges is driven by a variety of factors, such as CCE requirements, regional accreditation standards, national board examination content, institutional mission and philosophy, and scope of practice. This section focuses on the commonalities of chiropractic curricula.

Four main areas of study (basic sciences, clinical sciences, chiropractic practice, and associated clinical practice) will be covered as they relate to the national board examinations necessary for licensure in the United States. Chiropractic program curricula may closely follow the National Board of Chiropractic Examiners (NBCE) Part I through IV exams. Though the NBCE exam content provides structure to this chapter, this is not an exhaustive course and topic review for every institution. Course information can be found in the academic catalogs for each institution.

In addition to reviewing the four main areas of study, physiotherapy, chiropractic technique, and elective offerings will be covered in their respective sections. In the latter half of the curriculum, much of the content builds on the foundational concepts introduced earlier in the chiropractic program. This is reflected in the emphasis on clinical reasoning and case-based questions of the national board exam Parts III and IV and in the capstone clinical internship courses at each institution. *Clinical internship curriculum, requirements, and experiences are detailed in Chapter 5.*

Basic Sciences

The basic sciences coursework includes anatomy, physiology, neuroscience, biochemistry, histology, microbiology, pathophysiology, and embryology. Basic science education creates the foundation to understand the complexity of the structure and functions of the human body. Content is often covered in terms of normal structure and function, followed by abnormal or dysfunctional variations. Though the detail at a cellular level may overwhelm many students, this portion of the curriculum resurfaces throughout the clinical sciences in understanding human disease and patient presentation of signs and symptoms. Chiropractic follows a holistic model where the goal of patient care is to restore optimal function or optimal health, so understanding normal anatomy and physiology is as important as recognizing and understanding the expansive array of dysfunctional conditions.

The basic science subject areas are tested primarily on Part I of the NBCE examinations but are also interwoven throughout later exams. Part I board examinations are generally taken in the second year of full-time enrollment in an eligible chiropractic college program and require registrar approval. The NBCE groups the basic sciences into the following content areas: general anatomy, spinal anatomy, physiology, biochemistry, pathology, and microbiology.

Anatomy includes two overarching topic areas: general anatomy and spinal anatomy (neuroanatomy). This content may be integrated into four or more courses in the first year of study, depending on the institution. General anatomy encompasses anatomical terminology and topographic anatomy, which is the study of the regions of the body and the relationships between various structures, such as muscles, nerves, and blood vessels in the region. The main regions covered are the head, neck, back, thorax, abdomen, pelvis, and upper and lower limbs.

These regions are explored in terms of the bones (osteology), joints (arthrology), muscles (myology), ligaments and connective tissues (syndesmology), as well as related organ systems, including the cardiovascular, lymphatic, digestive, respiratory, urogenital, integumentary, and endocrine systems. For each region and system, both the histology (the microscopic anatomy of cells and tissues) and the developmental anatomy (the structural changes that take place from fertilization to maturity) are covered. Lecture content is explored in the laboratory with the use of human cadavers, specimens, and anatomical models, with students actively participating in structured dissections of the cadaver.

Spinal anatomy, or neuroanatomy, is a separate section from general anatomy for the NBCE Part I examinations. The content includes neuroscience as well as the osteology (study of bones), myology (study of muscles), arthrology (study of joints), syndesmology (study of ligaments), and developmental anatomy of the axial skeleton (bones of the skull and trunk, including the spine). Neuroscience has four main subtopics: the central nervous system (CNS), the peripheral nervous system (PNS), the autonomic nervous system (ANS), and special senses, such as hearing (audition), balance (equilibrium), vision, taste (gustation), and smell (olfaction). The CNS comprises the brain and spinal cord and refers to the nerve tissues that control most of the activities of the mind and body. The PNS consists of the nerve tissues outside of the brain and spinal cord, predominantly the sensory and motor neurons running from the CNS to muscles, organs, and glands. Involuntary nervous system activity, such as breathing, heart rate, pupil constriction and dilation, and stress response ("fight or flight") is controlled by the ANS, which is further divided into sympathetic and parasympathetic divisions. This particular material has significant implications on understanding the mechanisms and effects of chiropractic treatment on the nervous system.

Physiology courses are offered in the first year of chiropractic programs in conjunction with anatomy and are a prerequisite to pathology courses. The physiology section of the NBCE Part I examination includes the following systems: neuromusculoskeletal, cardiorespiratory, renal and fluid balance, gastrointestinal, reproductive, and endocrine.

Where anatomy is focused primarily on structure and development, physiology is focused on function. By understanding normal expected function from a cellular to a system level, chiropractic students learn how cells and tissues are intimately dependent yet adaptable in order to sustain life. One example of a normal adaptation is the physiological effects of exercise. Though many of these concepts are covered at the system level, students most often learn the impact of these systems on each other when one is not functioning properly, which relates to the next topic, pathology.

Pathology is the medical science focused on disease—the deviation from the healthy, normal, efficient structural and functional conditions. The term comes from the Greek *pathos*, which means "suffering," and *-logia*, which means "study." The fundamentals of pathology covered on the Part I NBCE examination include disease at the cellular level, inflammation and repair, neoplasia (cancer or uncontrolled cellular growth), and hemodynamic disorders (dysfunction in blood flow and thus the balances of fluid and oxygen in the body). Also included in pathology curricula and the pathology section of the NBCE are genetic and congenital disorders, immune system disorders, environmental and nutritional diseases, musculoskeletal and nervous system disorders, and disorders of the cardiovascular, gastrointestinal, respiratory, genitourinary, endocrine, blood, and lymphatic systems.

Pathology coursework typically follows courses in anatomy, physiology, histology, and embryology. Concepts of pathology are used later in the curriculum through physical and laboratory diagnosis, differential diagnosis, and diagnostic imaging courses.

Biochemistry, the study of chemical processes and characteristics in living organisms, comprises its own section of Part I of the NBCE exam and is often covered in multiple courses. Biochemistry topics include food sources, digestion, metabolism, structure, properties, function, and transport and storage of macronutrients (carbohydrates, fats, and proteins) and micronutrients (vitamins and minerals). Discussed within these topics are enzymes, hormones, nucleotides, and nucleic acids. Another key concept in biochemistry is biochemical energetics, which is how the body produces and stores energy. Biochemical energetics involves the Krebs cycle, oxidation-reduction reactions, oxidative phosphorylation, and electron transport systems. This information is particularly useful in chiropractic practice to help explain energy (and fatigue) and nutrients to support healing processes. These courses prepare students for required nutrition courses that cover material related to the systems of the body and chronic diseases.

The last section of Part I is microbiology, which includes the physiology, cell biology, biochemistry, ecology, evolution, and clinical aspects of microorganisms and their effects on other living organisms. Microbiology courses cover the structural and biochemical characteristics, resistance, genetics, immunology, and pathogenicity of bacteria, viruses and prions, fungi, and parasites. Communicable and infectious diseases, reservoirs of infection, modes of transmission, and immunization and vaccination are also reviewed, along with public health concepts like epidemiology and disease control. Microbiology and public health courses provide a general introduction to public health initiatives that the majority of health professions incorporate into their daily practices. They also provide context and framework to many of the concepts touched on in pathology and diagnosis courses. Since chiropractors function within public health to report health issues that are tracked by government agencies, content also includes overviews of health agencies, reporting, monitoring, prevention, identification, and control methods for communicable disease and population health assessments.

Clinical Sciences

There are six main clinical science topic areas covered in the chiropractic program curriculum:

1. General diagnosis
2. Neuromusculoskeletal diagnosis
3. Diagnostic imaging

4. Principles of chiropractic
5. Chiropractic practice/technique
6. Associated clinical sciences

The first three will be addressed in this particular section. The latter are separated into a combined principles and practice section and an associated clinical sciences section, with instructional content and approaches for chiropractic technique further explained later in the chapter. These six topics are covered in Parts II to IV of the national board examinations, which are typically taken by students enrolled in their third or last year of a chiropractic program.

General diagnosis involves the identification of diseases and disorders based on history and examination findings. A patient history refers to questions that a health care provider asks patients in order to learn more about them and their condition. Patient visits typically begin with the patient being asked a series of questions to better understand why he or she has come for evaluation and treatment. History taking involves questions about the chief complaint of the patient (history of present illness) as well as family history, social history, current and past medical history, and a review of systems. A good history is essential in directing the examination portion of a patient visit. Many clues are given during the history that help a health care provider know what area to examine and to what extent. Included in examination procedures and findings are vital signs (blood pressure, pulse, temperature, etc.), inspection (observing the area), auscultation (listening to the area), percussion (tapping an area to determine hollow versus solid or fluid structures), and palpation (feeling the structure) of related areas. Examination may also include laboratory studies and interpretation. Laboratory studies cover urinalysis, hematology, chemistry, and serology and other special studies, like stool analysis and joint fluid analysis, that help identify internal disorders. Urinalysis examines the urine whereas hematology, chemistry, and serology all use blood samples to look at the composition and properties of various components of the blood, such as immune function. Though most chiropractors do not treat internal disorders, they must know how to identify them so they can refer a patient to the appropriate provider or facility.

General diagnosis is typically broken into regions covering head and neck, thorax (including heart and lungs), abdomen, and rectum. Instruction includes disorders of the eyes, ears, nose, throat, respiratory, cardiovascular, blood, lymph, gastrointestinal, genitourinary, endocrine, metabolic, and immune systems in addition to nutritional disorders and infectious diseases. Nutrition assessment and interventions are typically covered in a multicourse series.

Neuromusculoskeletal (NMS) diagnosis covers the spine and limbs, or extremities, and is a major focus of chiropractic education. There are particularly useful history questions that aid in NMS diagnosis, such as how the injury happened (mechanism), when it happened (onset), what it feels like (quality, severity, associated symptoms), and whether there were existing or prior injuries, among many others. NMS examination procedures include posture and gait analysis and orthopedic and neurological exams. Orthopedic exams are designed to help determine biomechanical or musculoskeletal pathologies. These exam procedures often re-create a patient's pain, which can aid in accurately diagnosing the patient's condition. Neurological exams can help identify neurological involvement and the specific component of the nervous system affected. The combination of the patient history with orthopedic and neurological examination findings help health care providers understand the mechanism and extent of the injury or dysfunction. The NMS history and examination findings provide a basis for the diagnoses of central and peripheral nervous system disorders, neurovascular disorders, muscular disorders, and bone and joint conditions.

Both general and neuromusculoskeletal diagnosis elements are typically split over multiple terms with courses in patient assessment and clinical science education. Students gain practice constructing differential diagnoses and clinical impressions through case scenarios and role play. Laboratory courses help students practice and improve their examination skills and efficiency. When students perform these exams on each other and take each other's history, they also learn how it feels to be a patient and can better understand how a patient may respond during those procedures. While students practice these skills on each other, some institutions also incorporate the use of trained actors, called standardized patients, to portray patients for history and examination procedures. Similar course material related to conditions and diagnosis may also be covered in diagnostic imaging, although that topic has its own section for national board examinations. There is some overlap between these courses, which reinforces key material and provides opportunity to reflect on the material from different perspectives.

Diagnostic imaging primarily focuses on radiographs and X-ray technology. Key content includes normal anatomy, reasons to order imaging (indications), imaging interpretation, diagnosis, and clinical impression. Radiology report writing is a key skill developed in these courses that is consistent across health care disciplines and helpful for future doctors to communicate findings in a logical and comprehensive manner. Clinical applications of special imaging, such as magnetic resonance imaging (MRI), computed tomography (CT), diagnostic ultrasound, and nuclear bone scans, are included in diagnostic imaging courses. Students in a chiropractic program learn about the history, physics, and principles of X-ray technology, including how images were traditionally generated on film.

Radiographic positioning and corresponding imaging equipment settings for all regions of the body are covered. Radiographic positioning is the proper preparation and setup of a patient before radiographs are taken. This is important not only for doctors who want to provide in-house imaging but also to provide correct interpretation when reading images taken at another facility, whether printed or digital. Other key content related to positioning includes radiologic protection for both the patient and doctor, image quality, and appropriate equipment handling. Describing and interpreting diagnostic imaging studies is an integral part of a chiropractic practice regardless of where the images are taken. Courses involving diagnostic imaging content are offered almost every term throughout a chiropractic program because the content is expansive and central to appropriate diagnosis and management of conditions presenting to a chiropractic office. Diagnostic imaging helps a chiropractor formulate treatment decisions, including when it is not appropriate to provide treatment to a patient and/or making a referral to another provider. Diagnostic imaging course content also helps reinforce material covered in other courses, connecting anatomy and spatial relationships to clinical reasoning.

Chiropractic Principles and Practice

Chiropractic principles form the foundation of the study of chiropractic practice and technique, which are all covered in Part II of the NBCE examination. The term "principles" refers to the historical and scientific foundation of chiropractic and its philosophical underpinnings. Anatomy, pathophysiology, and biomechanics are studied in relation to chiropractic practice. Additionally, the term "subluxation" is defined, generally as an altered or aberrant motion of a joint, historically referred to as a "bone out of place." The concept of subluxation is explored from various models, including but not limited to proprioceptive insult/somatosomatic reflex, neural compression/traction, visceral reflex, vascular insufficiency/trophic, neuroimmunomodulation, and biomechanical models. Potential mechanisms, or etiologies, of subluxations as well as the general effects of an adjustment or manipulation are reviewed. "Principles" courses identify and discuss key areas of debate in the chiropractic profession, including the use of the term "subluxation" and how that relates to the institution's philosophy.

Chiropractic practice topics build throughout the curriculum, with chiropractic technique courses serving as a cornerstone of this main content area. Chiropractic principles and practice topics are taught concurrently with basic science and diagnostic imaging courses, providing different perspectives on similar material. This enables students to visualize the body in all dimensions and layers. Technique courses typically start with palpation and psychomotor skills. Palpation refers to the use of the sense of touch for examination and diagnostic purposes. Psychomotor skills are the foundational movements that a doctor of chiropractic will use to deliver therapeutic adjustments, such as hand contacts, thrusts, or impulses and stances. These sensory skills are taught in a laboratory setting but often accompany lecture courses that discuss the landmarks, structure, and function of the spine and extremities, including biomechanics and tissue characteristics. Examination and treatment procedures are introduced, such as physical inspection, normal range of motion of the different body regions, and chiropractic adjustment positions. Students practice these skills on each other with the supervision and guidance of their laboratory instructor. More detail on different chiropractic techniques is discussed in the "Advanced Clinical Studies" section later in this chapter.

The chiropractic practice section of the Part II board examination encompasses the core subjects that permeate the daily practice of a chiropractor. These include spinal analysis and patient evaluation as well as chiropractic techniques and other modes of patient care. Chiropractic practice is also inclusive of community health and wellness as well as occupational and environmental health. Chiropractic practice evaluates the patient's current state of health as well as assessing issues such as lifestyle and genetic and environmental factors that influence overall health and well-being. Case history, observation findings, manual examination of the spine and extremities, and other diagnostic procedures through case management, home care, prevention, and rehabilitation comprise the key skill set obtained in a chiropractic program that translate directly to practice. Although Parts II and III are written examinations consisting of multiple-choice items, questions are structured to test the knowledge base and application of these concepts. The Part IV examination focuses on the performance of and critical thinking related to these skills.

The community health and wellness topics covered in chiropractic program curricula typically include U.S. public health organizations, Healthy

People initiatives (the national health promotion and disease prevention initiative in the United States that brings together individuals and agencies to improve health, quality of life, and life span and eliminate disparities for all Americans[14]), screening activities for health promotion, substance abuse, exercise and healthy diet, behavioral theories, lifestyle change, and wellness counseling. Complementing these topics are occupational and environmental health concepts, such as work-based health risks, worker protection and ergonomics, injury and violence, and the impact of environment on human health, including waste and pollution. Students also learn about integrative health care topics and how to form relationships with other health care providers.

Associated Clinical Topics

The remaining content on the Part II board examinations is considered "associated clinical sciences." This section spans coursework in dermatology, toxicology, pharmacology, emergency procedures, psychology, sexually transmitted diseases, women's health, gynecology and obstetrics, pediatrics, and geriatrics. Since chiropractors examine and contact a patient's skin, training in dermatology can give significant clinical information and even save a patient's life through early identification of cancerous skin lesions. Toxicology and pharmacology are incredibly useful in comanaging patients on medications, particularly in the identification of symptoms and side effects from toxic or pharmacological agents. Awareness and certification in emergency procedures, such as basic life support, including cardiopulmonary resuscitation (CPR) and first aid, are essential for health care providers and may be crucial for the well-being of a patient.

Additional topics that provide breadth and enhance clinical reasoning skills include psychology, sexually transmitted diseases, and special populations. Psychology content may cover abusive relationships, alcoholism, mood disorders, and chronic pain syndromes. The psychological state of the patient may affect the treatment outcome; therefore, chiropractors must be able to identify whether concomitant psychological disorders exist and make appropriate referrals. Another source of ongoing or unrelenting pain may be due to sexually transmitted diseases (STDs). Although chiropractors do not generally diagnose and manage urogenital conditions, STDs may be responsible for symptoms that appear to be spinal or musculoskeletal due to pain referral patterns. Discussion of proper management of and prevention of STDs requires tact by a health care provider and is practiced by students in role-playing settings during communication and clinical education courses. Finally, recognizing normal patterns as well as specific risk factors and disorders for all human developmental stages is covered in courses related to special populations, such as pediatrics, pregnant women, and geriatric patients. This coursework provides chiropractors with the capability to manage patients of any age, life stage, and gender.

Also included in this course series covering associated clinical topics are ethics, basic economics, and jurisprudence or laws pertaining to chiropractic practice in the United States. Jurisprudence varies by state, and as such, states often test this information separately in a state-specific examination. Related to this section, but not tested on the NBCE examination, are practice management concepts such as setting up a practice, making a business plan, marketing, billing and coding, staffing, office procedures, malpractice and liability, professional networking and relationship building, and career and business development.

Advanced Clinical Studies, NBCE Parts III and IV

The Part III NBCE examination is a more advanced, case-based testing of the concepts covered in Part II. This examination is taken in the last year of a chiropractic program, within nine months of graduation. In order to take Part III, a student must have completed the Part I examination. At this point in a chiropractic program, students are expected to select appropriate history questions and construct a case-appropriate examination and then synthesize findings to generate a clinical impression or diagnosis along with a clinically consistent case management plan. Treatments incorporate chiropractic techniques and supportive interventions, such as physiotherapy modalities, corrective exercises and rehabilitation, nutrition and diet, protective body mechanics and ergonomics, patient education and self-care, and wellness and lifestyle counseling.

By the third year of their chiropractic studies, students are able to formulate a treatment plan with prognosis, identify procedures for follow-up and tracking patient progress, refer or comanage patients, and provide clinical documentation, including informed consent for evaluation and treatment. Students are also trained to identify indications and contraindications with knowledge of underlying pathophysiologic mechanisms. Indications are the situations where a patient would benefit from the doctor providing treatment. Contraindications are the situations when a treatment should not be used or needs to be altered because it may cause harm to the patient. Often those situations warrant special attention in chart notes, a referral, or a modification of the treatment plan.

The NBCE Part IV exam is primarily a practical examination testing three main content areas: diagnostic imaging, chiropractic technique, and case management. This practical examination includes simulated patient encounters and post-encounter probes that assess skills and ability in management of a variety of patient cases. Embedded in case management are patient histories, physical examination procedures, and orthopedic and neurological testing. The chiropractic technique stations prompt students to demonstrate the setup for chiropractic adjustments. The setup includes appropriate doctor position, patient placement, hand contacts, and line of drive without administering the actual therapeutic manipulation. The five regions covered in this portion of the Part IV exam are cervical, thoracic, lumbar, pelvic/sacral, and extremity adjustments.

The examination and technique portions include actors portraying patients, called standardized patients, as well as an examiner to observe the performance on the standardized patient. The post-encounter probe (PEP) stations involve answering multiple-choice questions based on the interaction with the standardized patient in the prior station. Additional clinical information may be presented at the PEP stations, including physical examination findings, diagnostic imaging, and laboratory results.

Diagnostic imaging in Part IV of the NBCE exam involves case scenarios where students are asked to review radiographs or other diagnostic images. The scenarios represent cases commonly encountered in practice, present cautions or contraindications to chiropractic case management, or require early detection to preserve the life or health of the patient. The case may demonstrate normal radiographic anatomy, congenital anomalies, skeletal variants, intervertebral disc disease, spinal stenosis, traumatic skeletal disorders of the spine or extremities, arthritic disorders, tumors and tumor-like processes, bone infections, and other conditions.

Physiotherapy

Physiotherapy is the therapeutic use of physical agents or means for treatment of pain or physical disability. There are two main types of physiotherapy: passive care, which is what the doctor will do when the patient's active participation is unneeded; and active care, which requires the patient to be active in the treatment. The main topics covered in active and passive care coursework and on the NBCE examination in physiotherapy include thermotherapy, electrotherapy, phototherapy, mechanotherapy, functional assessment, exercise physiology, endurance training, neuromuscular rehabilitation, and disorder-specific rehabilitation. This coursework often includes lecture and lab components since these therapies are hands-on or require students to be able to perform the movements they would ask a patient to do.

Thermotherapy is the use of heat or cold in order to decrease pain and inflammation in joints and muscles, increase tissue metabolism and extensibility, and affect blood flow. Modalities of thermotherapy include infrared therapy, paraffin baths, moist hot packs, hydrotherapy, ultrasound, diathermy, and cryotherapy. Electrotherapy also works to decrease pain and inflammation and improve function through energy in the form of electricity or sound. Common modalities covered include therapeutic ultrasound, interferential current, transcutaneous electrical nerve stimulation (TENS), and high- and low-volt galvanism. Phototherapy may also be considered electrotherapy. Phototherapy uses light for therapeutic effect, such as that in low-level laser therapy (LLLT), and may also include ultraviolet and infrared light therapy. Thermotherapy, electrotherapy, and phototherapy are considered passive care modalities.

Mechanotherapy can include both exercise and soft tissue work or massage. This category can be considered either active or passive, depending on the type of treatment. Chiropractic programs often cover these topics separately, with a course or series of courses dedicated to rehabilitation, exercise, and soft tissue techniques. Treatment techniques may incorporate exercise in conjunction with soft tissue treatment and may be purely manual or may incorporate tools or instruments to assist with the treatment. Basic concepts are covered in the core curriculum, while more advanced or specialized soft tissue techniques may be offered as electives.

The final categories of physiotherapy are exercise and rehabilitation with content focusing on functional assessment, exercise physiology, endurance training, muscle rehabilitation, neuromuscular rehabilitation, and disorder-specific rehabilitation. Specific assessments and treatment protocols are learned that may include named techniques such as the McKenzie Method. Also covered are therapeutic stretching, balance training, extremity and spinal stabilization exercises, physioball exercises, functional capacity evaluations, aquatic therapy, and functional and fitness testing.

The physiotherapy (PT) board exam offered by the NBCE is a multiple-choice examination that requires completion of 120 hours of instruction in physiotherapy prior to registration for the exam. Not every state requires the PT board exam for doctors of chiropractic to be licensed and include rehabilitation and physiotherapy in their practice approach. Students may decide not to take this portion of the NBCE exam. However, coursework in physiotherapy is part of the core curriculum of chiropractic programs, and these concepts appear in other sections of the national board exams. Physiotherapy may be included as a clinical internship requirement for graduation.

Chiropractic Techniques

Chiropractic technique courses provide both an introduction to and the integration of the philosophy, science, and art of chiropractic. Lecture and lab courses provide both theoretical underpinnings and practical application of chiropractic techniques for assessment and treatment. Beginning coursework in chiropractic adjusting (or manipulation) starts with identification of anatomical landmarks and palpation, which is using touch to sense and appraise joint motion and soft tissue findings. Courses typically start with the thoracic spine. Students are instructed in methods of analysis, motion palpation, and joint pain provocation. They then progress to adjustive procedures, including fundamental concepts of doctor and patient positioning, hand placement, vectors or line of drive, and thrust depth and velocity. Through the practical work in technique courses, students develop interpersonal skills and understanding of doctor-patient relationships. Students also learn how to position a patient on and operate a variety of chiropractic tables.

After covering the basics, technique courses are organized by region and skill level, such as spinal or upper extremity and lower extremity adjusting courses. More advanced courses review and expand on prior coursework, synthesizing and adding to the foundational concepts. Adjustments may include mobilization, various manual thrusts (i.e., recoil), instrument-assisted adjustment options, and combined approaches that use the chiropractic table to facilitate the adjustment, such as drop or breakaway pieces (parts of the table that can move with the adjustment), flexion, distraction, or axial traction options.

The most common technique approach taught in chiropractic programs is "diversified."[15] The diversified technique is considered the generic manual adjusting technique that is the culmination of the adjustment methods of the early pioneers of chiropractic. It is characterized by a high-velocity, low-amplitude (HVLA) thrust, which means that speed is of greater importance than force. Much of the laboratory component of technique courses help build confidence and understanding of joint "lock-out," or the position where the joint has capacity to initiate full segmental range of motion. At this position, a quick thrust can successfully achieve restorative motion and function to the joint and surrounding tissues. Students learn to control their movements and achieve proper mechanics to prevent injury to both themselves and their patients. Also covered and experienced in the laboratory setting are modifications to adjustments influenced by patient body types and shapes, relative contraindications, doctor body type and height, and table construction and size.

A large portion of the lecture content for technique courses includes biomechanics, the relationship between structure and function, pain patterns, listings (documentation of subluxations for chart notes, which is also tested on NBCE exams), common and uncommon diagnoses and conditions, and clinical management. Other technique systems are also reviewed based on historical significance and the clinical application for that particular chiropractic program. Some chiropractic institutions preferentially select techniques to be taught in the core curriculum and offer other techniques through electives. In addition, students may gain exposure by taking continuing education seminars or attending on-campus clubs, seminars, or workshops. Ultimately, students may choose to focus on one technique in practice or incorporate multiple techniques. The *Practice Analysis of Chiropractic 2015*[15] found that a typical DC uses five or six different adjusting techniques in practice.

Elective Course Offerings

Depending on the institution, there may be extensive or limited elective options. Some programs have such an expansive and comprehensive core curriculum that minimal electives are offered. However, other institutions have crafted course schedules so that students have more freedom to select elective courses, enabling them to gain certification while completing the DC program. Elective offerings are listed in the institution's academic catalog and are often subject to change from term to term based on instructor availability and student interest.

The most common elective offerings are named technique courses, including Activator Technique, Blair Technique, Cox Flexion Distraction, Gonstead, Logan Basic, Pettibon Technique, and Thompson Technique. Other common technique elective offerings are applied kinesiology, atlas orthogonal technique, chiropractic biophysics (CBP), motion palpation, sacro-occipital technique (SOT), and upper cervical technique. Elective course offerings that are not focused on technique may include ergonomics, advanced nutrition concepts, sports injury management, rehabilitation, neurology, special populations (geriatric, pediatric, women's health), soft tissue techniques, and expanded practice management topics. Chiropractic programs may also offer independent studies or research internships as electives.

Other Considerations Affecting Curriculum

Besides the Council on Chiropractic Education and the national board examinations, there are other drivers of chiropractic program content. Programs develop curriculum in such a way as to provide instruction encompassing the broadest scope of practice in the United States. This is beneficial for students since they may not practice in the state where they attended their professional program. The curriculum may also be shaped, however, by limitations imposed by the state's scope of practice where the institution is located.

Some of the biggest differences in the academic curriculum between chiropractic programs are apparent in the philosophical approach, proportion and emphasis on the scientific aspect of chiropractic and clinical practice, electives, and practice management offerings. Opportunities to dual enroll, or take courses in other graduate programs at the institution or a partner institution, may influence curricular options. Internship and externship offerings, requirements, and limitations are discussed in the next chapter. Finally, faculty experiences, qualifications, research, and scholarship may play a role in shaping course content and the academic atmosphere.

The overall campus culture, beyond the academic and clinical coursework, can be vital to students' success and their perceptions about the value of the educational program. Students can supplement the course offerings by attending extracurricular activities such as clubs, lunch or evening seminars, and continuing education courses offered either on or off campus. Students can also network with local doctors and alumni. Career development staff can provide guidance beyond what is presented in the classroom environment. Additionally, library resources can be incredibly valuable in providing supplemental content, models, videos, research articles, and texts, both in hardcopy and digitally.

Although there are many aspects of the chiropractic curriculum that are similar across institutions and programs, each has characteristics that make it unique. Institutions offer complementary resources that enhance the in-class content, including seminars, club workshops, networking, and the library. Taking advantage of faculty office hours, tutoring, and building study skills alleviate the significant curricular load. From the core courses in basic science, chiropractic technique, clinical science, and associated clinical practice to the philosophical approach and electives, the didactic portion of a chiropractic program will provide students with the fundamentals for successful clinical practice. Academic training often profoundly shapes the lifelong behaviors of chiropractors and provides definition to their mission, vision, purpose, and practice style.

References

1. Association of Chiropractic Colleges. Academic Requirements, 2015. http://www.chirocolleges.org/prospective_students.html. Accessed November 17, 2015.

2. Keating JC, Jr. *B.J. Palmer of Davenport: The Early Years of Chiropractic.* Davenport, IA: Association for History of Chiropractic Publishing; 1997.

3. Wardwell WI. *Chiropractic History and Evolution of a New Profession.* St. Louis: Mosby; 1992.

4. Armstrong KS. *A Report on Chiropractic Politics and Education.* Atlanta, GA: The Chiropractic Foundation of America; 1979.

5. Coulter I, Adams AH, Sandefur R. Chiropractic training. In: Cherkin D, Mootz R., eds. *Chiropractic in the United States: Training, Practice, and Research*:17–28. AHCPR Publication No. 98-N002, 1997: 17–28.

6. Coulter I, Adams A, Coggan P, Wilkes M, Gonyea M. A comparative study of chiropractic and medical education. *Altern Ther Health Med.* 1998;4(5): 64–75.

7. Christensen M, Kollasch M, Ward R, Webb K. *Job Analysis of Chiropractic, 2005.* Greeley, CO: National Board of Chiropractic Examiners; 2005.

8. Cooperstein R. The leading edge research symposium of 1984: early attempts to achieve consensus of subluxation. *Chiropractic History.* 1984:32–54.

9. Mirtz TA, Perle SM. The prevalence of the term subluxation in North American English-language doctor of chiropractic programs. *Chiropr Man Therap.* 2011;19:14.

10. McGregor M, Puhl AA, Reinhart C, Injeyan HS, Soave D. Differentiating intraprofessional attitudes toward paradigms in health care delivery among chiropractic factions: results from a randomly sampled survey. *BMC Complement Altern Med.* 2014;14:51.

11. McDonald W. *How Chiropractors Think and Practice: The Survey of North American Chiropractors.* Ada, OH: Institute for Social Research; 2003.

12. Miller G. Chiropractic technique: a quantified comparison of chiropractic college curricula. *Chiropr Tech.* 1994;6:4.

13. Eva KW, Bordage G, Campbell C, et al. Towards a program of assessment for health professionals: from training into practice. *Adv Health Sci Educ Theory Pract.* 2015 Nov 21;1–17.

14. Office of Disease Prevention and Health Promotion. About Healthy People. 2015. http://www.healthypeople.gov/2020/About-Healthy-People. Accessed May 15, 2016.

15. Christensen M, Hyland J, Goertz C, Kollasch M. *Practice Analysis of Chiropractic, 2015.* Greeley, CO: National Board of Chiropractic Examiners; 2015.

CHAPTER FIVE

Chiropractic Clinical Education

Stefanie Krupp, DC, MS; Ruth Sandefur, DC, PhD;
Rachael Pandzik, DC

Chiropractic programs typically begin the transition from the academic foundational courses to clinic-focused courses two-thirds of the way through the program. As discussed in the previous chapter, students first start to practice clinical skills on one another in laboratory courses. The clinical preparatory courses begin to connect individual content areas, such as history taking, physical examination, laboratory, and diagnostic imaging procedures, with the formation of a diagnosis, patient management, and treatment using simulated cases. These sample cases help students prepare for the types of patients and conditions they are likely to encounter upon entry into the clinic experience, often called the clinical internship. Most on-campus chiropractic clinics initially allow interns to work with patients generated from within the college community (students, faculty, and staff). Later, interns may treat public patients who are eligible for pro-bono care in exchange for their willingness to allow the time necessary for new interns to perform their tasks with close supervision from attending clinicians.

Clinical Oversight

As students enter clinic courses, they are often assigned to an individual attending clinician. The attending clinician is the treating chiropractor under whose license the interns can gain practice and exposure to a number of different cases. Clinicians oversee patient care through either observing all of, or components of, the patient visit. They review the patients' chart notes and engage the interns in discussions about patient management. By being assigned to a specific attending clinician during the clinical experience, interns are guided throughout the patient encounter as they progress from intern to professional chiropractor. Clinicians must be able to identify and work with a variety of student personalities, attitudes, and preparedness, and to assist each intern in becoming the finest and most competent chiropractor possible. After an initial period working with one clinician, interns may be assigned to a number of different clinicians, enabling them to observe various approaches to patient care. This enriches the clinical experience and further prepares interns for the transition to public service as a chiropractic practitioner.

Attending clinicians often work full time in the clinical program; some work part time in the clinic as well as teach other courses or work in private practice. Often attending clinicians have attained additional specialties or qualifications, such as the master's degrees, diplomates, or certifications that are discussed in other chapters. As employees at the chiropractic institution, many have taken a wide variety of postgraduate and continuing education courses or participated in research, bringing that breadth and depth of education back to the clinic interns.

Many institutions offer new interns the chance to shadow senior interns who are further along in the program. This is an invaluable way for student interns to learn the basics of the chiropractic clinic environment, since it involves learning about patient flow, clinic paperwork, and other aspects of the clinical internship. There are many nuances of clinic functions that are specific to each facility, such as location of supplies, how laundry is handled, how patients are scheduled, which rooms to use, and specifics of consulting with clinicians. It is also necessary to learn both from the attending clinician and other interns how to manage documentation of patient visits, which procedure codes to use, how to format certain sections of the electronic medical records, how much detail to include, and the submission process so that chart notes can be reviewed in a timely manner.

Clinical Rotations and Patient Base

By the final year of their program, student interns will begin treating "outpatients," or patients from outside the campus community. Most chiropractic college clinics accept insurance or offer discounted rates to serve those patients who demonstrate financial hardship. Clinical experiences also consist of rotations in a variety of outpatient settings, which may include hospitals, community clinics, specialty clinics, and other higher education institutions. Interns have the opportunity to work with pediatric, geriatric, and athletic populations in these settings. They are also exposed to a broader patient base with comorbidities and risk factors for a wide assortment of conditions that represent what they will encounter as doctors. At some institutions, students can select which rotations they prefer, already specializing in a technique, patient population, or care approach in their last year of clinical education. There may be opportunities for students to travel abroad and work with disadvantaged populations needing musculoskeletal care in other countries.

Each term students are assigned increasing numbers of credit hours in the clinical environment as they progress through their internship courses. This time is spent not only directly engaged with patients but also completing chart notes, management plans, and preparatory work for upcoming visits. In addition to patient care, clinical courses offer structured assignments, providing exposure to more complex cases, which helps ensure consistency in the educational content of the clinical experience.

Documentation and Billing

Within the clinical internship courses, documentation of patient visits becomes exceedingly valuable as both a teaching tool and a practical skill. Students must be able to document exactly what occurred during the patient visit in a clear, concise, professional manner that accurately represents all elements of the patient visit necessary for medical and legal requirements. In addition to detailing the patient visit, often using electronic medical records, students must also be able to generate written narratives that describe the patient's story for insurance, medical, or legal purposes. Student interns also practice writing radiology reports, and many have the opportunity to compose reports for patients in the clinic.

Documentation is inclusive of not only patient visit notes and management plans but also diagnostic and billing codes. Diagnostic codes, called the "International Classification of Disease" or ICD codes, are an almost-exhaustive list of codes for the majority of potential diagnoses. These codes help standardize the language of disease between all types of health care practitioners and other health care–related agencies. Though students have some exposure to ICD codes while in academic courses, these codes come to life through patient visits, where the nuances of primary and secondary diagnoses become important. Students begin to understand the language of coding as it is often the only way a medical provider can communicate a patient's case to a third-party provider, such as an insurance company.

Services billed for patient care, called Current Procedural Terminology or CPT codes, communicate information not only about the patient but also about the doctor's practice protocols. CPT codes can represent the amount of time a doctor spent with a patient, the complexity of care the patient needed or the level of care provided, as well as the variety of treatment approaches used. For example, a doctor may use chiropractic manipulation as well as passive modalities, such as electric stimulation or ultrasound. Clinic interns learn coding in clinic preparatory courses and during the clinical internship while using electronic medical records. Even though billing and coding procedures are amply stressed during the educational experience, many graduates report that they do not fully appreciate their importance until used in practice, where reimbursement from insurance companies generates revenue for the practice.

Treatment Approaches

The chiropractic treatment and patient management approaches used in chiropractic program clinics typically follow what is offered in the curriculum. This may include a variety of chiropractic techniques, most often diversified adjusting, drop table, instrument-assisted adjusting, flexion-distraction, and mobilization. Additionally, passive modalities can be used, including but not limited to electric stimulation, ultrasound, low-level laser therapy, therapeutic heat and ice, and various soft tissue manipulation techniques. Approved techniques may be the result of attending clinician preference and/or certifications as well as the curricular content of the chiropractic institution.

Most chiropractic program clinics also offer physical rehabilitation options and may have a dedicated "rehab room." Physical therapy equipment includes resistance bands, balance balls, kettle bells, medicine balls, treadmills, stationary bicycles, and other options. Interns have the opportunity to incorporate therapeutic exercises and rehabilitation protocols as part of the patient visit. Sometimes the expertise of the intern can dictate physical rehabilitation approaches, since many chiropractic students have experience in personal training and kinesiology. Attending clinicians may also have advanced training in rehabilitation and require interns to offer rehab as part of the patient care plan.

Nutritional counseling is another treatment approach required for at least some patient cases as part of graduation requirements. Student interns can determine what dietary changes or supplements may be most beneficial for patients, often recommending anti-inflammatory diets, supplements, or other supports for overall wellness. The comorbidities of patients are considered when including dietary or other lifestyle recommendations, particularly for patients presenting with hypertension and/or diabetes.

Learning to coordinate patient care with other health care providers is a key component of interprofessional education and comanagement. Obtaining medical records from and writing narrative reports to other providers are essential practice communication and documentation skills that students must learn in order to function as health care providers. Understanding the practice parameters of other health care disciplines facilitates coordination efforts.

Additional Clinically Relevant Opportunities

While in clinic, student interns may have the opportunity to engage in other clinically relevant educational activities. For instance, shadowing local chiropractors may count as a portion of the required clinic hours. Student interns may also attend seminars, watch webinars, go to health fairs, or participate in professional networking opportunities, such as business groups, supplement company presentations, or chiropractic association meetings.

There may be opportunities for student interns to participate in research within their institution. It can be incredibly valuable to gain experience writing a case report or research paper. Being published in a peer-reviewed journal can have a positive impact on a résumé or curriculum vitae when applying for positions as a chiropractor, educator, or researcher. Being published also adds authority for lecturing to the general population or teaching continuing education courses.

Externships and Preceptorships

By the final term of the clinical education experience, after demonstrating competency in the chiropractic program's outpatient clinics, interns may have the opportunity to work with or observe an established chiropractic practice full time. This immersion experience affords soon-to-be doctors the chance to see a practice in action, experience an associate relationship, or enhance their skills and knowledge. Students typically select the location or practice. These "externships" are approved through the clinical staff at the institution, and student interns are given guidance about what is acceptable and what is required as part of the externship. The externship generally lasts a month or more, depending on the chiropractic institution's guidelines. Both the practitioner and the student extern are required to submit paperwork to the chiropractic institution documenting their experiences, which provides valuable feedback about the program's success.

Ideally, students begin searching for these opportunities by the time they enter clinic. Some externships are organized by chiropractic programs and may be competitive, such as those offered by the Veterans Affairs (VA) Hospitals across the United States. Additionally, specialty clinics may have many students vying for an externship position, so it is best to make connections early for areas such as pediatrics and sports chiropractic. Externships help broaden the clinical experience by providing additional mentorship and exposure to patient cases and the logistics of the business side of running a practice. These competitive programs are increasing in number and provide students with exciting interprofessional education opportunities.

Graduation Requirements

In order to complete the requirements for the doctor of chiropractic degree, chiropractic programs follow the guidelines set forth by the Council on Chiropractic Education (CCE) Meta-Competencies. These competencies are assessed throughout the curriculum but are particularly important as a student is determined "competent" approaching graduation. The most recent draft of the CCE Meta-Competencies identifies eight competency areas:[1]

1. Assessment and diagnosis
2. Management plan
3. Health promotion and disease prevention
4. Communication and record keeping
5. Professional ethics and jurisprudence
6. Information and technology literacy
7. Chiropractic adjustment/manipulation
8. Interprofessional education

Historically, clinical internships determined competency based on a skills count, where students completed certain numbers of requirements, such as patient exams, adjustments, diagnostic imaging and laboratory evaluations, and patient case type exposure. With the advent of the CCE Meta-Competencies, clinical internship patient care and educational structure in these core areas are more carefully planned and evaluated in addition to the numbers requirement. This means a student intern must not only achieve a minimum number of patient visits but also demonstrate a high degree of proficiency in managing those patients. Chiropractic institutions are currently in the process of interpreting the CCE Meta-Competencies and implementing protocol to meet those standards. It is likely the number and types of competencies set forth by CCE will continue to evolve over time to meet the changing needs of education, health care, and the profession.

Grades for performance in a clinical internship are often pass or fail. As long as minimum competency is demonstrated for the term, the intern moves on in the clinical internship courses. Assessment measures often include performance with patient care and documentation as well as supplementary assignments. These other assessments often incorporate case studies (live, simulated, or virtual), grand rounds involving specialty faculty (most commonly diagnostic imaging) or complex cases presented by clinicians, and performance on practical and written examinations that mimic parts of the National Board of Chiropractic Examiners (NBCE) examinations.

Conclusion

Because DCs have, as the majority of their patient visits, individuals with musculoskeletal complaints, chiropractic graduates indeed have ample opportunity to diagnose and treat the type of patients that they will encounter in their practices. The basic and diagnostic sciences in earlier coursework prepare students to make appropriate diagnoses and to recognize patients with conditions requiring additional medical intervention and, therefore, a referral. Chiropractic institutions strive to make the clinical internship education as effective and realistic as possible. Increasing responsibility is given to interns as they demonstrate proficiency in making clinical decisions. Exposure to practice-building approaches and business skills is also crucial to effectively navigate the private practice environment. By graduation, doctors of chiropractic are armed with the clinical and practical knowledge and the entry-level clinical experience to successfully begin treating patients. As the chiropractor's practice unfolds, these skills are honed year after year through ongoing patient care.

Reference

1. Council on Chiropractic Education. CCE Accreditation Standards Principles, Processes & Requirements for Accreditation. http://www.cce-usa.org /uploads/2016-08-01_Final_Draft_CCE_Accreditation_Standards_-_Clean _Version.pdf. Accessed August 11, 2016.

CHAPTER SIX

A Global Perspective on Chiropractic Education

Phillip Ebrall, BAppSci(Chiropractic), PhD

In many respects it is fair to suggest that today's chiropractic curriculum remains true to principles and content that were determined some 70 years ago[1] in an age when chiropractic education remained a peculiarly North American phenomenon. The basics of the curriculum originated in Nugent's 1943 text *Chiropractic Education: Outline of a Standard Course.*[2] The first college to adopt this model was the Canadian Memorial Chiropractic College, and when Nugent "fathered" the Council on Chiropractic Education in 1947, his curriculum became the de facto standard.[2]

After Canada, and using international equivalency as the benchmark, came England with the Anglo-European College in 1965, and Australia with the Phillip Institute of Technology in 1975. By the late 1990s, there were as many chiropractic colleges outside the United States as there were within, and this has pressured the curriculum to change, particularly in its sociocultural aspects.

However, change is not something that is easy for those who manage accreditation and hence by default direct the curriculum. It is equally difficult for those who run chiropractic educational institutions where a stable economic model, achieved by minimal change, is preferred. An appropriate descriptor of accreditation bodies and chiropractic institutions is "conservative traditionalists," reinforced by a mind-set built within their own model of learning, which in most cases is aged 30 or more years and littered with chalkboards and overhead projectors.

Chiropractic education is therefore at its most exciting time ever. It is, on the one hand, a traditional activity that follows the style of those old mechanical industries that now form the rust belt in a number of Western countries. On the other, it is an emerging force driven by the tigers of the world's new economy that is emerging within that sector of the globe that holds the greatest population, hence the greatest influence and most money. Dynamic growth is an incubator for change as it creates an environment that is the most accepting of change. In social terms, the contrast could not be greater. Between the North American traditionalists and the emerging Asian curricula lies the European educational environment. In spite of these vastly different environments, there is a remarkable uniformity among all chiropractic programs. It really is time to accept that chiropractic has no borders and is a global profession regardless of mind-sets that countries and regions create. A new global outlook embraces the dramatic growth and development of chiropractic in general and chiropractic education in particular in other countries, particularly East Asia.

The name of the game is not just to improve on what has been the modus operandi since 1945, but to totally reimagine it. This chapter is meant to contribute to the essential reimagination of chiropractic education in a global sense.

There is little doubt that the acceptance of such a new approach is likely to be significantly higher in East Asia and Asia than elsewhere. However, questions remain: Is a global approach to chiropractic education useful? Can it really do anything? Could it facilitate global transferability of students? Would it ensure standardization of teaching staff? Above all, will it result in better patient care?

Current Global Status

The quality of chiropractic education is managed globally by a number of semi-independent regional accrediting bodies. Some regional bodies fall loosely under a global representative body (Box 6.1). It must be understood the Councils on Chiropractic Education International (CCE-I) has no standards of its own, and thus there can be no claim of a current global accreditation standard.

The CCE-I performs a role in overseeing minimal standards for quality assurance within chiropractic education and provides the valuable "trust" factor that ensures that graduates from programs accredited by its member institutions are quality practitioners of chiropractic. However, it does not yet facilitate global portability.

Box 6.1

Agencies Associated with Accreditation of Chiropractic Programs

CCE. Council on Chiropractic Education, based in Arizona, United States. See http://cce-usa.org. Accredits 15 institutions with a total of 17 programs (in addition to its "home" program, an institution may conduct an "additional education site" or a "branch campus"). CCE also addresses residency programs and recently withdrew from CCEI.

CCEA. Council on Chiropractic Education Australasia, based in Australia. See http://www.ccea.com.au. Accredits eight programs in five countries delivered in three languages.

CCEI. Councils on Chiropractic Education International, based in Idaho, United States. See http://www.cceintl.org/Contacts.html.

ECCE. Council on Chiropractic Education, based in the United Kingdom. See http://www.cce-europe.com. Accredits seven programs in three main languages and some dialects, such as Welsh, and evaluates a further two programs.

FCC. Federation of Canadian Chiropractic, also known as **CFCREAB**, which was part known as CCEC until 2007, based in Toronto, Canada. See http://www.chirofed.ca/english/. Accredits two programs, in two languages and recognizes five colleges of specialty chiropractic practice.

This raises the question of how one achieves global portability while maintaining standards. For example, the Council on Chiropractic Education Australasia (CCEA) states that the objectives of their standards for undergraduate chiropractic education are to establish a system of evaluation and accreditation of institutions teaching chiropractic, to ensure minimum quality standards for chiropractic educational programs. However, standards vary in intent and interpretation in different countries.

The Advantages of Accreditation

Worldwide, every patient of a chiropractor has the right to know whether or not his or her practitioner has a level of training that is uniform with that which confers legitimate use of the title "chiropractor." While the responsibility for ensuring this in a legal sense falls on regulatory bodies, the duty to measure and comment falls to accrediting bodies.

The world is segmented into a number of accrediting bodies (see Box 6.1). These have a somewhat common although diverging agreement on what "makes" a chiropractor. On the one hand, there is a traditional aspect going back to Nugent's curriculum of the 1940s,[1] while on the other, there is an increasing emphasis on evidence-based education practice.

Regardless of these details, every person using the services of a chiropractor who has graduated from an accredited institution can be assured that the registered practitioner has a solid knowledge of basic and clinical sciences and a demonstrated competency to provide safe, effective chiropractic care.

The key is to ensure one's chiropractor has graduated from an accredited chiropractic program. In some countries, this may not be so, regardless of whether the practitioner states that he or she will perform "chiropractic manipulation." *A listing of accredited colleges and programs is given in Chapter 2*; however, while it is definitive at the time of publication, it must be appreciated this list is of necessity fluid as new institutions emerge. It also fails to account for persons "grandfathered" into registration as a chiropractor based on a variety of reasons, including time in practice regardless of the status of the institution from which the individual graduated.

Grandfathering is an appropriate step on the path to legal recognition as it does not discriminate against those with some form of training and a reasonable period of safe clinical practice where both were attained prior to new legislation being introduced. It was successfully applied in Australia, where in fact one such grandfathered practitioner rose to become chair of a state registration board. Grandfathering is currently being applied in Japan as that country moves to a government-recognized chiropractors' register. Concomitant with and essential to a country's shift to legislation is the emergence of high educational standards at an internationally recognized level.

Accreditation is therefore seen as a tool with the potential to equalize global chiropractic education and thus the professional practice of the discipline. Professional accreditation has two tines, one institutional and the other programmatic. While institutional accreditation may have value in countries where chiropractic education is delivered by private institutions, it is superfluous in countries where it is the government's responsibility to accredit institutions of higher education.

These concepts are founded on the precept of private colleges in the United States from which grew today's collection of U.S. institutions that are generally financially solid and self-sufficient with good governance. As the environment changes, so too must the measurement dimensions relevant to larger institutions adopting university status and delivering more programs in addition to solely chiropractic ones.

Notwithstanding differences in the details of institutional and pro-grammatic accreditation, it remains the only implement to achieve equality in global chiropractic education standards. It is still valuable for a patient to insist on knowing the provenance of his or her chiropractor. A graduate from an accredited institution may be considered competent with the application of chiropractic assessment and management. On the other hand, a practitioner with a weekend certificate from a fly-by-night entrepreneur is one demanding extreme care and caution if not avoidance. The applicable outcomes measurements must be quantitative and not qualitative. In this context, institutional and programmatic accreditation has value for the protection of the public.

New Directions in Accreditation

The most valuable direction for accreditation is to strengthen its potential to confer global equivalency. At this time it does not,[3] which suggests accreditation is currently like countries, in that it has borders. It remains difficult if not impossible for a student enrolled in a program in one country to undertake a term of study (semester or trimester) at a program in another country. There remains little to no chance of this potential for student mobility to occur even within one country, even though all programs in that country or region are accredited by the same body.

A surface reason for this is the individual institutions' approaches to learning and assessment, which allows for considerable variability in course (subject) sequencing, which in turn creates difficulties in credit transfer.

On the other hand, the broad commonality of accreditation competencies assures a relative commonality of skills and safe technique among graduates from all accredited institutions regardless of an individual institution's mission and trajectory to achieve this.

Significant strength would be added to the accreditation process by developing postgraduate programs to achieve skill sets specific to varying practice styles. In some respects, this would be a valuable first step in elevating aspects of practice to the level of specialty while achieving more thorough teaching at a "general practice" level. Specialty practice is accepted in some jurisdictions but not others. Quite simply, it should be global.

The Globalization of Learning Manual Skills

Given the complexity of the development of psychomotor skills, the building of mind maps to repeatedly deliver optimal performance of the most appropriate therapeutic intervention, and the development of capability with the clinical decision-making process, it seems prudent for a global curriculum to provide a standardized skill set suited to general practice.

Specialized techniques and any related analysis systems deserve to be learned at the highest level. Institutions would wisely either expand their curriculum to achieve this in addition to a standardized general-practice skill set or develop and facilitate postgraduate awards (qualifications) in various techniques or bridging programs to facilitate graduate entry into propriety programs leading to certification.

A Quantitative Approach to Accreditation

The sense in which "quantitative" is used in this section is not as an expression of the "number of tasks completed" such as "patient encounters." The use of elementary school summation as a performance measure has little meaning, and its only application in the real world is a discernment between a practitioner who may have performed 100 or more procedures versus one who has only completed several.

Within the accreditation process, "quantitative" refers to the manner in which the accrediting team gathers, documents, and ranks its evidence against individual standards or elements. The most meaningful measures are those that document how an institution achieves its mission as opposed to qualitative opinions of a particular mission.

As an example, an institution may have evidence that its mission is best achieved by using areas of "open practice" in the learning clinic or to refer to patients as "practice members." The measure to apply in such a scenario is whether use of a different term within an open-practice environment makes a positive contribution toward the institution's mission. Evidence would need to be documented to facilitate a quantitative measurement and to remove any qualitative bias about terminology and style of clinical learning.

The same principle applies to the 19th-century concept that learning attainment is "time and place" based. This means that learning can only occur within a lecture theater at a time suited to the whim of the academic and that there is some magical vector that suggests the duration students spend in that place, whether or not they are learning or sleeping, equates to knowledge attainment. Outcomes-based assessment of the means by which an institution attains its mission and meets the elements of accreditation is quantitative.

Industry Engagement

The chiropractic profession's global industry body is the World Federation of Chiropractic (WFC). It is an amalgamation of associations that idealistically represent the majority of chiropractors in each of some 85 or more countries around the world. One of its objectives, embedded in its bylaws (6, B), is to encourage improvement in educational issues.

Indeed, since 2000, the WFC has conducted a biannual conference on chiropractic education, covering current trends in health professions education as well as the changing health care environment. Although the most recent conference was North American–centric, it is to be expected that more global perspectives will be examined at future conferences.

In 2005, a past president of WFC wrote a set of guidelines on chiropractic education that, following expert review, became an endorsed document of the World Health Organization (WHO).[4] It may be downloaded in any of some 12 languages from the WFC's website (www.wfc.org).

An Overview of Minimum Competencies

A chiropractic program that may be recognized globally will graduate chiropractors who have demonstrated a passing grade (50 percent, a minimum level of competency) in the following learning areas:

- basic sciences, as in the common sciences that underpin medical training
- social sciences, to provide a humanistic context
- diagnostic sciences, as in the common sciences that underpin diagnosis and management (This is perhaps the area appropriate for greatest change, given the immense advances in diagnostic procedures that have occurred in health care over the past decade or two.)
- clinical sciences, the key area of differentiation between chiropractic as a paradigm of health and wellness care and contemporary medicine as a paradigm of disease care and trauma rectification

However, as no patient would want to trust her or his life in the hands of a practitioner who only demonstrated knowledge of half (50 percent) of what she or he should, it is common for chiropractic institutions to derive a passing grade from the demonstrated ability to deliver 7 out of 10 procedures in a safe, effective manner. The actual 70 percent passing grade is then scaled back to fit within the institution's regular grading system. When practical exams are written to include a crossover of assessment results, the 70 percent value actually approaches 95–100 percent, which more properly represents the zone of capable practice.

The following demonstrates the variations and vagaries of the minimum competency for two basic elements of accreditation relevant to safe clinical practice. The acronyms are drawn from Box 6.1.

Element A: The Number of Patient Encounters Required

- Council on Chiropractic Education (CCE): No number is readily found online; however, the institution must provide faculty, student, and clinic manuals or handbooks and a presumption is a clinic manual will identify not only how many patient encounters are considered appropriate by the institution but also define what constitutes a "patient encounter."

- Council on Chiropractic Education Australasia (CCEA): (5.4, Basic Standard—Student Performance, p. 18). Students must have performed at least 300 chiropractic care sessions directed toward the alleviation of an identifiable ailment.

- Federation of Canadian Chiropractic (FCC), previously known as Council on Chiropractic Education—Canada (CCEC) until 2007: Students must have performed chiropractic adjustments and/or manipulations, primarily spinal, during at least 250 separate patient care visits.

- European Council on Chiropractic Education (ECCE): Apart from suggesting a mere 35 new patients encounters are expected, the total number is not quantified but is measured in terms of numbers during the final year of training of (1) new patients (mean number per student cohort/range), and (2) (returning) patient treatment visits (mean number per student cohort/range).

Element B: Program Duration

- CCE: The entry requirement is "completed the equivalent of three academic years of undergraduate study (90 semester hours) at an institution(s) accredited by an agency recognized by the U.S. Department of Education or an equivalent foreign agency with a GPA for these 90 hours of not less than 3.0 on a 4.0 scale. The 90 hours will include a minimum of 24 semester hours in life and physical science courses" and the following chiropractic program is quantified as "the equivalent of 4,200 instructional hours which ensures that the program is commensurate with doctoral level professional training in a health science discipline, a portion of which incorporates this training into patient care settings."

- CCEA: An accredited chiropractic program will "have facilities, equipment and staff sufficient for teaching and training the student body in accordance with its educational objectives" previously stated as "expected to be a minimum of 10 semesters in duration." There is no mention of hours.

- FCC: Federation-accredited programs require a minimum of four to five academic years of full-time study totaling no less than 4,200 hours. This appears to be in addition to three years of full-time study at a relevant university program.

- ECCE: No duration seems to be given. Rather, the "ECCE defines the education and training of a chiropractor in terms of: (i) first qualification education and training, at the end of which the graduate is safe and competent to enter practice, and (ii) postgraduate education and training that normally immediately follows graduation for a defined period of time, at the end of which the chiropractor is fit to practice in an autonomous and independent manner."

- WHO: Highly variable between one and six or more years dependent on the qualifications of the entrant.

It is clear that for chiropractic education to truly exist without borders there must be global equivalency in that which constitutes minimum duration and quantitative measurement with evidence as to how this is demonstrated.

Diversity of Institutions

To this point, this chapter has offered a loose categorization of chiropractic institutions as being either private institutions that may or may not have evolved into private universities or public universities largely funded by government. The latter category makes chiropractic academics public servants, which comes with a very high level of accountability. Not only does this cover the expenditure of public money, it demands a very high responsiveness to ensure an evidence-based and innovative curriculum.

The listing of chiropractic institutions by country is given in Chapter 2 and has been referred to earlier in this chapter. A careful reading will reveal a range of models for a structure to deliver chiropractic education:

- stand-alone private institutions that teach only chiropractic
- stand-alone private institutions that teach chiropractic and related programs
- private institutions that have transitioned from stand-alone chiropractic-only status to be private universities through the addition of related programs in health education with appropriate government approvals
- autonomous institutions with close links to a formal university
- public universities delivering a chiropractic program in a faculty of health sciences, which may also deliver programs in osteopathy and Chinese medicine among others

- public universities delivering a chiropractic program in a faculty of medical sciences or similar, which may also deliver programs in nursing, radiography, paramedic training, and oral health among others
- public universities delivering a chiropractic program with content common to a medical program delivered by the same institution
- universities listed on the stock exchange with the provision for staff to buy shares in the institution and where the chiropractic program may be delivered parallel but separate to medical and oral health programs

Of course, the above list is not exhaustive and other combinations and structures exist. However, a key question relates to how one may identify any common thread. It may or may not be duration, as this is dependent on whether the program is delivered in a semester, trimester, or quarterly mode. Neither will the common thread be related to number of hours taught, as there are also differences in how these are counted. This includes how they may be weighted between the traditional lecture and traditional practical, tutorial, or laboratory classes. And of course, an additional aspect is the extent to which an institution uses technology for distance learning for appropriate support courses.

Tertiary education is measured by the concept of "volume of learning," and this is a very useful guide as to what is actually thought essential to achieve outcomes appropriate to differentiate, for example, between a bachelor's degree and a master's. Matching the concept of "volume of learning" with quantitative measurement of "learning attainment" expressed as capability development is perhaps the most powerful way forward for accreditation processes that should be borderless and equivalent.

The above underscores why global equivalency and the removal of borders is to a large degree dependent on revisiting the accreditation process. Change is most effective when it falls ahead of the curve, at the leading edge.

For chiropractic education to grow in the global space at the rate it has in East Asia, there must be a driver. Given the difficulties in global portability and the proven inability of accreditation to facilitate student movement, one must ask, what does it mean? Could not a licensing authority have simple criteria that define institutions as being government approved and producing graduates that meet needs specific to the country of graduation? Would such a radical innovation truly remove borders or enhance them?

A strong argument could be mounted that portability is a fallacy, because chiropractic practice is known to be very specific to the jurisdiction (country, state, or province) where it is legally practiced. This argument would maintain that chiropractic education should align more fully with chiropractic practice, and since practice varies by locality, education should not be internationally standardized. An example of how chiropractic education can vary due to local jurisdiction, and also an example of one of many possible directions in which the profession may move, is the chiropractic program in Switzerland (see Box 6.2).

This is not a suggestion for isolationism. Rather, it opens opportunities for institutions to work together and build their own pathways to facilitate mobility and portability of learning attainment. Students will be attracted to those institutions that facilitate mobility, such as one particular university in Malaysia where chiropractic education is experiencing a continued, strong growth phase. A founding principle of this institution

---

Box 6.2

Possible New Directions for Chiropractic Education: The Example of Switzerland

In 2007, it became law in Switzerland that a chiropractic program be incorporated into a Swiss university.[5] The University of Zurich became the site for the first Swiss chiropractic educational program. Chiropractic medicine is recognized by Swiss law to be one of five professions composing the field of medicine: human medicine, veterinary medicine, dentistry, pharmacy, and chiropractic medicine. Perhaps unique among global chiropractic programs, prospective chiropractic students at the University of Zurich are required to be accepted into the medical school first, at which time they may select either the medical program or the chiropractic program. Those who select the chiropractic pathway must not only complete the same coursework as medical students but also take specialized chiropractic coursework. Medical and chiropractic students take many courses together, establishing an atmosphere for future interdisciplinary collaboration. Unlike many older chiropractic programs in other countries, Swiss chiropractic students also complete a mandatory two-year residency. After graduation and licensure, chiropractic physicians have the right to order and/or perform the same diagnostic tests as medical physicians and also have some prescribing rights. Swiss chiropractors are already accustomed to being part of collaborative health care teams; in many other countries, this must be accomplished through individual practitioner efforts (*see Chapter 13 for examples*).[5]

is guaranteed student mobility, particularly in medical training, where Malaysian students transition to university in a local home environment and on successful completion of the initial half of their medical program transfer to any of 25 or so highly reputable medical universities worldwide to complete their qualification.

The Importance of Capability over Competency

A report by The Centre for the Edge warns that employers are beginning to look for applicants who are smart and curious rather than simply relying on credentials. While this may not be especially relevant when a chiropractic graduate establishes his or her own practice and becomes the principal of a small business delivering health care, it is certainly relevant when he or she seeks a position as an associate in an existing practice or a role in the health care or education systems.

More important, this report from Australia's research arm of Deloitte emphasizes the point that capabilities and learning abilities are valued over credentialed expertise. Credentials such as a full degree are being unbundled in the marketplace into evidence of achievements in smaller certificates. This leading-edge emphasis on capability associated with "just in time" learning demands attention by curriculum designers for chiropractic education.

Using the analogy of a cocktail party, competency can be seen as the ability to make conversation. On the other hand, capability is engaging in appropriate conversation knowing one does not talk about sex, race, religion, or politics.

In terms of learning attainment, competency is a trade-level outcome that can be measured and checked off—examples include a nursing student giving an injection and a chiropractic student taking an X-ray. On the other hand, capability adds the dimension of professional judgment, as in when to inject and where, or when to X-ray and how to position.

In short, capability adds critical qualitative judgment to task performance, while competency is simply the task performance.

The development of a capability-based chiropractic curriculum may remain an outlier for a few years, but it will eventually be accepted as a revolutionary breakthrough. Of course, it will require considerable effort to bring about this change in particular; however, if chiropractic educators continue to do today what they did yesterday, then tomorrow will be yesterday again.

The *British Medical Journal* has published some strong papers on this theme, among them a piece by two professors that makes the point that capability is the extent to which individuals can adapt to change, generate new knowledge, and continue to improve their performance.[6]

The beauty of capability-based learning is that when assessment is appropriately matched to a capability or group of capabilities, the learner is forced to actually think as opposed to simply remember, recall, and regurgitate. An additional and very necessary outcome of the transition to capabilities is the cessation of assessment using multiple-choice questions, as is occurring in progressive Australian universities. The implications for organizations such as the U.S. National Board of Chiropractic Examiners (NBCE) are profound.

Chiropractic Clinical Education

This chapter previously identified the total chiropractic curriculum as incorporating basic sciences, social sciences, diagnostic sciences, and clinical sciences. The basic and social sciences are able to sit within virtually any model of pre-chiropractic education while the specificity cycle starts broadly around diagnostic sciences and rises to the very specific clinical sciences.

The combination of diagnostic and clinical sciences generates the curriculum portion termed "clinical education," or depending on the perspective taken by the institution, "clinical learning." Although the clinical element is the core differentiator of a chiropractic curriculum over other health curricula, it may not have received the critical attention it warrants.

A global conference was held in 2015 on chiropractic clinical education by the Tokyo College of Chiropractic. The outcomes are summarized below. The next event in the series will explore the development of core values in chiropractic clinical education.

Outcomes from the First Global Conference and Workshop on Chiropractic Clinical Education: An International Meeting

Classroom Level

Improve understanding of one another's roles among academics, practitioners, and students.

Dissonance between classroom teaching staff and clinical teaching staff was a common theme. Awareness of this as a potential pathway to strengthen the clinical education experience is a significant step forward.

Focus on student self-awareness very early in the curriculum and build the confidence to underpin improved patient care.

Self-awareness needs to be instilled within students early in their specific chiropractic studies, and in turn it is expected this will help shape stronger outcomes as learners and practitioners in the institution's clinical environments.

Strengthen learning in technology.

The challenges with technology for the Wi-Fi generation go beyond the Apple/Android divide and include institutions working with e-processes such as email that no longer connect with contemporary learners, cumbersome distributed learning systems that vary significantly across institutions, library and support IT systems that attempt to blend "real-world" databases into "institution-style" formats and approaches while missing the best of both, and clinical recording systems that are disjointed with intraclinic information, such as the patient health record, the imaging systems, and the patient scheduling systems.

Improve availability of and access to mobile technology.

Mobility of technology has the potential to significantly enhance the clinical learning experience. The various ways to achieve this remain works in progress.

Improve availability of and access to databases and Web-based knowledge.

New ways of leading the learning experience in the preclinic and clinic environments need to be explored to ensure all learners have optimal access to an institution's resources and portals to external resources.

Improve access to technology-assisted learning, such as force-plate fitted mannequins.

Technology is about more than managing access and learning support for students. An example of embedding technology into learning aids is mannequins for adjusting skills, and not only the wealth of information this provides but also the documented improvements in learner performance that such higher-level activities are able to achieve.

Clinic Level

Facilitate the sourcing of knowledge for more complex case mix.

This outcome builds on the previously mentioned need to improve database access for clinical learners, where "improved access" means also to improve and enhance institution sites, such as library portals. Clinics also need Wi-Fi printers so student clinicians can print relevant studies for inclusion in any hardcopy patient file.

Develop a better understanding of patients' health information needs.

This builds on the preceding comment and deserves institution-based analysis and improvement.

Concentrate on emergent themes: work-integrated learning (WIL), improved campus communications with external institutions and agencies, increased diversity of the range of learning experiences students are exposed to.

> This thought resonated within the group. All institutions are actually providing a very broad range of experiences. The intention of this outcome is to encourage all institutions to review the enriching experiences that are offered and identify ways in which they may be expanded and enhanced.

Support and incentivize research and scholarship.

> Incentives for research and scholarly productivity should be substantial to provide motivation (e.g., $5,000 cash as opposed to a $50 book voucher).

Professional (Practitioner) Level

Strengthen mentorship by the institution by establishing a database of expertise to assist practitioners wanting to research and write.

> Institutions should be repositories of peak clinical knowledge, understanding, and application. This resource could be better managed, perhaps on a multi-institutional basis, to provide a "genius" level of service (after the Apple model) to both clinical students and alumni.

Retain access to the institution library. Position the institution in a leadership role for practitioners.

> To support the "genius" concept as an integral part of the institution, access to library databases, included pregraduation, could be extended for no cost for the first year of practice and at a nominal cost for a library card in subsequent years. This would allow graduating students appropriate access to support the finalization for publication of their pregraduation projects and then build a long-term alumni benefit.

Practice-based clinical research hubs can become a crucial point of facilitation in the practice/academic community.

> There is a strong sense that the Practice-Based Research Network (PBRN) is a useful future direction, and the development of such should include the institution and its staff members, given most academic staff maintain some level of clinical practice. Academic staff must become exemplars, and this point closes the circle back to the first outcome of removing dissonance within the institution, strengthened by reducing institutional dissonance with the external clinical world.

In summary, this inaugural meeting called for a greater integration between practitioners and educators and proposed mechanisms to achieve this. It recognized the nature of engagement possible at the classroom, clinical, and professional levels.

Diversity of Models of Clinical Learning

Just as there is diversity in the nature of the institutions that deliver chiropractic education, there is a related diversity in the manner in which clinical learning is provided, including the following:

- the traditional model of a university/college-managed clinic
- the model of a multidisciplinary complementary and traditional hospital setting
- the model of a houseman (resident) year in a busy hospital
- placement in real-world clinics external to the institution
- placement in specialty clinics, such as sports chiropractic, child and maternal health, and advanced clinical neurology
- outreach activities both within and beyond the jurisdiction in which the institution operates
- variants and combinations of the above

The preclinical curriculum and coursework must be sufficiently attuned to the needs of learners specific to the model of clinical learning they will be entering. For example, a learner entering a model centered on a houseman year will require knowledge of hospital protocols, including rights and responsibilities. Not only will these be different to the protocols required for those entering a single-discipline (chiropractic) clinic managed by the chiropractic institution, they will differ to reflect the characteristics of the specific hospital in which they will undertake their houseman year.

To achieve increased student mobility in the global context, an elective course (subject) will be required that is tailored to specifically prepare learners for transition to their chosen clinical learning environment or country.

As the inaugural meeting/workshop on chiropractic clinical education agreed, there must be a theme, preferably starting in the preclinic program, that leads learners to appreciate the importance and value of clinical research and ways for students to contribute. It was felt academics should be exemplars and mentors, including part-time academics who primarily work in their own clinics.

Such academics are valuable assets to any chiropractic program in that they are perfectly placed to write and publish case reports and case series based on their own private patients. In this regard, they can lead by example and enhance their credibility as clinical educators.

The Tokyo meeting in 2015 also identified postgraduate learning as an important component of chiropractic education. It is reasonable to include this within the concept of advanced chiropractic education as continuing professional learning (CPL), which is critical to the ongoing development of individual and group practice. This field of learning is also considered as being postprofessional-qualification learning and includes the following:

- The need to develop effective, nonproprietary models for clinically based CPL for graduate practitioners.

- Ways in which such learning may be documented and quantified; these may already be in place in some jurisdictions, such as Australia, where practitioners are required to maintain a log of ongoing self-development together with reflections on the nature of the learning experiences as applicable to the individual practitioner.

- The perspective of students, which is the juncture between pre- and post-professional learning and occurs during another period named by the contemporary term "work integrated learning." Students are able to bring a variety of contemporary knowledge into practice during their period of clinical placement with a practitioner. Learners may actually be the ones who write a publishable case report with the practitioner as second author, drawing together a case based on that practitioner's clinical records.

- The perspective of an expert observer, which has a reverse effect to that described immediately above. As first presented at the Tokyo meeting, this could be implemented by adopting the Apple genius model where the practitioner is the "genius" and the student the learner. Appropriate practitioners who are recognized "experts" in particular fields of practice can schedule a weekly block of time to either attend an institution in person or use technology such as FaceTime for global accessibility. This latter approach would better serve the global improvement of chiropractic clinical education by providing a vast range of knowledge and experience that can be readily accessed by learners. This model is under development by an Australian private practitioner of chiropractic, Dr. Donald McDowall.

The models of clinical learning given above range from placement in an institution-managed clinic to outreach activities and must be used with an awareness of the patient case mix a learner will experience. Institution clinics can be thought of as more likely to attract the "worried well" patient, while outreach carries the danger of being more a "freebie feel-good" activity for the student when conducted as a time-limited visit to a location or country where chiropractic care is provided and then withdrawn.

Outreach activities provide greater learning and community benefits when managed by the institution in an ongoing manner, such as a charity clinic conducted in a less-fortunate community. Not only is the community continually served with chiropractic care, learners have a higher level of certainty that they will be able to include an outreach activity in their case mix of learning environments.

Such a case mix is essential to strengthen the clinical learning experience. The term "case mix" is used here with two meanings. The first relates to the range of patient encounters presented to the student. Several hundred presentations by the "worried-well" patient in a middle-class environment is unlikely to present the student with a reasonable spread of clinical conditions likely to be encountered in real-world practice. A record of the patient case mix should be kept to provide evidence the learning clinician has managed a variety of common presentations within a variety of demographic groups.

A "learning environment" case mix record will provide evidence that the learner has attained his or her patient case mix in a variety of environments. For example, if all patient encounters are undertaken as a houseman in a hospital setting, then there is a selection bias regarding the type of cases available and the patient case mix will suffer as it would with placement only in an institution-managed clinic. A mix of learning environments can be reasonably expected to provide a greater case mix of patient presentations and thus a broader and more complete clinical learning experience.

Global Mobility of Students

Student mobility will start with a handful of institutions around the globe whose leaders have the foresight to appreciate the benefits and then sit down together to make it work. Chiropractic education will benefit from a mobility program that engages with a number of universities worldwide. The engagement and pathways do not have to be with every one of the world's chiropractic institutions, just those that have the ability to work together for the greater benefit of enhanced patient care. Therefore, it is quite likely that a mobility program for chiropractic learners could include just some five or so institutions globally. This alone would place enormous pressure on those remaining institutions that failed to appreciate the benefits of a mobility approach. In many respects, this can be seen as disruption of the status quo, and it should not be suggested that those institutions that remain outside this relationship will not form a second and perhaps a third relationship with like-minded institutions.

The commonality among institutions within any one such mobility program is a curriculum that achieves agreed outcomes such that mobility is seamless. This means similar institutions will work together to achieve portability with mutual recognition of skills and capability attainment.

Similarly, chiropractic education is rapidly moving toward the clinical placement of learners in approved environments in other countries. Some governments provide funds to support this approach to work-integrated learning, and a growing number of universities are appreciating its benefits. One example is the placement of paramedic students enrolled in an Australian university program into ambulances in New York City.

As chiropractic institutions develop new resources in their home countries, such as a private hospital in Kuala Lumpur, a hospital of integrative medicine in Tokyo, or a center of chiropractic clinical excellence in East Asia, there will be new opportunities for multidirectional mobility between countries. Where an autonomous university agrees that the placement of its students offshore in such sites attracts learning credits equal to those able to be earned onshore, there is no role for an accrediting body to deny that credit. There is, after all, no difference in learning outcomes between placement in an institution's own clinic on the other side of town or in an approved clinic or other environment on the other side of the world. Distance in learning and assessment is no longer a barrier.

A Futurist's View of Where Chiropractic Education Is Headed

Chiropractic education will continue to evolve more rapidly than external accreditation standards, hence the argument that accrediting bodies will shift to establish guidelines and principles while institutions determine the elements and capabilities and their measurement. One would hope the two will be synergistic. In other words, the details of accreditation will be driven by institutions, not by outdated external organizational structures. All accrediting bodies will cease to exist in their current forms within 5 to 10 years.

There will be a rapid uptake of simulated learning, such as with mannequins in which force transducers are embedded to develop higher levels of manual skills[7] and other mannequins[8,9] that facilitate bidirectional conversation between the mannequin-as-patient and student-as-learner. High-end mannequins are able to simulate negative responses to intervention. Central Queensland University in Australia is a world leader in this approach designed to dramatically improve learners' skills in risk reduction and optimal clinical management.

Mobile devices such as the Apple Watch will become mandatory clinical tools and replace some measuring devices that date from the 19th and

20th centuries. New outcome measures of chiropractic intervention will emerge within five years and include personalized, wrist-driven heart rate variability and pulse oximetry. In turn, this will provide opportunities for new research projects to test the validity and specificity of these measurements and their meaning in the chiropractic clinical setting. Examples of similar devices already in use in some programs of chiropractic clinical education are infrared devices for measuring body temperature and finger or wrist devices for measuring blood pressure.

The concept of "anywhere, anytime" learning, facilitated by mobile devices, will drive the ability to reduce face-to-face contact hours and allow new forms of learning where lectures are chunked into smaller pieces that will, with supportive discussion and direction to appropriate online content, drive the parallel removal of face-to-face sessions that are currently considered "skills practicals." Instead, the chiropractic skills and basic science laboratory components of the chiropractic curriculum will be delivered in interactive face-to-face small-group learning where a learning object that was once part of a 50- or 100-minute "lecture" delivered remotely from any attendant skills practicals will be delivered as a short chunk, discussed, and then immediately put into practice in the same learning space. This requires the redesign of all chiropractic learning spaces and new courses for academics on how to maximize this Wi-Fi generational approach to learning.

As learning shifts into the "anywhere, anytime" mode of delivery, so too will practical assessment. Learners will no longer be corralled into a "time and place" event to sit an examination in unison. Such examinations are not tests of learning; they are tests of memory and perseverance with a dash of cunning to know what the examiner prefers to see written. In contrast, learners will select a task from a prepared list that recognizes the variations in individual learning styles and at "anytime, anyplace" create a portfolio with a much greater use of video that demonstrates their understanding and application of the desired learning outcomes.

A more dramatic transition that is now in development is the use of virtual reality (VR) to create personal spaces in which students can achieve quantitative and qualitative learning outcomes. Within a few years it will be common to see learners wearing VR glasses and using hand gestures to air-tap within a virtual learning space, perhaps an optimized clinic room, to bring up a patient health record and read through it, to load the simulated patient's diagnostic images, and even to have a simulated patient who can be dissected by air-swipes to illustrate the highest possible anatomical detail.

The step beyond this is the inclusion of voice recognition to interpret the conversation of the learner and synthesize answers from the virtual patient that direct the learning outcomes embedded in the specific scenario.

A final transition will be the end of class timetabling as it is now known. There should be no strictures on learning and the demand, for example, that "Year 2 students will be present at this time in that space to all learn a task predetermined by the academic" will become an artifact. In its place will be the concept of learner-driven attainment, and the role of the academic will shift to one of creating a preferred yet flexible matrix of learning objects to be mastered to allow progression in a logical and sequential manner.

There will no longer be a demand that all learners in any one class undertake a common task, meaning one small group from Year 1 may wish to work on postural assessment while another works on gait analysis. Further, the concept that an interactive skills tutorial will be limited by year level will cease, and in the foregoing example a small group of learners from Year 2 may be in the same space to learn assessment of the ankle.

In effect, this is the learning principle that underpins the success of the Apple stores, where the learner determines his or her own needs then selects from a roster of when that need may be addressed, either in a structured learning format (equivalent to a small group in chiropractic education working on a common topic) or open training where at one table half a dozen people of all ages are each working on their own project (equivalent to several small groups in the one learning space working with different learning objects).

Conclusion

Learners are increasingly mobile, and this is driving the imperative of global standardization of the chiropractic curriculum, particularly that for clinical education. However, at this point students are unable to freely move within different chiropractic programs around the world.

The benefit of a somewhat common accreditation process for chiropractic education is an assurance of standards of safety and effectiveness for chiropractic patients.

Chiropractic education is moving into a period of change that will see stronger use of advanced technology. Current technology, such as electronic greeting stations in clinics, automated management of patients' iPad-based education clips, and digital imaging stations will rapidly be integrated into whole-of-clinic electronic environments, which will require specialized training at the pregraduate level in the world's chiropractic programs.

The prime intent of every chiropractic institution's efforts, that of providing a variety of learning experiences to produce well-qualified graduates, will remain paramount and the hallmark of chiropractic as a paradigm of health and wellness care.

References

1. Watkins CO. *The Basic Principles of Chiropractic Government.* 1944, reproduced by the National Institute of Chiropractic Research, Phoenix, Arizona, 1992.

2. Gibbons RW. Chiropractic's Abraham Flexner: the lonely journey of John J. Nugent, 1935–1963. *Chiropr Hist.* 1985;6:45–51.

3. Ebrall PS, Takeyachi K. International equivalency for first-professional programs and chiropractic education. *Chiropr J Aust.* 2004;34:103–112.

4. World Health Organization. *WHO Guidelines on Basic Training and Safety in Chiropractic.* Geneva: World Health Organization; 2005.

5. Conversation with Dr. Kim Humphreys. *Primary Contact.* 2016;Spring:14–16.

6. Fraser SW, Greenhalgh T. Coping with complexity: educating for capability. *BMJ.* 2001;323(7316):799–803.

7. Triano JJ, Descarreaux M, Dugas C. Biomechanics—review of approaches for performance training in spinal manipulation. *J Electromyography Kinesiology.* 2012;22(5):732–739.

8. McGregor M, Giuliano D. Manikin-based clinical simulation in chiropractic education. *J Chiropr Educ.* 2012;26:14–23. doi:10.7899/1042-5055-26.1.14.

9. Giuliano DA, McGregor M. Assessment of a generalizable methodology to assess learning from manikin-based simulation technology. *J Chiropr Educ.* 2014;28:16–20.

CHAPTER SEVEN

Opportunities for Additional Training and Experience

Clinton Daniels, DC, MS, DAAPM; Stefanie Krupp, DC, MS; Shawn Hatch, DC

There are a variety of possibilities for professional and academic advancement available to chiropractic physicians. Providers can continue their education through on-site residency programs, graduate degree programs, diplomate training, and/or a multitude of certifications. The decision of which avenue to follow depends largely on personal motivation, willingness to invest time and money, and clinical interest. Each form of training can further enrich individual providers and the chiropractic profession.

Resident training programs are available to new and recent graduates. They require substantial time commitment (one to four years) and dedication to on-site training and may include the opportunity to obtain an additional graduate degree or certification. These positions are paid a small annual stipend and are typically accompanied by health care benefits. Resident programs can be very competitive and commonly lead to academic positions or other occupational opportunities both within and beyond chiropractic.

Graduate degree programs require a willingness to make a large financial and time investment in education. The length of programs varies based on individual pursuits; however, many chiropractic colleges offer graduate degrees that can be completed concurrently with doctor of chiropractic programs. Graduate degrees are typically considered academic and are the most widely recognized of all chiropractic postgraduate education. Academic degrees (such as MS, PhD) are most commonly used to gain employment in a university setting, whereas professional degrees (such as DC, MD, PT) generally consist of specialized training for licensure.

Diplomates allow for specialization and advanced training but typically involve a large financial investment in attending and traveling to weekend continuing education seminars. However, this training typically does not require on-site dedicated residency training and can be well suited to working practitioners. These programs also tend to be very clinically oriented, whereas residency and graduate programs bend toward a large academic influence.

Certifications are typically the easiest form of continuing education to achieve and generally require the smallest time and financial investment. There are lots of organizations offering certification-level training that is very practical and at times may be applied toward diplomate training.

Residency Programs

Resident training programs serve as competitive postdoctoral training for chiropractic physicians. Residencies differ from student clinical rotations and student externships in that they are paid full-time positions. There are many advanced training programs that require a one- to three-year commitment. At this time, chiropractic colleges and universities fund the vast majority of programs.

Resident training opportunities at chiropractic colleges and universities include diagnostic imaging, chiropractic orthopedics, primary spine care provider, clinical sciences, clinical rehabilitation, and sports medicine/rehabilitation. The Department of Veterans Affairs offers training in integrative clinical practice. More information can be found in the human resource or employment section of a chiropractic institution's website or may be included with the academic programs.

Diagnostic Imaging

Diagnostic imaging residencies are three-year, full-time, on-campus academic training programs, commonly known as chiropractic radiology residencies. These programs are offered at eight chiropractic colleges within the United States and Canada. Several programs award a master's of science degree in diagnostic imaging, and all programs qualify successful candidates to sit for examination by the American Chiropractic Board of Radiology.

Table 7.1 Chiropractic Resident Training Programs and Their University Affiliations

Residency Institutions	Diagnostic Imaging	Sports Medicine	Primary Spine Care Provider	Rehabilitation	Clinical Sciences	Clinical Research	Chiropractic Orthopedics	VA Integrative Clinical Practices
Canadian Memorial Chiropractic College	X	X			X			
Logan University	X	X						X
National University of Health Sciences	X					X		
New York Chiropractic College								X
Northwestern University of Health Sciences		X						
Palmer College of Chiropractic (Davenport)	X			X				
Parker College of Chiropractic	X							
Southern California University of Health Sciences	X	X	X					X
University of Bridgeport, College of Chiropractic							X	X
University of Western States	X	X						
Department of Veterans Affairs								X

Chiropractic radiologists function as supervisors and interpreters of routine radiology as well as consultants on complex imaging procedures. Their training puts them in a position to advise referring physicians on the necessity and appropriateness of radiology services and to assist in clinical decision making. Radiology training includes, but is not limited to, plain films, fluoroscopy, computed tomography, magnetic resonance imaging, and diagnostic ultrasound. The programs develop chiropractic radiologists who have acquired advanced skills and competencies in diagnosis of pathologies, contraindications to spinal manipulative therapy, and expertise in the diagnosis of the mechanics of the locomotor systems via radiographs. Training consists of modules covering areas of subspecialty: musculoskeletal imaging, neuroradiology, imaging of the gastrointestinal and genitourinary systems, thoracic radiology, and fundamental imaging physics. Training includes the auditing and teaching of radiology classes to doctor of chiropractic candidates, practical training in all aspects of radiology, research, clinical involvement, consultation, assigned study, testing, and other endeavors.

The minimum program eligibility requires a doctor of chiropractic degree from an institution accredited by the Council on Chiropractic Education, active license in the appropriate state, minimum 3.0 GPA in a chiropractic professional program, and 3.0 GPA in diagnostic imaging courses. Diagnostic imaging resident selection is based on curriculum vitae, letters of recommendation, and transcripts from the chiropractic institution and National Board of Chiropractic Examiners.

Residency committees review applications, and interview opportunities are provided to selected candidates. Interviews typically consist of an on-campus interview with residency committee representatives, oral examination with the chair of the radiology department, and a presentation of a clinical radiology case.

Chiropractic Sports Medicine

Sports science resident programs provide advanced clinical experience concentrated in sports injuries and advancing human performance. Canadian Memorial Chiropractic College, Logan University, University of Western States, Northwestern University of Health Sciences, and Southern California University of Health Sciences all offer two-year, full-time resident training programs. Residents are mentored by senior sports medicine chiropractors and undergo hands-on and academic didactics consisting of clinical and field experience, doctoral student mentoring, and scholarly research. Residents participate in a wide array of exciting real-world sports and integrated health care settings. Emphasis is placed on providing care for all levels of athletes from high school to world-class professionals. The residents are involved not only in learning for themselves but serve as teaching assistants and guest lecturers for doctor of chiropractic courses. Some programs have a heavy emphasis in providing on-field care for local high school, college, and professional teams. At Logan University, the residents are concurrently enrolled in the master's degree program for sports science and rehabilitation as part of their compensation. NWHS offers its residents an optional third-year fellowship, and UWS offers a one-year fellowship to individuals who have completed both a doctor of chiropractic and a master's of sports science program.

Training is designed to provide residents with an advanced skill set for sports injury and performance management. They are prepared to evaluate, treat, and rehabilitate acute and chronic sports injuries as well as musculoskeletal pathology. Graduates understand the musculoskeletal anatomy and biomechanics that influence human performance and can apply exercise physiology principles to muscle, cardiovascular, and respiratory function to enhance human performance. Additionally, they demonstrate knowledge of sound nutritional concepts and basic emergency procedures within their scope of practice, and they develop safe and effective exercise and rehabilitation programs for athletic, normal, and special populations.

Residents are selected on a competitive basis, and openings are limited. Upon completion of these programs, residents are eligible to sit for credentialing as a certified chiropractic sports physician (CCSP) and board certification from the American Chiropractic Board of Sports Physicians (ACBSP). Residents are well positioned for nonchiropractic-specific credentialing examinations, such as certified strength and conditioning specialist (CSCS), performance enhancement specialist (PES), corrective exercise specialist (CES), and/or certifications from the American College of Sports Medicine (ACSM).

Primary Spine Care Provider

At the time of this writing, Southern California University of Health Sciences is the only academic institution to offer a primary spine care provider resident training. This is a two-year, full-time residency designed to provide advanced training in the diagnosis and management of the majority of spine-related disorders using evidence-based methods. Instruction emphasizes clinical training and experience in an interdisciplinary setting. These providers would ideally function as first contact for patients with spine-related disorders and could coordinate the referral and follow-up of the minority of patients who require special tests (e.g., radiographs, MRI, or electrodiagnosis) or invasive procedures (e.g., injection and surgery).[1] The pillars of the program include completing relevant academic courses, self-directed research, publication, and teaching. Primary spine care practitioners are positioned to act as clinicians, consultants, and researchers and are capable of participating in and leading integrative health care teams.

Upon completion of the training, these residents are skilled in differential diagnosis and management of patients with spine pain and have a wide-ranging understanding of spinal pain and the psychological factors that may contribute to suffering and disability. The first-line treatments that a primary spine care practitioner would employ include manual therapies, manipulation and mobilization, McKenzie Method, neural mobilization techniques, various forms of exercise, evidence-based education, and use of nonsteroidal anti-inflammatory and nonopioid analgesics.

Residents are selected on a competitive basis with limited openings. They receive an annual stipend with health benefits, excellent learning and teaching experiences, off-campus interdisciplinary rotations, and eligibility to sit for a specialty experience examination. In addition, a six-month to one-year fully funded fellowship may be arranged in a clinic caring for underserved populations in the developing world.

Rehabilitation

Palmer College of Chiropractic Davenport offers a three-year postgraduate residency in rehabilitation. This is an intensive clinical experience with a focus on incorporating rehabilitation into an interdisciplinary setting. Attention is paid to educating residents on the latest treatments and applying evidence-based rehabilitation techniques in helping patients attain their best level of health and mobility. Training meets the requirements of the American Chiropractic Association Council of Chiropractic Rehabilitation, and graduates are eligible to sit for board certification from the American Chiropractic Rehabilitation Board.

Clinical Sciences

Resident training in clinical sciences is available through Canadian Memorial Chiropractic College. The clinical sciences training consists of coursework, practicum, teaching, and research. Trainees are placed in multidisciplinary community and hospital-based environments, participate in external rotations, and work as chiropractic college teaching assistants. They must complete an independent original thesis project and systematic review of publishable quality, which is approved by the graduate student's faculty research mentor and the program coordinator. Program graduates often pursue careers in the areas of clinical consulting, research, and as scholars capable of participating in a multidisciplinary environment, including hospital settings.

Clinical Research

National University of Health Sciences offers a resident training program in clinical research. The residency is a full-time, three-year program and is completed in conjunction with a master's of public health (MPH) degree through the University of Illinois Chicago (UIC). Enrollment and completion of the MPH is an integral and mandatory part of the program. Residents are full-time employees and are paid an annual stipend. Working as a research assistant for UIC can offset the cost of tuition in the MPH program.

Chiropractic Orthopedics

Resident training in chiropractic orthopedics is available only to graduates of the University of Bridgeport College of Chiropractic. This is a three-year resident program and, at the time of this writing, is the only chiropractic orthopedic resident training available. University of Bridgeport has an agreement with a federally qualified health center (FQHC) to provide medical services for their patients, which subsequently generates revenue and funds the program. Residents are full-time employees of UB. As an added benefit for individuals that complete a residency as well as fellowship training and continue to serve as UB clinical faculty and/or providers for an additional four years, their chiropractic student loan balance is forgiven.

Training is offered through the University of Bridgeport Health Sciences postgraduate department. Residents are concurrently enrolled in orthopedic and neuromusculoskeletal medicine (NMSM) programs, which are open to all practicing chiropractors.

Orthopedic and neuromusculoskeletal medicine training topics include the following:

- neurosciences for chiropractic clinicians
- evidence-based chiropractic medicine

- neuromusculoskeletal medicine
  - orthopedic, neurologic, and pain evaluation and management
  - diagnostic imaging
  - neurodiagnostics
- understanding primary care medicine for the chiropractor
  - integrative medicine
  - patient-centered care
  - evidence-based medicine
  - patient-centered medical home
  - community health care

A single new resident is hired each year. Upon completion of the three-year residency, graduates that become board certified in chiropractic orthopedics will have the opportunity to participate in a three-year fellowship in neuromusculoskeletal medicine. This fellowship would consist of providing clinical services in community health centers and mentoring newer residents. Orthopedic and NMSM specialists are well positioned to become members of an integrated health care team within a FQHC or a patient-centered medical home.

Veteran Affairs Integrated Clinical Practice

The Veterans Affairs (VA) chiropractic residency program was introduced in July 2014 with funding for a three-year pilot program. VA Central Office establishes national policy and parameters of the training program, and a group of five VA facilities was selected to implement the program locally. It is designed to focus on integrated clinical practice—specifically emphasizing incorporation of chiropractic care in hospital-based health care systems. Collaboration and communication with primary care physicians, specialty care, and associated health providers are key components of these programs. Training is for one year, extending from July 1 to June 30 the following year.[2]

The vast majority of patient encounters within the VA are for musculoskeletal-related conditions. A survey of VA chiropractors ranked low back pain as the most common patient complaint, followed by neck pain.[3] VA training provides residents with extensive exposure to managing complex cases. A study at the VA of Western New York Health Care System revealed that 16.44 percent of patients had a diagnosis of post-traumatic stress disorder, 79.11 percent of patients were classified as obese by BMI, and 51.56 percent had a service-connected disability.[4]

Table 7.2   Location of VA Chiropractic Resident Programs and Their Respective Academic Affiliates

VA Facility	Academic Affiliate
VA Connecticut Health Care System, West Haven, CT	University of Bridgeport College of Chiropractic
VA Western New York Health Care System, Buffalo, NY	New York Chiropractic College
Canandaigua VA Medical Center, Canandaigua, NY	New York Chiropractic College
VA St. Louis Health Care System	Logan University College of Chiropractic
VA Greater Los Angeles Health Care System, Los Angeles, CA	Southern California University of Health Sciences, Los Angeles College of Chiropractic

Table 7.3   Frequency of Conditions Seen within the Past Week in 33 Chiropractic Clinics within the VA System[3]

Chief Complaint	Percentage
Low back	48
Neck	21
Thoracic	10
Lower limb (hip, knee, ankle, foot)	7
Headache	6
Upper limb (shoulder, elbow, wrist, hand)	6
Wellness	1
Visceral complaint	<1

In addition, VA training requires the residents to rotate through other medical and associated health clinics and participate in scholarly activities. The particular clinical rotations vary somewhat based on the individual nature of the respective hospitals. Some of the specialties and clinics observed by the inaugural resident class included primary care, physical medicine and rehabilitation, pain management, spinal cord injury, rheumatology, neurology, emergency care, mental health, orthopedic clinic and surgery, neurosurgery, acupuncture, dietetics, radiology, geriatrics, and musculoskeletal diagnostic ultrasound.

Potential applicants are required to have earned their doctor of chiropractic before entering the residency program on July 1 and must meet VA requirements for employment, including U.S. citizenship. The program is aimed at new graduates or early-career chiropractors interested in practicing in a comprehensive medical setting, contributing to research, and applying an active health care model.

Chiropractic college and graduate school transcripts, professional experiences, letters of recommendation, and interviews are all used to guide the resident selection committees. A call for applications is issued each year on the second Monday of January. Applications are only accepted during the open call. Through this program, residents will develop their knowledge of hospital practice, policies, and procedures and are better prepared for employment in VA or other health care systems.

Board Certifications

A diplomate is a board-certified credential that signifies the provider has demonstrated competency in a particular specialty. The American Chiropractic Association officially recognizes 11 specialties with diplomate status. Board certification typically consists of postgraduate study encompassing 300 to 400 hours of coursework, completed through online courses, weekend seminars, or often a hybrid of the two. Some, like radiology, require commitment to an on-campus residency program. Coursework is usually administered through the postgraduate department of an accredited chiropractic college or by a college holding status with an accrediting agency recognized by the U.S. Department of Education or with similar reciprocity. While most diplomate certifications are gained with a series of lectures and hands-on workshops, each certifying board has its own qualifications. A candidate must have taken the required number of hours of additional education in that specialty—some require that their own specific coursework be completed in order to test for certification, and others do not offer a set curriculum. Many also have other requirements in addition to the coursework, and all require that the candidate pass an examination. Examinations may be written, practical (hands-on), and/or oral.

Acupuncture

The Council of Chiropractic Acupuncture (CCA) offers postgraduate training and board certification status as a diplomate of the American Board of Chiropractic Acupuncture (DABCA). Training provided by the CCA is based on international standards and follows the recommendations of the World Health Organization (WHO) guidelines for acupuncture.

Formal board certification in chiropractic acupuncture is available through the American Chiropractic Association. To be eligible for board

---

Box 7.1

Chiropractic Specialty Programs Approved by American Chiropractic Association (ACA)

- Acupuncture
- Clinical neurology
- Diagnostic imaging
- Diagnosis and management of internal disorders
- Forensic sciences
- Nutrition
- Occupational health and applied ergonomics
- Orthopedics
- Pediatrics
- Rehabilitation
- Sports medicine

---

certification, the CCA has a 300-hour didactic and clinical training requirement. Many chiropractic colleges offer acupuncture training, and candidates have the option of completing their hours at multiple colleges and with multiple instructors. Postgraduate education must include clinical training and education in clean needle technique and patient safety. Examination for the DABCA involves rigorous written and practical examination.

To maintain diplomate status, the provider must obtain 24 hours of additional accredited continuing education hours in chiropractic acupuncture every two years and must attend the ACA-CCA symposium biannually. Chiropractors interested in providing acupuncture services need to contact their local state board, as acupuncture regulation varies from state to state, and chiropractors cannot perform acupuncture in all states—even with diplomate-level education.

Clinical Neurology

Chiropractic neurologists use the musculoskeletal and sensory systems as they interact with the neurological system to improve quality of life. They use a variety of treatment modalities, including chiropractic manipulation and other sensory-based modalities, to bring about improvements in health. There are two different organizations that certify chiropractors in neurology— American Chiropractic Neurology Board (ACNB) and International Academy of Chiropractic Neurology (IACN).

To be eligible for certification by the ACNB, a chiropractor must have taken 300 postdoctoral hours of coursework in functional neurology from a chiropractic college, university, institution, foundation, or agency whose program is approved by the Commission for Accreditation of Graduate Education in Neurology (CAGEN). Upon completion of coursework, they may sit for written and performance examinations and if successful are granted the designation diplomate of the American Chiropractic Neurology Board (DACNB). In order to maintain competency, all diplomates must complete a minimum of 30 classroom credit hours of continuing education in neurology each year in a program of study accredited by the CAGEN. Credit hours must include training in the areas of weakness identified at the time of initial certification.

The International Academy of Chiropractic Neurology (IACN) governs administration of the diplomate of the International Board of Chiropractic Neurology (DIBCN). Their certification requires a minimum of 300 hours of coursework in neurology with a passing grade of 80 percent in the program. DIBCN examination consists of written and practical exams.

Diagnostic Imaging

Chiropractic radiology is a referral specialty that provides consultation services at the request of other qualified doctors. Chiropractic radiologists provide consultation in health care facilities (private offices, hospitals, and teaching institutions) to meet the needs of referring doctors and their patients.

The American Chiropractic Board of Radiology (ACBR) provides recognized status to individuals who have successfully passed the Part I and Part II examinations leading to the designation diplomate of the American Chiropractic Board of Radiology (DACBR). Applicants must be enrolled in the final year, or have completed a three- or four-year full-time postgraduate radiology residency program as established by the host facility. A chiropractic college that holds status with a national chiropractic accrediting agency recognized by the U.S. Department of Education, or an agency having a reciprocal agreement with the recognized agency, must sponsor the postgraduate residency. The postgraduate residency in radiology must be taught by a DACBR or equivalent (medical or osteopathic board-certified radiologist) and should follow a comprehensive multisystem curriculum prescribed by the host facility.

Providers must gain recertification every five years. This may be done by either fulfilling certain educational activities, such as publishing scientific papers or attending annual symposia, or by retaking and passing an ACBR certification examination.

Diagnosis and Management of Internal Disorders

Chiropractors who wish to become better trained in modern medical diagnosis, functional medicine, and natural therapeutics can pursue certification from the American Board of Chiropractic Internists (ABCI). Chiropractic physicians who are diplomates of the ABCI (DABCI) use conventional medical diagnostics, specialized functional testing, and holistic medicine diagnostic evaluations. They incorporate therapeutic methods that emphasize conservative and minimally invasive approaches, such as clinical nutrition, exercise, vitamin and mineral supplementation, homeopathic medicine, botanical medicine, acupuncture, natural hormone replacement, and pharmacologic counseling.

In order to achieve diplomate status, a chiropractor must complete 300 hours of coursework in one of the approved DABCI programs and must successfully pass a written exam for each module. Upon completion of the coursework, they must successfully pass the American Board of Chiropractic Internists examination.

In order to maintain certification, a DABCI must obtain at least 12 hours per year of continuing education that meets the criteria of the accrediting board. They are required to attend an annual symposium once every two years.

Forensic Sciences

The practice of forensics involves the application of medical facts to legal issues. Chiropractic forensic experts have the ability to do independent medical examinations, testify in medical legal cases, and determine disability and impairment ratings. They have a focused awareness of injury and disability evaluation, data analysis, concise and well-written reporting processes, and an ability to testify on forensic conclusions. Chiropractors who wish to distinguish themselves through education and training in forensics may seek certification through the American Board of Forensic Professionals (ABFP). Diplomate training incorporates advanced instruction on disability determination systems, impairment rating systems, independent medical examinations, federal functional (work) capacity and physical assessment systems, Department of Transportation return-to-work and fitness-for-duty assessment, fraud and abuse investigation, maximum medical improvement, and causation.

A provider seeking to be credentialed as a diplomate of the American Board of Forensic Professionals (DABFP) must satisfactorily complete a minimum of 300 postgraduate hours in prescribed educational areas and successfully pass the oral and written certification examinations. Part I of the educational program must include a minimum of 40 hours in orthopedics, 40 hours in diagnostic imaging, 50 hours in clinical diagnosis, 30 hours in rehabilitation and physical medicine modalities and procedures, and 30 hours in forensic examiner responsibilities. Part II consists of 100 hours of forensics courses approved by the ABFP.

Nutrition

There are two different organizations that provide a nutrition diplomate certification for chiropractors—the American Clinical Board of Nutrition (ACBN) and the Chiropractic Board of Clinical Nutrition (CBCN). The ACBN is the only certifying agency in nutrition to offer diplomate status to all doctorate-level professionals in health care. Credentialed members of the ACBN hold the distinction of diplomate of the American Clinical Board of Nutrition (DACBN).

All applicants interested in sitting for the ACBN examination must be licensed professional health care providers that have successfully completed 300 hours of specialized postgraduate training in nutrition, or health care providers who have completed a 300-hour residency program. Candidates must write a nutrition-oriented article or paper acceptable for publication in board-approved journals and have a minimum of two years' practice experience in nutrition prior to sitting for the ACBN examination.

For diplomate certification by the CBCN, a candidate must hold the degree of doctor of chiropractic from a CCE-accredited college or its equivalent and must show evidence of having successfully completed at least 300 hours of coursework. The applicant must also submit two written case histories from real patient files in the format provided by the CBCN and possess a license or registration to practice chiropractic in good standing for a minimum of two years.

Occupational Health

Experts in occupational health are positioned to provide services directly to business and corporate clients, occupational nurses, human resource directors, engineers, and other health care professionals to improve workplace environment. Postgraduate training focuses on applying skills to consult with businesses and industries regarding occupational safety, evaluation, and treatment of injured workers; developing preventative interventions; and providing employee education.

The American Chiropractic Board on Occupational Health (ACBOH) provides diplomate credentialing. Training comprises three phases, each phase accounting for 120 hours of specialized education for a total of 360 hours. The diplomate program includes the completion of a project conducted on-site at a workplace or completion of a research project relevant to the specialty.

Diplomate training is also available through 228 hours of distance learning via DVD. In addition to the DVD training, 16 hours of online Department of Transportation (DOT) examination courses are required. For the distance-learning option, 72 hours are awarded for completion of a field study or research paper. Upon completion of the minimum 300 hours, doctors may apply to sit for a proficiency examination. To maintain certification, providers must complete 12 hours of continuing education every two years.

Orthopedics

Chiropractic orthopedics is a branch of chiropractic that concentrates on normal functions and diseases of the body as they relate to the neuromusculoskeletal and referred organ systems. Advanced proficiency in orthopedic evaluation and nonoperative management of a broad range of injuries, conditions, and disorders of the neuromusculoskeletal system can be attained from two different organizations—the Academy of Chiropractic Orthopedics (ACO) and the American Board of Chiropractic Orthopedists (ABCO).

To become board certified by the ACO, the chiropractor is required to provide certification from an accredited chiropractic college or university noting that the candidate has successfully completed a course of education specific to orthopedics. To be eligible for the diplomate examination, chiropractors must complete a minimum of 300 hours of ACO coursework. To maintain certification, a diplomate must attend 60 hours of continuing education in the area of orthopedics over a three-year period.

The ABCO requires 360 hours of coursework. It does not require specific modules or curricula components within the 360 hours. Coursework must be in chiropractic orthopedic content, which must be verified by an accredited school. The candidate is permitted to complete the 360 academic hours at more than one chiropractic college, but ABCO will require verification of hours from each school attended to make up the total required hours.

Pediatrics

There are two organizations that offer diplomate certification for chiropractors in pediatrics—the International Chiropractic Association Council on Chiropractic Pediatrics and the International Chiropractic Pediatric Association. These programs position providers as experts in the drugless care of children and women before, during, and after pregnancy.

The diplomate in clinical chiropractic pediatrics (DICCP) is a certification program offered through the International Chiropractic Association Council on Chiropractic Pediatrics. It consists of 360 classroom hours in all aspects of pediatrics—prenatal, pregnancy, birth, and infancy to adolescence. Each stage of pregnancy and of a child's development are covered in depth so the practicing doctor of chiropractic acquires greater skills and competencies in a wide range of evaluative, diagnostic, and assessment procedures, as well as manual treatment skills for different stages of development. Curriculum includes expanded modules on radiology, nutrition, functional medicine and immunology, sports injuries, orthopedics, neurology, and special needs. Chiropractors with a pediatric diplomate report commonly managing back or neck pain, asthma, birth trauma, colic, constipation, ear infections, head or chest colds, and upper respiratory infections.[5] Writing research papers is a mandatory requirement for diplomate status. The ICA Council on Chiropractic Pediatrics publishes the *Journal of Clinical Chiropractic Pediatrics.*

Candidates must complete the full three-year program, all assignments and projects, and pass a final internal exam to be eligible to sit for the DICCP board examination. To maintain certification, diplomates must complete 24 hours of continuing education in chiropractic pediatrics every three years. They must also attend at least one annual conference or symposium presented by the ICA Pediatrics Council every three years.

The International Chiropractic Pediatric Association (ICPA) also offers a diplomate certification in chiropractic pediatrics. It consists of a two-part series of coursework and projects totaling 400 hours. Part I is a 200-hour certification program that includes 14 classroom modules, two in-office Practiced Based Research Network (PBRN) projects, and successful completion of the comprehensive certification final exam. Part II is a 200-hour advanced competency program. Most requirements are in-office clinical and research projects. This format is intended to show clinical implications of the Part I curriculum.

Rehabilitation

Active care and physical rehabilitation play a large role in many chiropractic practices. This includes in-office rehabilitation as well as prescribed home exercises. For chiropractors who want to specialize in rehabilitation, the American Chiropractic Rehabilitation Board (ACRB) offers a program leading to board-certified status as a diplomate of the American Chiropractic Rehabilitation Board (DACRB).

The program consists of online reading material and exams, 150 hours of rehabilitation seminar attendance, completion of the oral practical examination, and submission of a case study. Of the 150 hours of rehabilitation seminars, 45 hours must be related to spine, 45 hours related to extremities, 48 hours of electives, and an online McKenzie Method Overview course must be completed. There is no set curriculum for diplomate training in rehabilitation. Rather, a provider may choose from a variety of organizations and instructors. A recertification examination must be completed annually to maintain diplomate credentialing.

Chiropractic Sports Medicine

The American Chiropractic Board of Sports Physicians (ACBSP) offers certifications for chiropractors wanting to work as team physicians and

---

Box 7.2

Courses Offered by American Chiropractic Rehabilitation Board (ACRB) Organizations and Instructors Approved toward Diplomate Hours

Dr. Dan Reyes—123Rehab
Dr. Craig Liebenson
Dr. Corey Campbell—Motion Palpation Institute
Steven Weinger—PosturePractice
Active Release Techniques
NY Chiropractic College
Midwest Rehabilitation Institute
Clinical Rehabilitation Seminars: Sessions 1–4
The McKenzie Institute, USA

sideline doctors or who just want to specialize in treating athletes. In some states, only chiropractors with the certified chiropractic sports physician (CCSP) credential or a diplomate of the American Chiropractic Board of Sports Physicians (DACBSP) may return an athlete to play after he or she is diagnosed with a concussion. The ACBSP governs the administration of the examinations and certifications.

The CCSP certification, which consists of at least 100 hours of coursework and a written examination, is a prerequisite to the DACBSP certification. Various accredited chiropractic colleges offer the curricula and training leading to qualification for taking the certification exams. Earning the DACBSP certification requires an additional 200 hours of coursework, successful completion of a written exam, a six-station practical exam, a written project, and 100 hours of practical experience in the field. Completion of a sports medicine residency program in its entirety may also qualify a candidate to take the diplomate exams.

Once certification has been achieved, a DACBSP must complete at least 24 hours per year of continuing education in coursework related to sports medicine in order to maintain an active certification. A diplomate must also maintain an active health care provider CPR certification.

Graduate Degree Programs

This section focuses on the curriculum, admissions requirements, career options, and applicable professional certifications of various graduate specialties offered at chiropractic institutions in the United States. There are many graduate degrees that complement a doctor of chiropractic degree, ranging from dual-degree master's to doctoral options that provide advancement or specialization. (See Table 7.4.) Graduate degree programs may be offered online, in person, or a combination of both (hybrid) depending on the program and institution. The majority of these programs can be completed concomitant to a doctor of chiropractic program with some courses potentially double-counting for both degree programs. The graduate programs that offer fellowships or residency programs are primarily postprofessional and require the completion of a doctor of chiropractic degree for entry to the program.

Many chiropractic colleges and universities offer options for furthering education and professional opportunities through dual and postprofessional master's degrees. Master's degrees provide a credential that is recognized across disciplines, which may facilitate collaborative professional opportunities, particularly in health care. Master's degrees can serve to

Table 7.4 Graduate Degree Programs Offered at Chiropractic Institutions (the Majority of Programs Offered Are Master's Degree Level)

Graduate Degree Institutions	Nutrition	Exercise, Rehabilitation, and Sports	Acupuncture and Oriental Medicine	Diagnostic Imaging	Other Degrees Available
Canadian Memorial Chiropractic College					■
Cleveland University					■
D'Youville College					■
Life University	■	■			■
Logan University College of Chiropractic		■		■	■
National University of Health Sciences			■	■	■
New York Chiropractic College	■				
Northwestern University of Health Sciences					■
Palmer College of Chiropractic (Davenport)					■
Parker College of Chiropractic					■
Southern California University of Health Sciences, Los Angeles College of Chiropractic		■	■		
Texas Chiropractic College		■	■		
University of Bridgeport College of Chiropractic	■	■	■		■
University of Western States				■	■

expand or focus a professional career. For instance, obtaining a master's degree in sports science will allow a chiropractor to focus his or her practice on helping athletes attain optimal performance, whereas a master's in nutrition may expand a clinical practice to include more in-depth supplement and diet recommendations for a range of conditions and optimal health.

The most common degree options will be reviewed in detail and include nutrition, sports science, acupuncture and Oriental medicine, and diagnostic imaging. Other graduate degree options also complement a doctorate in chiropractic, such as doctoral degrees in education (EdD); health science (DHSc); biomechanics, research, or health promotion (PhD); or public health (DrPH). Additional beneficial master's degree credentials include business administration (MBA) or public health (MPH) as well as the master's of science (MS) options included in this section. Health care degrees that expand the scope of practice for chiropractic in many states include physician assistant (MSPA); nurse practitioner (NP), which can be achieved through a master's in nursing (MSN) or a doctor of nursing practice (DNP); doctor of medicine (MD); doctor of osteopathy (DO); doctor of naturopathy (ND); doctor of physical therapy (DPT); and even doctor of veterinary medicine (DVM). Some chiropractic programs offer dual-degree opportunities for these graduate programs within their institution or in partnership with another institution.

Nutrition

Graduate degrees in nutrition are predominantly clinically focused and provide chiropractic students and doctors with evidence-informed diet and lifestyle strategies to prevent and manage disease and metabolic dysfunction. Most programs teach a functional medicine approach, which encompasses understanding root causes of dysfunction through biochemical and physiological mechanisms. Programs are offered on campus, online, or in hybrid format depending on the institution and typically run about two years depending on course load.

Foundational courses for master's programs in nutrition include biochemistry and physiology focusing on metabolic processes and pathways. Courses typically include elements of clinical assessment, diagnosis, and/or patient management. Nutritional plans and supplement recommendations are often woven through the majority of the curriculum. Graduates will be able to apply their practical knowledge to create a holistic and personalized therapeutic approach.

Typical nutrition program topics include the following:

- macronutrients (carbohydrates, lipids, proteins and amino acids, fiber, etc.)
- micronutrients (vitamins and minerals)
- nutrigenetics and nutrigenomics
- herbology/botanical medicine
- nutritional therapeutics and neutraceuticals
- food as medicine
- interconnectedness of critical systems of the human body, such as:
  - gastrointestinal and urogenital systems, including detoxification
  - endocrine and metabolic systems
  - cardiorespiratory
  - neurological, including pain
  - immunological, including inflammation
  - musculoskeletal system and structural integrity
- human developmental and life cycle nutrition
- nutrition epidemiology (incidence, causes, distribution, and prevention of disease in populations)
- food industry concepts, including food labels, product development, marketing, food safety, food science, and agricultural practices

Key assessment methods covered in most nutrition graduate programs include the following:

- health history and symptom surveys
- family history and genetic predispositions
- analysis of diet for micro- and macronutrient deficiencies
- lifestyle and physical activity evaluation
- food allergies and intolerances
- physical examination
- anthropometric measurements
- environmental factors
- functional laboratory testing, including blood, stool, urine, and saliva testing

Supplemental topics covered in a nutrition program include the following:

- pharmacology, herb/drug and food/drug interactions, and drug-induced nutrient depletion

- exercise physiology and nutrients for recovery and enhanced human performance
- communication skills, counseling, and behavior modification techniques
- mind-body medicine and psychology of well-being
- community health issues, including policy making, food insecurity, and health disparities influenced by economic, social, and cultural factors
- practice management concepts, such as business practices, marketing, social media, and consumer behavior theory
- professionalism and ethics, including scope of practice, credentialing, HIPAA, and risk management
- Some programs offer internships, research projects, and independent study opportunities

Information literacy is also woven through much of the curriculum for nutrition graduate programs and is a critical component of generating evidence-informed management plans. Evidence-based care integrates clinical experiences and patient values with the best available research information.[6] Evidence-based nutrition courses cover research methodologies, experimental design, data analysis including biostatistics, data integrity, and research bias. Graduates will know how to appropriately navigate the many health and nutrition claims that abound in the media and on the Internet as well as from supplement companies to provide sound evidence-informed care and advice for their patients.

Programs often cover integrative approaches so that graduates can work as part of a health care team. In an integrative environment, it is important to understand the role of supportive or adjunctive care in working with other licensed professionals. Additionally, understanding the standards of care for particular conditions will also facilitate collaboration for the patient's best interest.

Nutrition programs require prior coursework in anatomy and physiology, chemistry, biochemistry, and nutrition for admission, which is met by most chiropractic curricula in the first year of study. An institution may have additional requirements not mentioned here.

Completion of graduate degree programs in nutrition typically satisfy all or most of the educational requirements to sit for national certification exams, including the certified nutrition specialist (CNS), the certified clinical nutritionist (CCN) through the Clinical Nutrition Certification Board (CNCB), certified sports nutritionist (CISSN) through the International Society of Sports Nutrition (ISSN), the diplomate of the American Clinical Board of Nutrition (DACBN), and the diplomate of Chiropractic

Board of Clinical Nutrition (DCBCN). Those wishing to obtain certifications should review requirements by their local state board to determine licensing, registration, and scope of practice.

Those with master's degrees in nutrition can work in integrative health care settings such as physicians' offices and hospitals. Their knowledge base also affords them opportunities in public health programs, school systems, health clubs, nursing homes, and food companies, with a focus on research, development, sales, marketing, public relations, and public education. Other avenues to use this specialty include nutrition and health communication, consulting, corporate wellness programs, and nutrition-related business ventures in the private and public sectors. The master's-level degree also opens doors to teach courses in nutrition, biochemistry, anatomy and physiology, and biology in higher education.

Exercise, Rehabilitation, and Sports Studies

Graduate programs in sports science, exercise, and rehabilitation focus on enhancing human performance through the evaluation, treatment, and rehabilitation of acute and chronic injuries and musculoskeletal pathologies. Programs are often collaborative and integrative, and practical experiences are typically offered with local athletic teams. Due to the clinical requirements of these programs, they are primarily hybrid or on-campus programs, particularly for those dual-enrolled in a doctor of chiropractic program. Prerequisites for admission into a sports science graduate program are typically satisfied by the chiropractic curriculum, including anatomy and physiology, chemistry, and physics. Programs may require a minimum grade point average (GPA), the Graduate Record Examination (GRE), letters of intent, and recommendations and may have technical standards for admission.

Sports science programs provide training in the physiological responses and adaptations to exercise, including human performance limitations, training effects, and health benefits of physical fitness. The main topics covered by a sports-oriented master's program include the following:

- neuromuscular skeletal anatomy, biomechanics, and arthrokinematics
- exercise physiology covering neuromuscular, cardiovascular, and respiratory systems
- examination, testing methods, and protocols with focus on biomechanics of sports injuries
- sports-oriented nutrition and psychology

- emergency procedures (within scope of practice)
- communication and professionalism as an allied health team member
- evidence-based and integrative management strategies
- exercise and rehabilitation plans and treatment approaches for athletes and normal and special populations, such as children or geriatrics

Sports science has the most certification opportunities based on the areas of study and interest, including the following:

American Chiropractic Board of Sports Physicians (ACBSP)
  ○ certified chiropractic sports physician (CCSP)
  ○ diplomate American Chiropractic Board of Sports physicians (DACBSP)

American College of Sports Medicine (ACSM)
  ○ health fitness specialist (HFS)

International Federation of Sports Chiropractic (IFSC)
  ○ international certified chiropractic sports physician (ICCSP)

International Society of Sports Nutrition (ISSN)
  ○ certified sports nutritionist (CISSN)

National Academy of Sports Medicine (NASM)
  ○ corrective exercise specialization (CES)

National Strength and Conditioning Association (NSCA)
  ○ certified personal trainer (NSCA-CPT)
  ○ certified strength and conditioning specialist (CSCS)
  ○ tactical strength and conditioning facilitators (TSAC-F)
  ○ certified special population specialist (CSPS)

Advanced training in sports science is essential for chiropractic graduates to pursue careers as clinical exercise physiologists, strength and conditioning coaches, health club managers, corporate fitness providers, sports media consultants, sports nutritionists, athletic coaches and directors, and team managers. The additional training and related credentials may open doors to integrative health care settings and higher education career opportunities.

Acupuncture and Oriental Medicine

Acupuncture is a system of diagnosis and treatment that uses stimulation of prescribed points on the body known as meridians, which directs the flow of "qi," or energy, in order to restore balance and health. Acupuncturists use a variety of treatment techniques, including traditional acupuncture (ultra-fine needles inserted into meridians), electroacupuncture (electrical current), moxibustion (therapeutic application of heat), cupping (vacuum pressure), tui na (massage), and exercise and breathing practices. Acupuncture is one of the most well-researched complementary and alternative medicine (CAM) therapies.

Oriental medicine, or traditional Chinese medicine (TCM), is a system of pattern identification used to assess patients and generate individualized treatment plans using acupuncture as well as Chinese herbs. The Oriental medicine master's programs typically start with the acupuncture curriculum and then include coursework in traditional Chinese herbal medicine, such as the study of the Materia Medica and herbal dispensary management.

The typical acupuncture program curriculum includes the following:

- cultural and philosophical foundations of traditional Chinese medicine, including Chinese language and nei jing
- anatomy and physiology
- needling anatomy, point location, and point energetics
- biomedical sciences, including radiology, pathology, microbiology, and public health
- patient assessment and diagnostics
- acupuncture treatment principles and practical skills
- oriental bodywork (tuina or tui na)
- exercise and breathing practices (tai ji/tai chi/taijiquan and qi gong)
- qi development
- nutrition and oriental food therapy
- herbal formulas and treatment strategies
- pharmacology (indications, contraindications, mechanism of action, side effects, and interactions)
- health psychology and patient communication
- evidence-informed practice and information literacy
- Western medical screening, emergency care, and basic life support
- medical law, ethics, and risk management
- business, marketing, and practice management
- clinical experience (typically in the last year of the program)

Acupuncture and Oriental medicine (AOM) programs typically require coursework in biology, chemistry, physics, and psychology for admission, which is met by most chiropractic curricula in the first year of study. An institution may have additional requirements, such as a minimum GPA. AOM degree programs are primarily full time and on campus due to the vigorous course load and practical and clinical experiences required for competency. Courses may be offered in the evening or on weekends to accommodate working professionals or allow for dual enrollment with a chiropractic program. Acupuncture and Oriental medicine graduate programs often take at least two years to complete, depending on course load, degree (master's or higher), and concentration(s).

Certification in acupuncture is voluntary, but most states require certification for licensure. Additionally, licensure is a criterion to provide care in health insurance networks. Graduates of master's degrees in acupuncture and Oriental medicine programs are eligible to sit for the licensing examinations conducted by the National Certification Commission for Acupuncture and Oriental Medicine (NCCAOM) as well as the National Board of Chiropractic Examiners (NBCE). There are four modules for NCCAOM certification:

- foundations of Oriental medicine
- acupuncture with point location
- biomedicine
- Chinese herbology (Oriental medicine programs only)

Licensure requirements vary by state with some states not offering licensure. Practitioners can consult the NCCAOM for more details.

Master's degrees in acupuncture and/or Oriental medicine allow chiropractors to offer treatment approaches for patients that may not have responded to traditional chiropractic care. The additional specialty degrees and certification may expand practice options, with graduates working in hospitals and integrative settings that may have excluded chiropractors otherwise. The demand for acupuncture and Oriental medicine has steadily increased in recent decades, particularly due to evidence supporting the relatively low risk to treatment.

Diagnostic Imaging

Diagnostic imaging is the use of machines and techniques to create pictures of the structure and function of the human body for examination. Imaging techniques may include radiography, nuclear medicine scans, magnetic resonance imaging (MRI), computed tomography (CT or CAT scan), and ultrasound. Diagnostic imaging residency programs often include a master's of science degree in diagnostic imaging. Residency means that these programs require completion of the doctor of chiropractic degree prior to application. Institutions offering the master's degree as part of the residency program include National University of Health Sciences, New York Chiropractic College, and the University of Western States.

Core topics for diagnostic imaging master's programs include the following:

- musculoskeletal pathology and disorders (arthritis, blood-vascular, congenital/dysplasias, infection, internal derangement, metabolic and endocrine, nutritional, trauma, tumors)
- neuroimaging
- chest and intrathoracic pathology and disorders (cardiovascular, pulmonary)
- gastrointestinal pathology and disorders
- genitourinary pathology and disorders
- medical physics, radiation health and safety
- instructional methodology

Programs include auditing and teaching radiology classes to DC students, practical training in all aspects of radiology, research, clinical involvement, consultation, and independent study. Rotations with radiology departments of local hospitals and medical imaging centers add practical experience beyond a purely chiropractic setting. Residency programs in diagnostic imaging are the only way a doctor of chiropractic may become eligible for examinations leading to the professional certification diplomate of the American Chiropractic Board of Radiology. Graduates function as imaging specialists, educators, and administrators in chiropractic institutions.

Because of the limited opportunities for this type of residency and master's program, the requirements for selection are competitive and may include interviews and examinations by the institution. Applications typically go through the human resources department rather than admissions office since this is a salaried position with teaching responsibilities. The cost of the master's degree is waived. Programs are full time and on site and typically last three years.

Other Graduate Degree Options

Many chiropractic institutions are expanding or already offering broader options for students and practicing chiropractors to pursue graduate opportunities for additional master's and doctorate credentials to work in higher education, research, business, consulting, public health and policy, and integrative environments. Institutions with traditional college or university systems offer many other graduate options than are mentioned here.

Certificate Programs

There are countless certifications for postgraduate education available to chiropractic physicians and health care providers in general. Summaries of all certification programs are beyond the scope of this chapter. A sample of the most well-known certifications is highlighted in this section. Certifications often provide increased practice exposure since certifying programs often have patient and provider resources, including a "find a certified practitioner" section of their website.

Certified Chiropractic Sports Physician

Completion of the certified chiropractic sports physician program (CCSP) is the first step toward earning diplomate status from the American Chiropractic Board of Sports Physicians. The program consists of 100 hours of postgraduate education covering diverse topics in sports medicine, such as concussion management and emergency procedures in sports. Individuals that possess an athletic trainer certification (ATC) or master's of science in exercise and sport science may sit for CCSP examination without completing postgraduate courses. All candidates must have completed a hands-on training emergency procedures course and have a health care–provider-level CPR certification.

Motion Palpation Institute Certification

The Motion Palpation Institute (MPI) offers postgraduate courses on a broad array of topics, including, but not limited to, spine analysis and adjusting, extremity adjusting, shoulder rehabilitation, disc injury management, upper extremity and lower extremity dynamic assessment, and gait analysis. Seminars are concentrated on an active care model of chiropractic. MPI provides certification to doctors who have attended a spine, extremity, and two dynamic movement assessment classes.

Certified Chiropractic Extremity Practitioner

The Council on Chiropractic Extremity Adjusting (CCEA) offers certified chiropractic extremity practitioner (CCEP) certification for doctors who have completed seven weekend seminars (105 hours) of CCEA training. Course topics include principles of temporomandibular joints (TMJ), ribs and shoulder girdle; upper extremity adjusting; lower extremity adjusting; extremity rehabilitation; principles of foot, gait, and orthotics; and soft tissue methods for spine and extremities. Providers must pass an examination at each seminar as well as a practical examination upon program completion.

Functional and Kinetic Treatment with Rehab

Functional and kinetic treatment with rehab (FAKTR) is a concept for evaluation and treatment that can be used with virtually any technique. FAKTR incorporates static, motion, resistance, functional, and proprioceptive treatment approaches. Training is designed for use by manual and instrument-assisted practitioners within all health care specialties. There are two parts for certification—a 12-hour hands-on course that contains didactic materials based on the latest research, and a 6.5-hour online course expanding on research from the International Fascial Congresses, upper extremity neural mobilization, and functional taping. After completion of the online course, the provider may sit for the certification examination.

Certified Strength and Conditioning Specialist

The National Strength and Conditioning Association offers the certified strength and conditioning specialists (CSCS) certification. Certified providers are professionals who apply scientific knowledge to train athletes for the primary goal of improving athletic performance. They conduct sport-specific testing sessions, design and implement safe and effective strength training and conditioning programs, and provide guidance regarding nutrition and injury prevention. To be eligible for certification, trainers must have a bachelor's degree or an advanced professional degree and pass written examination.

Selective Functional Movement Assessment

The selective functional movement assessment (SFMA) is the movement-based diagnostic system designed to clinically identify fundamental movement patterns in patients with musculoskeletal pain. The assessment provides an efficient method to systematically find the cause of symptoms, not just the source, by logically breaking down dysfunctional patterns and diagnosing their root cause as either a mobility problem or a stability/ motor control problem. This model integrates the concepts of altered motor control, the neurodevelopmental perspective, and regional interdependence. There are three levels of certification that involve completion of three courses and subsequent exams.

Mechanical Diagnostic Technique

The McKenzie Method of mechanical diagnostic technique (MDT) is an assessment process intended for musculoskeletal problems involving the spine and extremities. The McKenzie assessment explores different positions and movements, how the patient performs them, and the response to various movements and integrates this information to guide treatment practices. McKenzie Institute International recognizes and credentials providers with basic competency in MDT. To be eligible for certification, providers need to complete courses A–D and pass written and performance examinations.

Certified Kinesio Taping Practitioner

Kinesio taping method is a therapeutic taping technique designed to reeducate the neuromuscular system, reduce pain, and optimize performance. Kinesio Taping Association International (KTAI) is a leading certifying organization for proprioceptive taping. To become certified, practitioners must complete KT1 (Fundamental Concepts), KT2 (Advanced Concepts and Corrective Techniques), and KT3 (Clinical Concepts and Advanced Taping Methods) approved seminars and pass the CKTP examination. There are no recertification requirements, but annual membership must be maintained.

References

1. Murphy D, Justice B, Paskowski I, Perle S, Schneider M. The establishment of a primary spine care practitioner and its benefit to health care reform in the United States. *Chiropr Man Ther.* 2011;19(17).

2. Daniels C, Dluzneiwski A, Golley D, Liang B, Perrucci R. Q&A with the first VA chiropractic residents: inaugural class of 2015 shares their residency experiences. *Dynamic Chiropr.* 2015;33(13).

3. Lisi AJ, Goertz C, Lawrence DJ, Satyanarayana P. Characteristics of Veterans Health Administration chiropractors and chiropractic clinics. *J Rehabil Res Dev.* 2009;46(8):997–1002.

4. Dunn AS, Passmore SR. Consultation request patterns, patient characteristics, and utilization of services within a Veterans Affairs Medical Center chiropractic clinic. *Mil Med.* 2008;173(6):599–603.

5. Pohlman KA, Hondras MA, Long CR, Haan AG. Practice patterns of doctors of chiropractic with a pediatric diplomate: a cross-sectional survey. *BMC Complement Altern Med.* 2010;10(26).

6. Masic I, Miokovic M, Muhamedagic B. Evidence based medicine—new approaches and challenges. *Acta Informatica Medica.* 2008;16(4):219–225. doi:10.5455/aim.2008.16.219-225.

CHAPTER EIGHT

Starting a Chiropractic Practice

Ronald J. Farabaugh, DC

The most common dream of a chiropractic college graduate is to one day establish his or her very own practice. There are many steps in the process leading to ownership, and it's important to review and analyze each step of this exciting journey. Before forging ahead, there are issues to consider, including knowledge and recognition of the systems required to run a successful business. The issues can be divided primarily into two categories: business decisions and clinical decisions. Within those two categories are seven subsets of business systems that every business owner must master to be successful: leadership, management, money, marketing, new patient generation, conversion, and fulfillment. The *E-Myth* by Michael Gerber provides in-depth knowledge regarding the seven systems of a business.[1] It takes skill and finesse to wear all seven hats related to those systems, but the more familiar one becomes with each required category, the better the chances for financial and personal satisfaction and overall success.

This chapter will explore each side of the practice matrix, both pre- and post-start-up, and offer suggestions to help the reader open his or her first chiropractic office. The information in this chapter can also be used by experienced clinicians wishing to review and refine their own office systems. The following issues represent only the beginning of the information gathering needed to establish and grow a practice. This is a long journey, not a sprint.

Clinical Decisions

Before obtaining financing and opening the doors, there are many questions to answer about the clinical side of the practice. Consider the following list a starting point only. Well-thought-out answers to the questions below will construct an organized and solid framework upon which to build a new business.

1. Where is the practice located?
2. What is the type or focus of the practice (for example, evidence-based, workers' compensation, personal injury, family practice, pediatrics)?
3. What specific techniques and services are provided?
4. What is the atmosphere in the office (casual, formal)?
5. How will new patients be attracted to the practice?
6. How will new patients become established (regular) patients?
7. How will patients' expectations be met?
8. How will the practice be distinct from other practices? What makes it unique?

Key Business Decisions

There are as many business decisions as clinical decisions in starting a practice. The following list is a step-by-step roadmap to construct a new practice. Even the very best chiropractors may experience unnecessary stress or even fail if they are not organized and efficient in business matters. These considerations will be discussed in detail in this chapter:

1. Getting started; possibilities are: work for another doctor of chiropractic (DC) as an associate, open a solo practice, incorporate the practice, enter into a shared rental agreement with another DC, or employment in an integrated health care clinic
2. The business plan; financing for the office
3. Demonstrating leadership
4. Marketing considerations
   a. Mission, vision, strategic objective
   b. Target market
   c. Logo, color scheme
   d. Website
   e. Social networking strategy
   f. Décor/sensory analysis of interior and exterior of practice

5. Management considerations, both managing staff and patients

   a. Employee handbook

   b. Personality types

   c. Salary strategies

   d. Staff size

   e. Organizing the computer system

6. Financial considerations

   a. Financial basics

   b. Business control systems

   c. Financial intelligence

   d. Hiring/firing/training staff

   e. Setting goals

Key Clinical Questions

Location of the Practice

One of the most important decisions is the location of the practice. Building a practice takes years, so it is essential that the country, region, city, and neighborhood be chosen only after careful deliberation. Once financially and emotionally vested in an office, community, and lifestyle, it is very difficult to move.

The new practitioner must decide on the geographic area and then zero in on an actual physical address. Interviewing several chiropractors and other health professionals in that area is helpful, but these doctors should be chosen carefully; seek out mentors who have an "abundance" mentality. It is not easy to succeed in this era of health care, but it can be done with proper planning and persistence. There are no get-rich-quick schemes in chiropractic—or life in general—so be leery of consultants who promise this.

These three principles are the foundation for achieving success in an ethical manner:

1. Provide patients what they need, and only what they need—nothing more and nothing less—always.

2. Tell patients if you can help them, and tell them if you cannot help them—and make a proper referral!

3. Be patient centered, evidence based, outcomes driven, and cost conscious.

Society in general will seek out those doctors who get the best results, in the shortest period of time, with the lowest cost.

Type or Focus of the Practice

The focus of a practice is not the same as specializing. It is more of an emphasis, for example, on a particular condition, treatment, or patient population. Bottom line: this emphasis will determine the way the office is designed and equipped, so it must be decided before seeking financing or opening the doors for patient care. Some issues include type of equipment needed, techniques to be used, and philosophical approach. Beginning with the end in mind (the opening of a practice), the decision about techniques and practice style is ideally considered within the first one to two years of chiropractic school.

There is a wide variety of practice themes and associated therapies to consider. The vast majority of practices are a blend of several techniques and therapeutic modalities. One thing is for certain, an effective DC has to have a lot of tools in his or her toolbox. What works for one patient may not work for another. The spinal manipulation therapy/adjustment (hereafter referred to as simply "SMT") for a toddler is vastly different than the SMT for a 290-pound dock worker or a 90-year-old osteoporotic woman. However, there is no need to access every therapeutic modality under the sun to start a practice. Begin with the basics and add tools as the need arises. Examples of themes and modalities/services are listed below:

- pain relief practice
- wellness clinic
- functional medicine and nutrition practice
- personal injury practice
- workers' compensation (work comp) practice
- sports practice
- extremity practice
- occupational medicine practice
- rehabilitation practice
- nonsurgical spinal decompression practice
- open versus private treatment areas
- neck pain/headache practice
- pediatric practice

- spa-style chiropractic
- multidisciplinary/integrated practice
- subluxation-based theme
- academic-evidence-based theme
- acupuncture practice and/or massage therapy practice
- traditional manual adjusting
- instrument-assisted adjusting (Activator, ArthroStim, PulStar, etc.)
- free clinic
- mobile clinic

The range of potential office themes and services varies greatly and is often influenced by state or country scope of practice. It is essential to investigate the specific laws governing chiropractic in the practice location. A little research in the beginning could save thousands of dollars and months or years of heartache and frustration.

Box 8.1

Controversy: Chiropractic as a Pain-Relief Specialty

Since the inception of chiropractic in 1895, there has been an unfortunate philosophical dilemma that continues to affect the development of the chiropractic profession. It is related to a battle between the extremes, the "pain relief" versus "subluxation correction" philosophical camps.

Opponent's viewpoint of "pain relief" practice: Critics of pain relief–only patient care tend to be vocal and very critical of DCs who primarily provide pain relief. These critics believe that it is a disservice to the patient to focus on treating pain rather than on "correcting" the spine. In terms of pain relief, this is actually only a difference in attitude and perspective, since pain reduction generally occurs with either approach.

Opponent's viewpoint of "correction care" and/or "spinal-remodeling" practice: Critics of "correction-care" or "spinal-remodeling" care often suggest that providing care beyond pain relief, at multiple visits per week for extended periods, is not supported by quality literature, and it breeds overtreatment and excessive expense to the patient, employers, or third-party payors. There is much controversy about the objective identity of a subluxation and no definitive way to know when it is corrected. Thus, each doctor must determine this for him- or herself, since patient symptoms are not integral to determining the need for an adjustment. For example, selling 60 visits

---

per year for thousands of dollars prepay based on just the initial examination, all in the name of "principled chiropractic," continues to erode the public trust in chiropractic, making it harder for all DCs to thrive in the current health care market.

Sandwiched in the middle are the silent majority of DCs who simply want to provide the best care they can for their patients and go home at the end of the day with their head held high. Contemporary chiropractors understand that society will reward those doctors who achieve *the best outcome in the shortest period of time with the least amount of cost*. It is highly recommended that the philosophical war that has plagued this profession be avoided; instead, practitioners should focus squarely on the needs and desires of the patient. From a practical viewpoint, the argument is not worth the time and effort given the reality of practice. Therefore, the remainder of this chapter will avoid the issues related to philosophy. The business realities of daily practice do not vary much regardless of philosophy. That is, regardless of philosophical preference, the average DC consults, examines, and diagnoses the patient. And then the DC does what? Answer: He or she provides a spinal adjustment. So what is there really to argue about? We have much more that binds us than we have separating us.

Over the course of one's career, there will be a naturally increasing percentage of wellness patients in the overall patient matrix. The vast majority of those considered "wellness" patients are in reality "chronic pain" patients. Those patients return monthly since care helps them control pain and makes them feel better. Few true "wellness" patients (those with absolutely no pain) visit the average chiropractic office. The best news is that there is some evidence supporting monthly care for chronic pain management.[2,3]

Services and Techniques

There is a wide range of potential services that might be provided, depending on the laws of the local jurisdiction. Before succumbing to the sales presentation by a manufacturer's rep, be sure to request quality evidence of effectiveness of the potential therapy. Simply ask: "Do you have any literature on this therapy, reported in a peer-reviewed journal, versus the manufacturer's own marketing material?" Be sure to perform due diligence. A doctor's reputation depends on the decisions he or she makes related to the therapies offered. The following therapies are in use by DCs and other medical professionals. Some are appropriate and evidence based, while others are less well documented. Practitioners need to decide which are legitimate after doing their own research. They also need to check with the state board to ensure the therapy is compatible with state law because chiropractic scope of practice is defined by laws in each state and country and can vary greatly. Below are lists of commonly used diagnostic and treatment procedures and practices by chiropractors in the United States.

Treatments

- acupuncture and/or dry needling
- Active Release Technique (ART)
- bracing
- exercise and lifestyle modification
- massage therapy
- nutrition advice and food supplements
- orthotics (specially made shoe inserts)
- physical modalities used for pain management and to promote healing
- physio-taping
- rehabilitation programs

Diagnostic procedures and activities

- athletic physicals
- Department of Transportation (DOT) exams
- laboratory diagnostics
- pre-employment screening
- scoliosis screening
- X-ray (diagnostic imaging)

The lists above represent an array of potential services chiropractors might incorporate into practice. It would be wise to discuss with experienced practitioners before deciding whether it is more feasible to use these techniques or refer patients elsewhere for these services.

One practitioner cannot be all things to all people, so the direction of the practice, and the appropriate services to include, is a serious decision.

It's worth spending time considering the business decisions described in the next section. A practice career can be divided into three phases: The *foundation phase*, the *growth phase*, and *preparing the practice for sale phase*. Done properly, a practice will be a valuable asset in 20 to 30 years, providing options for retirement. This chapter focuses on the *foundation* stage of practice.

Getting Started: Start Small, Think Large!

What are the minimum requirements to start a practice? Based on the most current evidence related to quality outcomes, there are three musculoskeletal issues and three services that, combined with the initial patient evaluation and management, form the basis of a small but successful chiropractic practice.

Musculoskeletal Issues

1. *Joint mobility*: The services best suited for treating joints with impaired mobility are high-velocity, low-amplitude (HVLA) SMT and instrument-assisted SMT, which is appropriate for patients who are not candidates for HVLA SMT.
2. *Muscle flexibility and strength*: The service best suited for improving these is instruction to the patient using exercise/rehabilitation equipment (such as bands, balls, and balance boards).
3. *Soft tissue healing*: The service best suited to this is use of physical modalities, such as electrical stimulation, ultrasound, ice, and heat.

To provide the basic services mentioned above, it is recommended to start with just a few items to keep costs low:

1. *Adjusting table:* A static pelvic bench will suffice to adequately adjust most patients. As soon as feasible, a "hi/lo" chiropractic table with drop pieces and a flexion-distraction table are recommended.
2. *Rehab/exercise room:* A few exercise balls, resistance bands, and foam-rubber balancing pads will be adequate initially.
3. *Therapeutic modalities:* Electric stimulation, ultrasound, ice, and heat. Buy a small refrigerator to store the ice packs.

Working out of one room, with an open exercise area, will provide enough resources and space to effectively treat patients and to develop a very profitable practice with minimal financial exposure. The list in Table 8.1 identifies the clinical and office equipment and supplies needed to open a chiropractic office.

Open versus Closed Treatment Areas

This is a topic unique to chiropractic practice and is somewhat controversial, with proponents and opponents on both sides of the issue. The basic issue is this: Do patients prefer privacy or to be treated in front

Table 8.1 Equipment List, by Room

Room	Items
Reception	Six reception-room chairs
	Coffee table and end table(s)
	Lamp
	Magazines and chiropractic-related educational material
	Credenza
	Television—use for educational videos
	Wall posters with health-related educational materials
	Shelf or cabinet with examples of products available in office (pillows, lumbar supports, supplements, etc.)
	Hand sanitizer—wall mounted is best
Front desk and billing	Desk and/or built-in work station
	Office chair
	Computer/monitor
	Battery backup/surge protector
	Software/EHR
	Telephone
	Digital camera
	Office supplies
	Copier with scanning and fax functions
Hallway	Educational posters
	Pamphlet rack
	Bulletin board
Treatment room	Adjusting table
	Flexion-distraction table
	Headrest paper
	Stool
	Mechanical adjusting device (Activator, ArthroStim, Impulse, etc.)
	Computer/monitor for EHR
	Battery backup
	Pamphlet rack
	Wall file holders
	Pens/paper clips/sticky notes, etc.
	Educational posters

(Continued)

Table 8.1   (Continued)

Room	Items
	Office chair
	Exam equipment: sphygmomanometer, stethoscope, otoscope and ophthalmoscope, penlight, pinwheel, reflex hammer, dynamometer, eye chart, tuning fork, measuring tape
	Trash can
	Hand sanitizer
	Mirror
	Coat rack
Rehabilitation room	Therapy table
	Headrest paper
	Cervical pillow
	Exercise balls
	Balance trainer/balance board
	Foam roller
	Therabands
	Posture pulley
	Trash can
	Office chair
	Mirror
	Coat rack
Therapy room	Therapy tables
	Headrest paper
	Face rest pillows
	Trash can
	Posters
	Bulletin board
	Pamphlet rack
	Mirror
	Coat rack
	Therapy equipment
	Electric stim/ultrasound unit
	Mechanical traction table (optional)
	Small freezer
	Ice packs

of other patients? It is common for patients to transfer from clinics with open-style treatment areas to clinics with more private settings if they feel uncomfortable with the experience of being treated in front of other patients. Opponents of open adjusting areas feel that privacy is not protected and believe many patients feel uncomfortable with the experience. What are the odds of a patient switching from a clinic with private treatment rooms to a clinic with open treatment areas because they want less privacy? Not likely!

Opponent's viewpoint: Open treatment areas for spinal manipulation do not maintain the privacy that society expects. Patients often feel uncomfortable with the experience of open adjusting, and females wearing dresses feel exposed. Doctors are not able to discuss individual needs with patients when other patients are within close proximity. Patients often will not reveal details of their case due to lack of privacy and possible embarrassment, particularly on sensitive issues. This type of setting is doctor centered, not patient centered.

Proponent's viewpoint: Open treatment rooms prevent unnecessary discussion that causes inefficiencies in patient/office flow; allows the doctor to educate several patients at once; creates a friendly, relaxed, and energetic atmosphere; allows for private conversations to take place in another room when requested; and takes less space and less equipment and office furniture so keeps costs down.

It is conventional within society and the health care system in general to conduct exercises and rehabilitation in an open setting. However, individualized treatment is another issue altogether. In making this choice, it is paramount that the issue be considered from the perspective of the patient's interest rather than the doctor's convenience.

Doctor and Staff Attire

The very second patients step inside a clinic they are evaluating and deciding, even on a subconscious level, whether office, staff, and doctor are trustworthy. Appearance has important and long-term implications and can affect patients' confidence in the doctor. Therefore, take some time to consider appropriate office attire. Some practitioners like to say that patients really do not care about attire as long as they are improving and feeling less pain. However, attire contributes to the doctor's and the practice's overall credibility, even if on a subliminal level.

Recommendations for men: Dress professionally with clean black shoes, black socks, black wrinkle-free pants, black leather belt, white shirt, conservative tie, monogrammed white waist-length lab jacket with full-length sleeves, minimal cologne, minimal jewelry, and simple wristwatch. Men should have well-groomed hair and be clean shaven with fresh breath, no visible tattoos or body piercings, and clean nails.

Recommendations for women: Dress professionally in dress slacks, monogrammed polo shirt or professional-looking blouse, monogrammed waist-length lab jacket with full-length sleeves, minimal perfume, minimal jewelry, and a simple wristwatch. Women's hair should be neat, polished, and easy to maintain, and they should have fresh breath, manicured but short nails, and no visible tattoos or body piercings.

If the preferred office atmosphere is more casual, doctors may consider monogrammed scrubs. They are still very professional looking, comfortable to work in, and portray a respected clinical image. Have clean clinic tennis or running/walking shoes on site to wear only in the office. Avoid wearing clinic shoes outside. Poor personal grooming like bad breath, wrinkled clothing, and dirty shoes diminish one's credibility. Patients understand and appreciate the clinical look of scrubs. A professional appearance that is congruent with patients' concept of "doctor" reinforces their confidence—and underscores that a licensed DC is a part of the medical health care team.

It has become trendy in chiropractic to wear dress pants and a monogrammed polo shirt. However, although this is certainly acceptable attire, it is no different from the used-car salesperson down the street and may make it difficult for patients to recognize the difference. A colleague once noticed that he went to the same bank for over a year without being recognized as a doctor because he looked no different than anyone else entering the bank. However, if the entire clinic wears polo shirts that are color coordinated and monogrammed with the clinic name and logo, this can give patients the impression that the practice is well organized and credible.

New Patient Generation

Since new patient generation is a topic worthy of its own textbook, this chapter will only cover a few highlights. One thing is for certain: it is impossible to develop a solid base of patients if the doctor cocoons in his or her new office. The biggest mistake new doctors make is related to office hours. In order to be available for any patient who may call, many new doctors schedule office hours each day, morning to night, including evening hours, thereby minimizing the time available for personal marketing. A better strategy is to consider being open for patient care only three days per week initially (for example, Monday, Wednesday, Friday, 8:00 a.m. to 12:00 p.m., and 3:00 p.m. to 6:00 p.m.).

Be sure that one staff person is present to answer the phone every day, open to close. The DC should use Tuesday, Thursday, Saturday, Sunday, and the extended lunch hours to network and integrate into the community. A practice can only grow if potential patients are aware of its existence and have a positive impression of it. Consider the following ideas:

- *Medical professional referral system:* Create a snail-mail and email list of local health care professionals, which may include primary care providers (PCPs), medical specialists (orthopedic and neurosurgeons, dermatologists, obstetricians/gynecologists, neurologists, pain management specialists, etc.), doctors of osteopathic medicine (Dos), physical therapists (PTs), massage therapists, acupuncturists, dentists, optometrists, podiatrists, psychologists, and athletic trainers.

  Send them a monthly summary of a current and topical research paper with a cover letter explaining its relevance to the receiver. The topic should be neuromusculoskeletal-related research, as the most relevant to typical chiropractic practice. After six months, reduce the frequency to quarterly intervals. This establishes the DC's reputation as an evidence-based practitioner and provides useful information to local providers.

  After obtaining signed permission from the patient, begin to send initial, interim, and discharge summaries to his or her primary care provider (PCP), whether or not the doctor referred the patient. This increases the DC's recognition by the PCPs in a positive way. Why? When their patients inquire about chiropractic, they will tend to refer to a DC with whom they are familiar and know to be conscientious about patient care. Awareness often translates into referrals.

- *Attorney referral system:* The same strategy used for medical professionals can be used to familiarize local attorneys with the practice by sending research summaries of topics relevant to their practice, such as motor vehicle accidents and work injuries.

- *Social networking:* Social media sites like Facebook should be used regularly, even daily. Messages should be short, positive, and informative, avoiding negativity, controversy, and heavy promotion. The goal is to achieve positive, professional visibility.

- *Website/blogging:* The practice's website must be contemporary and professional looking and should include blogging capability.

- *Community involvement:* Volunteering for community activities out of genuine interest in their causes helps not only the cause but also the doctor who is volunteering. It makes the volunteer a part of the community and will naturally result in community members referring themselves and others to the practice. There are many opportunities to give back to the community, and those that are most congruent with the doctor's principles and beliefs should be chosen. These could include Rotary and/or any other service organization; church, synagogue, or temple; local food pantry; or local gym.

- *Donations of equipment:* An example is to donate high-quality medical weight scales to the local gym, with a plaque with the practice name, phone, and website.

- *Phone calls:* Consider placing a personal call to each new patient at the end of the day with a reminder to use ice (or other instructions given at the visit). Ask how the patient feels. Reinforce that this is a process, not a quick fix. Another call should be made to the referral source (after seeking permission from the patient) to thank her or him for referring that patient.

- *Grand rounds:* Local hospitals often have grand rounds or lectures, and this is an excellent way to get to know local medical practitioners.

- *Open house:* Soon after the practice opens, an open house should be scheduled. However, the attendees should not be left to chance; invite local dignitaries (mayor, legislators, city council) and other key townspeople.

- *Business to business:* Taking the initiative to visit local businesses personally will help you become integrated into the community. Reinforce your message by taking along a healthy snack with a note on the outside that reads, for example, "Breakfast provided by Dr. John and the staff at Westside Chiropractic. Enjoy!"

There are dozens of other ways to become an integral part of the community. These are marketing strategies, but they should always come from a professional and ethical position. Marketing efforts fall into four categories:

1. Community programs (off site), low cost (for example, on-site shoulder massage therapy, spinal exams, public lectures)

2. Community programs (off site), high cost (for example, patient appreciation dinners, radio/TV advertising, social networking/Google ranking initiatives)

3. On-site (in-office) programs, low cost (for example, spinal care class, gift certificates, patient appreciation days)

4. On-site (in-office) programs, high cost (for example, professional practice analysis, pay per click Internet ads)

Use a variety of marketing techniques, and record statistics on how well each one worked, including the cost and time, how many people were reached, and how many patients were referred from each activity. A ratio of 3–5:1 return on investment indicates success.

New Patient Conversion

The term "new patient conversion" simply means that a new patient will return whenever he or she needs chiropractic care in the future. It is vitally important to have systems in place to create an extraordinary experience and build confidence. How is that accomplished? To do this, the chiropractor needs to be proficient in six clinical systems:

1. New patient consultation
2. New patient examination
3. Report of findings/treatment plan
4. Reexamination and reexamination report
5. Discharge to wellness explanation
6. Daily patient education

1. *New patient consultation system.* The main goals of the new patient consultation are to gain a full understanding of the patient's complaint and to help the patient see a little further down the road in the "process of care." This will make a good first impression and build the patient's confidence in the doctor. The initial consultation is also a good time to recognize the referral source and impress upon the patient that referrals are welcome. To facilitate these goals, repeatable systems must be in place. The patient primarily wants to know four things: (1) What is wrong? (2) Can the doctor help? (3) How long will it take? and (4) What is it going to cost? These four items must be addressed in the consultation. This process includes the following:

- The doctor must be prepared for the consultation and be familiar with the patient's chart, chief complaint, and referral source.
- The doctor should enter the room with a warm smile and firm handshake.
- Patients should be addressed as Mr. or Ms., unless they express otherwise, regardless of their age.
- Sitting facing the patient, knee to knee, rather than behind the desk establishes an attitude of partnership rather than authoritarianism.
- Explain the visit's agenda.
- A thorough consultation includes investigation of the main complaint, mechanism of injury, location of pain, severity, quality, what makes it worse, what makes it better, previous treatment, associated signs and symptoms, secondary complaint, and tertiary complaint.

  If the patient's complaint stems from an accident or workers' compensation injury, include questions specific to the research related to personal injury (PI) and/or workers' compensation (WC). Examples of PI terminology and issues include rear-end collision versus side-swipe, awareness of impending crash, back versus front seat, seat belt worn or not, head impact on object inside of car, and so on. Examples of WC questions to ask include: Was the injury reported at work? Was there pain prior to the injury? What is the patient's job description? Did the patient take time off from work due to injury? Are there complications with the injury in terms of job requirements?

- After interviewing the patient on his or her complaint and history, the doctor should summarize the main issues so that the patient knows that he or she has been heard and the condition understood. Patients will put the greatest faith in those they believe understand their problem the most.

- The doctor should explain the gowning and examination process and then leave the room and reenter when the patient is ready.

2. *New patient examination system.* The goal of the examination is to zero in on the diagnosis and build on the confidence being established with the patient by performing the most thorough examination he or she has ever had. Be professional at all times and recognize the vulnerability the patient feels while wearing a gown. It's always best to have another female in the room if the DC is a male, and vice versa. At the very least, offer the patient the option of exam monitoring. The examination procedure is as follows:

- Always perform vitals on a new patient.

- If red flags or concerns exist, be sure to include examination of the cranial nerves.

- Begin with static and motion palpation of the main area of complaint, then move to secondary and tertiary areas.

- Examine the patient first in a seated position, then supine; finish in a standing position.

- Perform a thorough battery of regional-appropriate diagnostic orthopedic and neurological tests, and be sure to examine the entire spine when appropriate.

- Review any diagnostic tests provided by the patient or any X-rays taken by your office.

- When finished, sit down with the patient and provide a brief explanation of your findings, your preliminary diagnosis, and a treatment plan.

- Give the patient his or her first treatment when possible.

- Provide first-day discharge instructions.

- Relate what will happen during the next visit (i.e., review the treatment plan).

3. *Report of findings (ROF) system.* The goal of the report of findings is to educate and motivate patients and help them understand what it will take to accomplish their stated goals. Remember that the term "report of findings"

is somewhat unique to chiropractic. Therefore, at the end of the examination, state the following: "On your next visit we will discuss your treatment plan, what is wrong, whether or not I can help, how long it will take, and how much it will cost." A ROF should last no longer than 5 to 10 minutes, because the patient will not be able to absorb and remember more than this. A good ROF contributes to better patient compliance. Recommended resources to help educate patients during the ROF include the following:

- nervous system chart
- autonomic nervous system chart
- spinal degeneration chart (illustrating degenerative changes in the spinal segments)
- video graphics/animation program to demonstrate spinal pathology
- informed consent form
- guidelines for patient review, for example, guidelines by the Council on Chiropractic Guidelines and Practice Parameters (CCGPP) and/or the American College of Physicians/American Pain Society.)[4,5]

The ROF system is as follows:

1. Review the examination findings.
2. Review the diagnosis.
3. Discuss the causes of low back pain using wall charts.
4. Review signs and symptoms related to spine dysfunction using the nervous system and autonomic nervous system charts.
5. Discuss pain relief with medication versus correction of the underlying problem/spinal dysfunction.
6. Discuss short- and long-term goals of care, including frequency of visit over the next two to four weeks, which will be followed by reexamination.
7. Discuss informed consent, and then have patient sign consent form.
8. Treat patient.
9. Provide discharge instructions.

4. *Reexamination system.* The reexamination is one of the most important systems to master to ensure not only that patients are improving as expected but to reset the treatment plan and remotivate the patient. In an evidence-based practice, short-term treatment planning with periodic progress examinations are critical. Contemporary guidelines suggest that examinations should be performed approximately every 6 to 12 visits to monitor the success or failure of treatment. The system is exceptionally important, yet one of the easiest to implement.

   1. Front desk chiropractic assistant (CA) has the patient complete an updated pain chart and/or outcome assessment form (OAT).

2. Examine the patient. Be very thorough, performing all appropriate tests consistent with patient complaints.

3. DC reviews the pain chart and OAT with the patient.

4. Remind patient of original pain score versus updated pain score.

5. Provide update on overall progress of care.

6. Reset the treatment plan based on the progress to date.

7. Treat and then discharge the patient.

Be sure to make the reexamination an "event" so that the patient realizes its importance. The reexamination system begins on the visit before the reexamination when the doctor states, for example: "John, on your next visit we are going to conduct another very thorough examination. The purpose of the examination is to evaluate your progress and decide on which exercises you may be able to upgrade to and what the next step is. It will take about 10 minutes, and I'll give you an idea of the updated treatment plan at that time. Sound okay?"

5. *Discharge to wellness system.* The goal of the discharge to wellness system is to provide patients with options for future case management—not to coerce them into lifelong care. Once a plateau in recovery is reached, the question becomes "What's next?" Providing options neutralizes the main criticism and fear of chiropractic: "Once you go to a chiropractor you always have to go to a chiropractor!" In reality, only a small proportion of patients actually transition to monthly ongoing care. The vast majority of patients come in, get treated, get well, and terminate care, treating only if the pain returns, regardless of attempts to educate them otherwise. Offering options at the point of maximum therapeutic benefit (i.e., plateau in recovery) fosters greater respect and trust in doctors of chiropractic. If patients are confident they are not going to be lectured for opting for pain-relief care, they are more likely to have confidence and trust in their doctor, return for care when necessary, and refer others.

The discharge to wellness system begins when a plateau in care is reached. At that point, perform an examination (including pain chart and/or other outcome assessment) and review those findings with the patient, reminding him or her of the initial scores versus the current scores. When patients understand the following four issues, they are better prepared to make a rational decision about their future health care:

1. Negative effects of joint tightness

2. Positive effects of joint flexibility

3. Research related to ongoing care

4. Costs of care

Consider the following steps during the office visit in which options for care will be discussed:

1. The chiropractic assistant has the patient complete an updated patient-based outcome measure, such as a pain chart or visual analog scale for pain.
2. The doctor performs a thorough examination.
3. The doctor reviews, with the patient, her or his initial symptoms and pain score compared to the current pain score.
4. The doctor reviews, with the patient, the current exam findings.
5. Together they discuss treatment options (pain relief versus wellness care/chronic pain management), when the patient reaches maximum therapeutic benefit (MTB).
6. Together they discuss payment options.
7. Treatment is administered.
8. The front desk assistant asks the patient which program he or she would prefer: pain relief or wellness/chronic pain management, which is generally scheduled about once per month.
9. The assistant explains payment options and schedules the next visit or visits.

By allowing the patient to make the decision regarding episodic pain relief care and/or wellness care/chronic pain management, the patient is placed in charge of his or her health and will be more compliant with greater confidence in the doctor.

Patient Education

If you desire a strong evidence-based practice built on internal referrals, there are several topics you must be able to confidently discuss with patients. In order to create a strong evidence-based reputation, become familiar with the literature related to these topics and questions. Examples include the following:

1. Dosaging: Why is the treatment frequency important?
2. Recovery: Why do I feel bad some days and good on other days?
3. X-ray: Don't I need an X-ray before treatment?
4. Cervical manipulation: Are adjustments to the neck safe? Don't they cause stroke?
5. Nonsteroidal anti-inflammatory drugs (NSAIDs, such as ibuprofen): Is it okay to take NSAIDs while I'm being treated?
6. Electrical stimulation (e-stim): Why do I need e-stim? Is it really necessary?

7. Nonmusculoskeletal conditions: Can you help colic [insert any other non-MSK condition]?
8. Exercise: Can't I just exercise to cure my back pain?
9. Etiology: What is causing my pain?
10. Surgery: Why can't I just have surgery to fix this once and for all?

There are many common questions that patients routinely ask in practice. DCs must be familiar with the research to address each question. The 10 questions above represent a starting point and remain some of the more routine questions posed on a daily basis regardless of practice type or philosophy.

Chiropractors as Pain-Relief Experts

The loggerhead between chiropractic extremes continues to stymie the growth of chiropractic. On one side of the equation are pain-relief, condition-focused, evidence-based practitioners who understand the role of guidelines and cost-effective chiropractic. On the polar opposite are those who believe that pain-relief doctors are actually doing patients a disservice if they do not further "correct" the subluxation and restore the spinal curves to a theoretical "normal" or ideal degree. The latter group are criticized by the pain-relief doctors for providing unnecessary care and often sell patients treatment time (for example, 60 visits for the year, $5,000 prepay) regardless of the diagnosis or mechanism of injury. It is time to move beyond the fray and focus on what patients need, not what chiropractors need. If we serve our patients well, chiropractic will thrive well into the future.

The reality is that most patients seek chiropractic care for pain relief. If every patient accepted the philosophical message of lifelong chiropractic care, average patient visits (number of patient visits/total number of new patients) would be greater than 1,000 over the course of a 30-year career. However, most DCs realize an average of less than 20. Why? Despite all the rhetoric about wellness, when it comes to chiropractic care most patients just want out of pain. Given that reality, does it not make sense to work with the patient to increase the odds that when pain again rears its ugly head, the patient returns?

The reality discussed above does not negate the need for patient education. As medical professionals with a mission to help people, chiropractors have an obligation to explain the truth about health care, including the stark reality that the present health care system focused primarily on symptom relief has been a colossal failure. The United States has higher health care costs than any other country on the planet, and Americans' life expectancy and quality of life are below that of other industrialized countries.[6] Much of this has to do with health behavior—poor lifestyle habits—and overuse of expensive medical procedures and medications when prevention of disease and disability would be less expensive in terms of human suffering as well as finances.

New Patient Fulfillment

New patient fulfillment relates to those systems that promote excellent service to patients. The goal: create an extraordinary experience for the patient that begins with the new patient phone call, extends through the five systems of new patient processing and management (consultation, examination, report of findings, reexamination, and discharge to wellness), and continues to the point of discharge, extending for decades throughout the patient's life. How can that be accomplished? By adhering to two key practice values and never straying from that commitment:

1. Give patients what they need and only what they need—nothing more and nothing less—always!
2. If you can help your patient, tell him or her. If you cannot help the patient, tell him or her that as well, and make an appropriate referral.

New patient fulfillment becomes rather automatic, creating a practice that runs on auto-pilot, if these two values are consistently maintained, combined with five other practice qualities:

1. *Evidence based:* This means a commitment to making clinical decisions based on the best-quality evidence/research available, not just because "that's the way I've always done it." Time to become familiar with current guidelines like those developed by the Council on Chiropractic Guidelines and Practice Parameters.[4]
2. *Patient centered:* This means that all office systems are designed to meet the needs of the patient versus the needs of the doctor. Example 1: Systems designed to treat 300 patients per day while ignoring the unique needs of each patient are the opposite of patient centered. Example 2: Continuing to treat a patient multiple times per week for months or years while the real cause of their spinal dysfunction is overconsumption of diet soda and other negative nutritional habits is not being patient centered.
3. *Outcomes driven:* This means that care is designed to achieve the greatest result in the shortest period of time. The practice is committed to measuring the progress of care and adjusting treatment recommendations based on

progress. Avoid long-term treatment plans based on the first examination. No one can predict how fast an individual patient will recover or respond; therefore, it is not possible to recommend a specific number of visits for the next year based on just the initial examination.

4. *Value based:* This means a commitment to providing the best service at the most reasonable cost, and all decisions are made with full disclosure to the patient about the costs of those services. From the patient's perspective, receiving a trial of 6 to 12 chiropractic adjustments, at very low cost, certainly makes more sense than submitting to spinal injections and/or surgery, which costs exponentially more money. Patients deserve to know the costs and benefits of all treatment, a message that should equally apply to all medical providers.

5. *Ethics based:* This means that the doctor and everyone in the practice will respect the sanctity of the doctor-patient relationship at all times and create systems that protect the patient in every way. It is helpful for beginning DCs to take a live or online course on ethics before beginning practice to ensure they are current on contemporary issues related to the doctor-patient relationship.

Exceptional patient fulfillment systems result in exceptional patient compliance and increased new patient referrals, stimulated by satisfied, loyal, and motivated patients. Doctors need to keep their promise of providing the best care possible via the establishment of solid patient care systems, caring and competent staff, and good patient outcomes. However, even in the best of circumstances, there are often three key reasons patients may not finish their recommended treatment plans: time, belief, and money.

Patients will follow through with care if the DC adequately addresses these three issues. Deep exploration of each topic is beyond the scope of this chapter. *Time* refers to the patient's time: How can the office be run efficiently so that the patient feels satisfied with the time he or she has invested? *Belief* refers to the "placebo effect," in that people's belief in, and expectations for, a treatment greatly affect treatment outcomes.[7] *Money* obviously refers to costs of care. Working with patients' insurance plans and being willing to discuss costs is part of working through this issue.

Clinical Decisions Summary

DCs are required to make innumerable clinical decisions in practice; although the information provided above of the basic principles that guide clinical decisions just skims the surface, it should help new DCs setting up practice. Still, it is highly advisable to seek out a mentor in chiropractic practice. Where can one find a mentor? The best sources are local, state, or national chiropractic professional organizations. DCs who belong to associations are quite likely more familiar with current trends, laws, rules, and procedures related to building a strong and successful practice. Mentors tend to be givers in life and would love nothing more than to see new doctors succeed. Seeking out a practice manager is another option and potential time saver and stress reducer. However, in the chiropractic profession, it's important to consider the values and qualities of the consultant/practice manager.

Questions to ask a practice manager/consultant include the following:

1. Are you evidence based?
2. Why do you consider yourself evidence based?
3. Have there been complaints about you, or have you ever lost your license? If so, why?
4. What are your fees?
5. Do you require a long-term contract?
6. Do you require a percentage of my growth as a fee?
7. Have you ever sued clients? If so, why?
8. Do you belong to local, state, and/or national associations? Which ones?
9. Do you believe in long-term treatment plans based on just the first evaluation (e.g., 60–80 visits for the year, $5,000 prepay)?
10. What was the last research paper you read?
11. Are you familiar with CCGPP and do you support them?
12. Have you read the CCGPP guidelines?
13. Do your fees include staff?
14. Do you offer live seminars, webinars, personal coaching, and on-site visitation?

Practice consultants can be valuable sources of information. However, buyers beware. Historically, some practice consultants provided bad advice, luring young, impressionable, and desperate students in with promises of quick wealth and unrealistic incomes. The result of questionable practice strategies and false practice promises continue to erode both student and public trust in the chiropractic profession. In stark contrast, other practice consultants focus on patient-centered, outcomes-driven, and evidence-based practices built on solid and efficient office systems, linked together with ethical standards that result in new DCs growing respectable and successful practices. It can be done. However, one must never lower one's personal or ethical standards in search of a get-rich-quick chiropractic practice.

Key Business Questions

Starting a Practice

Starting a chiropractic practice is a challenge. The goal of this section is to minimize the barriers to getting started. One of the first issues to consider is the type of employment: Associate or self-employment? Incorporation? Shared rental agreement with another DC? Employment in an integrated medical clinic?

There are many options, but the most practical course of action is to work with another experienced DC for one or two years to learn the business. One of the weaknesses in chiropractic education is the lack of a postgraduate internship or residency program. Therefore, new graduates are faced with the uncertainty of starting their own practice or taking a position as an associate with another DC, often working for relatively low wages for a few years. Chiropractic is not yet thoroughly integrated into the health care system, so there are very few well-paid positions for new graduates. This situation is what lures many recent graduates into get-rich-quick schemes with some exceptionally high-priced practice management programs. Building an ethical practice is a slow walk, not a sprint. But if done properly, even as an associate, one can earn a good living before transitioning into a solo practice. It is essential for those interested in associateships to perform due diligence and investigate each potential employer carefully.

- Call the state board to inquire about complaints.
- Ask about any past or pending malpractice actions.
- Determine the pay schedule.
- Inquire as to why they are seeking an associate.
- Are there enough new patients to provide the associate with a full schedule?
- Have the contract reviewed by an attorney or trusted adviser.
- Is the senior doctor involved in his or her local, state, and/or national chiropractic association?
- Doe the clinic owner follow an evidence-based model with nationally accepted guidelines, or does he or she recommend dozens of visits and high prepay amounts at the initial examination?
- What is the theme of the clinic: personal injury, work comp, family practice, pain relief?
- How does the clinic owner generate new patients?
- What are the associate's hours?

- Does the contract include a noncompete clause? Is so, what is the specified distance from the clinic one must be to set up a practice?
- Most important, what kind of training program is in place to teach associates the business?

While considering whether to associate with an established practice, be realistic about income.

After accepting the position, treat it as a learning experience to help with the desired end point of owning a practice.

Financing a New Office: The Business Plan

Financial capital is the lifeblood of any business. In fact, running out of money before the business gains self-sustaining traction often results in business failure and extreme stress. It is highly recommended that the recent graduate begin with enough money to finance the business for the first six months. If all goes well, after approximately six months, funds collected from patient care should be able to finance the day-to-day operations of the clinic. The financial stress associated with running a business can ruin one's life—or it can realize one's childhood dream.

Start Small and Build Slowly but Steadily

The lifestyle more experienced DCs lead may have taken decades to acquire, so new practitioners must be patient and live a frugal life initially. In order to determine the amount of capital needed to sustain the first six months, complete a business plan. This requires considerable time and effort before approaching a bank for funding. The remainder of this chapter will focus on the basics related to the creation of a business plan. There are many opinions, resources, books, and consultants that can help in this area. This chapter represents just one approach. There is no substitute for a mentor who can personally advise on this step in the process. The following outline can be used to structure a business plan. Answer the following questions and consider the issues listed below in order to produce a plan you can confidently present to a banker.

What are financial institutions looking for when considering a loan to a chiropractor for a new practice?

- clearly defined marketing strategy to differentiate the practice from the competition

- assumptions regarding market saturation (for example, is the market saturated or is there room for growth?)
- market analysis of the location, zip codes, and so on
- description of the social media strategy and methods to create search engine optimization (SEO)

Create a Business Plan

Much of the information below was provided by experts in the banking industry, along with the U.S. Small Business Administration website (https://www.sba.gov/writing-business-plan). A typical business plan can be divided into the following sections.

Part I: Executive summary.

The executive summary is a snapshot of the business plan as a whole and touches on the company profile and goals.

- *The mission and vision statements:* Brief statements that describe the overall purpose of the business and the owner's perception of where it will be in the future.
- *Company information:* A short statement that covers (1) when the business was formed or incorporated; (2) names of the founders and their roles; (3) estimated number of employees; (4) business location.
- *Growth highlights:* Graphs and charts to describe the anticipated growth of the business.
- *Products/services:* Description of the products or services the practice will offer.
- *Financial information:* Summary of your current financial information and anticipated financial needs for the next five years.
- *Future projections:* An estimate of income and expenses for the next five years.
- *Other issues:* Short paragraphs describing the
  - strategic objective;
  - unique selling proposition;
  - personnel/costs;
  - practice manager; and
  - office structure (such as solo, group, shared rental agreement).

Part II: Organization and management.

The organizational structure of the practice needs to be developed.

- Management: Will there be a president/CEO?
- Legal structure: Will the business be a sole proprietorship, a limited liability company (LLC), an S-corp, or a C-corp? Health care professionals can also form profession corporations (PCs). Obtain the advice of an accountant before making these decisions.
- Number of employees anticipated from year one to year five, along with salaries and benefits.
- Provide an "org board" describing the company.

Part III: Company description.

A brief description of the business, including planned products and services.

- What is the target market?
- What differentiates this business from the competition?

Part IV: Market analysis.

This is an analysis of the health care industry in general, the local health care market, and anticipated competitors. Include the following items:

- industry description and outlook
- information about the target market (for example, work comp, personal injury, family practice, low back pain, neck pain, headaches, pediatrics, sports, occupational health)
- distinguishing characteristics of the practice's services
- size of the primary target market and anticipated market share
- fee schedule and gross income targets
- competitive analysis: description of competitors, market share, strengths and weaknesses, potential barriers (for example, changing technology, high investment cost, lack of quality personnel), and regulatory restrictions

Part V: Services offered.

Provide an itemized list of all planned services, with a brief description of each. Use the lists offered earlier in this chapter as a guide.

Part VI: Marketing sales projection.

Explain the marketing strategy.

- Provide sales projections for each of the first five years.
- Provide estimated numbers of new patients and established patients in each of the first six months. Graphs and charts are helpful to visually demonstrate the anticipated growth of the practice.

Part VII: Financial projections.

These are necessary to support the application for funding.

Creditors usually require a five-year plan. This includes forecasted income statements, balance sheets, cash flow statements, and capital expenditure budgets. For the first year, monthly or quarterly projections are needed. For years two through five, the projections may be quarterly or annual.

Part VIII: Funding request.

The request should be specific. The following items will help develop this part of the business plan:

- total funds requested
- explanation of the specific funding request
- list of necessary equipment and office needs, including approximate costs
- if renting, include address and monthly rental amount
- if renting, estimate capital improvement expenses for building out the space
- if renting, estimate additional monthly expenses (such as utilities)
- source of the 20 percent down payment typically required to obtain the loan

Part IX: Strengths and weaknesses.

Provide a paragraph to describe the practice's areas of strength and another paragraph to describe the practice's areas of weakness.

Part X: How to make the business plan stand out.

Explain the unique aspects of the practice.

- Be clear and specific about the practice's services and products.
- Characterize the practice's anticipated niche in the community.

Part XI: Appendix.

The appendix provides supplemental information that strengthens the application, for example:

- photos of the business, exterior and interior, and of the practitioner
- résumé or curriculum vitae
- a short biography of the practitioner applying for the loan
- a copy of the rental/lease agreement
- copies of any applicable permits
- photos of office equipment required to start the practice

Side note: Red flags.

What are the red flags that bankers or investors look for when considering a loan to a new doctor?

- lack of industry knowledge
- lack of assets (although it is usually acceptable to borrow money from the applicant's parents for the 20 percent down payment, this needs to be reflected in the balance sheet to be repaid)
- poor personal credit history
- lack of credit history

In summary, applications for loans are scrutinized more carefully now than they were 20 years ago. New practitioners need to be prepared and present a professional and confident image. The more detailed the business plan, the greater the chances of securing a loan.

Leadership

The doctor who owns the practice is responsible for setting the tone, providing the vision, and putting the action plan in motion. He or she provides the "why" of the office. Clearly, the entire staff is necessary to support the doctor's success. Staff will remain loyal, dedicated, and motivated when they function in an atmosphere of appreciation, approval, and love. They want to work in an environment in which they respect the owner. How does she or he garner respect? While an old cliché, the following statement is true: People do not care how much you know until they know how much you care. Leadership flows from the top down. The leader of the practice must impart his or her vision for the office so that staff members realize they are vital components in the formula for success. And, financial incentives must align with office growth in order to accomplish set goals. Remember, leaders are readers. Please refer to the reading list at the end of this chapter to review topics such as leadership, business-financial intelligence, and clinical excellence. Read current published papers related to treatment guidelines developed with a chiropractic perspective.

Consider the following leadership issues:

1. Is there a clear vision for the practice?
2. Are the right people working in the office?
3. Are the right people in the right positions, based on position requirements, personalities, and skills?
4. Does everyone in the office know the mission and vision?
5. Are there clear and acknowledged goals?
6. Are all staff members aware of the five-year strategic objectives, including how they fit into the formula for practice success?
7. Have staff members been empowered to participate in the development of the mission statement, position contracts, roles, responsibilities, and financial incentives?

The preceding ideas represent just the tip of the iceberg of what a successful practitioner needs to learn about leadership. While some people seem to be born leaders, the vital characteristics of effective leadership are learned skills. Those who actively pursue excellence in leadership throughout their careers will rise to the top and realize greater success compared to those who allow life to just happen to them. Be sure not to get stuck in the habits of the past.

Management

While leadership is related to the "why" of the business side of the practice, management is related to the "how." Remember that systems run the business, but people run the systems. No one person in any organization should have the ability to change a system on his or her own, under any circumstances. If a system needs to be changed, have a mechanism in place to change it. The following three-step process can guide development of such a mechanism:

1. What is the problem?
2. Why is it a problem?
3. What are the possible solutions?

Answers to these questions are submitted to the company president/ CEO. The process must be considered in the overall context of the office. One system may affect another, and the law of unintended consequences should always be considered. It is the job of the person in charge to first establish, then document and record all systems as an operations manual. The operations manual can effectively be divided into seven major sections:[1]

1. Leadership
2. Management
3. Money
4. Marketing
5. New patient generation
6. New patient conversion
7. New patient fulfillment

Each of these seven major system categories have been addressed briefly in this chapter. Developing operations manuals, employee handbooks, safety, Health Information Portability and Accountability Act (HIPAA), and compliance manuals, along with a sound financial profit-and-loss and balance sheet are essential throughout the life of the practice.

Like the other systems, the topic of management is extensive, so this section will identify just a few highlights in an effort to provide clear direction for doctors beginning their careers.

Employee Handbook/Human Resources

The importance of an employee handbook cannot be overstated. It is possible to purchase an existing employment handbook, develop one's own using resources found on the Internet, or develop a basic handbook and keep adding to it as issues requiring a formal policy develop. Whatever the source, the handbook must be reviewed by an attorney to be sure all applicable local, state, and federal laws are followed and policies are well within the standards of employment rules and regulations. An employee handbook effectively takes the pressure off the practice owner regarding questions posed by staff. Once a policy is developed, it must be followed by all staff. The practice should also have manuals for operations and administration, compliance, safety, and the facility.

Salary Strategies

Small businesses should set the stage early on with every employee regarding the realities of salary. Small businesses cannot compete with large corporations. As a result, sooner or later, staff will reach an artificial (or documented) ceiling or salary cap. At that point, if they want to make more money or have access to better benefits they may have to transition into a corporate environment. On the other hand, an excellent office environment can offset the necessarily lower salary, and staff may remain very happy and loyal despite the salary cap and wish to stay rather than deal with the impersonal nature of a large corporation.

It is advisable to develop a salary grid showing possible salary increases at predetermined intervals, as long as goals and benchmarks of the employee are attained. For example, if an employee starts out at $12 per hour, with standard cost-of-living increases and periodic salary increases and/or performance bonuses each year, along with vacation increases, after 10 years the employee's salary may have surpassed what the position is really worth, with more vacation than is practical. A matrix showing scheduled salary increases every six months until a salary cap is reached will prevent this. Furthermore, salary increases should be based on performance, with no automatic or "entitled" salary increases. The benchmarks in time remain goals for the employee; it is the owner's job to make sure employees understand what must be done to qualify for the salary increase or bonus.

Staff Size

A beginning practice may need only one staff person. The largest line items in the budget will be related to staff and rent, so these items are best minimized until the practice grows. A general rule of thumb: employ one staff member per 50 patient visits per week. Therefore, a practice seeing 150 patients per week may have one staff member at the front desk, another in billing/front desk backup, and another in therapy/exercise/rehab.

Add staff as the practice grows. It is wise to have a part-time staff member available as soon as possible so there is redundancy in case of illness. Taking a positive attitude with employees—focusing on what they do right rather than on mistakes—will increase staff loyalty and motivation and decrease turnover.

Organizing Electronic Information

One of the most important issues regarding organization is how and where to store the massive amount of information related even to the beginning practice. Not being able to locate electronic documents easily wastes time and causes stress. File folders in the computer system should be set up in a logical manner from the very beginning of the practice.

Finances

Financial Basics

Managing the financial side of practice remains one of the most important skills to master. A common statement made by financial advisers is to "pay yourself first." However, this is impossible without first considering the necessary financial commitments of the practice. One of the biggest challenges to success is the self-destruction brought on by living beyond one's means early in the development of the practice. One simple strategy to prevent unnecessary financial stress is to follow this formula:

From collections:

1. Pay oneself a very small salary.
2. Pay the employees.
3. Pay all office bills.
4. Put at least 5 percent into an emergency account until six months of expenses are covered in the bank account.
5. Put 5 percent into a "wealth" account to be used to fund, and pay cash for, new equipment, repairs, and investment into the practice. Save until there is at least $20,000 in an account to fund large expenditures like capital investments and equipment.
6. Set aside money for taxes, unless the business is incorporated and taxes are withheld automatically.
7. The owner only takes a monthly bonus when there is money left over after accomplishing the first five items.

The next step in financial responsibility is related to how the owner uses the income he or she generates. The process is the same:

1. Out of each paycheck, give back to the world via tithing (5–10 percent) or some other form of giving.

2. Place 10 percent of net salary into an emergency fund until there is at least six months of living expenses saved.

3. Place 10 percent of net salary into a retirement account.

4. Calculate personal tax liability and put those funds aside.

5. Only spend the remainder.

In summary, this means that personal expenses should stay within the formulas above. This will avoid the financial stress of living beyond one's means. Be patient and remember that money always follows service.

Business Control Systems

Business control systems (BCS) are behind-the-scenes allies. Develop systems related to the following:

*   bank deposits
*   inventory
*   ordering supplies
*   payroll
*   staff performance bonus schedule
*   pay raise limits/expectations
*   billing
*   collections
*   data entry
*   financial reports review

The beauty of BCSs is that they help the business run smoothly and free the practitioner and employees to concentrate on more important matters. BCSs form the information link between business activities and accounting and help the practice run smoothly.

*   *Rule #1:* Never assume that everyone is using source documents correctly! (For example, patient ledger, electronic health records data input, Current Procedural Terminology [CPT] coding, explanation of benefits reconciliation, etc.) Train employees consistently, and reinforce training at regular intervals.

*   *Rule #2:* When it comes to money, always have two people involved.

*   *Rule #3:* Lock up signature stamp and checks every night and assign only one other staff person with authority over the signature stamp.

- *Rule #4:* Use a business checking account to pay all business expenses. Never use the office checkbook to pay personal expenses.

- *Rule #5:* Document all business systems in writing. Systems are the glue that hold the business together.

Financial Intelligence

Understanding financial concepts and gaining financial intelligence should be a priority. For example, what is the difference between a profit-and-loss statement and a balance sheet?

Quiz: When financing a car, does the value of the car belong in the asset or liability column?

- Profit/loss statement = income minus expenses
- Balance sheet = assets minus liabilities

When starting a practice, the DC wears two financial hats:

- Owner: the investor = income/benefits
- Chief executive officer (CEO): charged with running the business properly

Within those two roles, one finds an inherent conflict between current income versus long-term wealth. The tradeoff: *The more one pays him- or herself as an employee, the less money there is to fuel the growth of the business, which reduces its ultimate market value.* The personal conflict touched on previously is one's current standard of living versus higher market value for the business.

Hiring, Firing, and Training Staff

Ask this question: Do I have the right people on the bus? When it comes to staff, the basic rule of thumb is "hire slow, fire fast." It is a disservice both to the business and to employees to keep them in positions to which they are not ideally suited.

The greatest challenge related to staff is the time it takes to train the new chiropractic assistant versus the very short notification of termination provided by staff who quit. When a staff person quits unexpectedly, the new person needs to be recruited, interviewed, hired, and trained within a two-week time frame. As a result, many DCs settle for employees they can find quickly instead of implementing a lengthy hiring process to ensure the right person is hired for the open position.

The best way to hire and retain staff, preventing the revolving door of turnover, is outlined below:

- Develop a *hiring process* that includes position contracts, company and position standards, position-specific minimum competency requirements, references, complete employee application, desired salary, basic math test, filing test, personality test, and position-specific interview questions.
- Hire the best *personality* to match the position available.
- Take genuine *interest* in staff members. They need to know the owner cares about them before they'll be loyal to the practice.
- *Train* continuously.
- Be *realistic and forgiving,* to a point. Micromanaging staff does not inspire loyalty or develop competence.
- Make *personal notes* all week, and in a weekly staff meeting review the issues from a systems perspective instead of putting individual staff on the hot seat, which is embarrassing.
- Follow the *95 percent rule.* Accept that any employee will get 95 percent of the job done appropriately. The owner can enjoy the 95 percent and train for the 5 percent, or allow the 5 percent to destroy the relationship. It's valuable to teach the staff this rule as well.
- Conduct *meetings* consistently. There are several types of meeting: (1) individual staff meetings, (2) weekly staff meetings, (3) daily team huddles, and (4) quarterly business development meetings.
- *Termination.* If it is necessary to let an employee go, it should be done gently, professionally, and sympathetically. However, once the decision is made, it shouldn't be postponed.

Setting Goals

Clearly written goals help one move forward in a strategic manner. Having a dream board, a visual representation of goals, is even more important, according to some motivational speakers. Set 1-, 3-, 5-, and 10-year professional/office goals and share them with the staff. Monitor the journey. Make adjustments when necessary and give specific incentives for achieving specific benchmarks.

Marketing

Marketing is necessary to build a strong and profitable business. This chapter will review a few key topics related to marketing and branding.

Branding and marketing efforts will continue to evolve as the practice grows and matures. The key issues include the following:

- branding versus marketing
- mission and vision statements
- strategic objective
- logo
- website
- social networking strategy
- décor/sensory analysis (internal and external)

Branding versus Marketing

Too often people confuse branding with marketing. In a nutshell, branding relates to the image for the practice. It is the "why" of the practice. Essentially, branding is strategic, whereas marketing is tactical. Branding is the declaration of the essence or value of the practice. It communicates key characteristics and values that clarify what the practice is and is not. Marketing, on the other hand, includes the systems used to promote the practice.

In order to create a brand and develop marketing strategies, answer the following questions:

- Why does this practice exist?
- What does it bring to the patients served?
- How does it differ from similar practices?
- What characteristics of the practice will bring the owner and employees joy and passion every day?
- Would the staff support the purpose of the practice?
- Would patients appreciate and recognize the "why" behind the formation of the practice?

Mission versus Vision Statements

The mission statement is related to the present. The vision statement is created more for internal use and is related to the future. All the preceding questions must be considered before creating a clear mission, vision, and strategic objective. Once created, the mission statement should be displayed openly and shared with the public in all communications (for example, letterhead, social media, advertising, business cards). The vision statement is the rallying point for the staff.

Mission statement.

A mission statement is a brief statement used to communicate the purpose of your company. It is more related to the present.

Vision statement.

A vision statement is an aspirational description of the future of the practice. It provides a compass to guide strategic decisions leading toward growth (for example, "We will be *the* resource for evidence-based chiropractic in our community and grow into the premier multidisciplinary integrated health center in Springfield.")

Strategic Objective

Strategic objectives are long-term organizational goals that help convert a mission statement from a broad vision into more specific plans and projects. A properly developed strategic objective includes 1-, 3-, 5-, and 10-year benchmarks. Once defined, the strategic objective drives the actions and activities leading toward growth and accomplishment of goals. Without a strategic objective, most offices grow into the future by sheer happenstance.

Logo

A logo is the graphic symbol that represents a person, company, or organization. If the logo is well known, such as the Nike swoosh, you may even see it used without the name of the business with which it is associated. Work with a graphics designer to create a logo to be used in all marketing efforts.

Website

There are myriad options regarding websites. It's best if the owner of the practice owns the website rather than having the company that designs the website own the domain name and content, which will often mean a commitment Websites provided by web design companies are often tied to mandatory search engine optimization (SEO) programs. The web design company may terminate the contract if the practice owner decides he or she doesn't want the SEO function. There are a few simple rules and characteristics related to websites:

- The site should be contemporary looking.
- It should include a section for new patients with new patient paperwork.
- The mission statement should be displayed prominently.
- The logo should also be prominent.
- Include directions to the office.
- The site should be easy to navigate.
- The office phone number should be readily located on the home page.
- It should be filled with meta-tags (but be sure to check with an expert since ranking on Google is a moving target).
- Provide the company "story," staff bios and information, office hours, and complete contact information.
- A virtual tour with photos of the doctor, staff, and office (interior and exterior) is very helpful.
- A one-to-three-minute introductory video is helpful.
- If the doctor will keep it well written and current, include a blog function.
- Provide links to social networking pages.
- Testimonials may be included if the patients have given written permission.

It's possible to start with a low-cost, simple website. Additional functionality can be added as the practice grows. Even the most impressive website will still not be as great a referral source as direct referrals from other satisfied patients and area health care professionals. Patients often visit the website merely to obtain your phone number and directions once they've already made their decision. Other patients explore the Internet looking for a quality DC to visit, so a presence on the Web is essential. There are a few items to avoid when creating a website:

- Do not promise a cure or make unsubstantiated claims on the far-reaching effects of spinal manipulation. Wild claims erode the credibility of the profession and the practice making them.
- Keep the site evidence based.
- Do not include videos of painful- or strange-looking spinal manipulative techniques.
- Be sure the site complies with state and federal regulations.

- Avoid bait-and-switch schemes (for example, don't offer a free exam but bill the insurance company). These are illegal and unethical.
- Do not discuss fees on the site.

Social Networking

Like the website, social networking is important, but it should not be your main strategy to generate new patients. As stated earlier, the majority of patients come from direct established patient referrals and referrals from area health care professionals. However, patients are increasingly using the Internet to research health care providers. Therefore, it's beneficial to have a consistent social network presence.

- The website should link to common social networking sites like Facebook, Twitter, LinkedIn, Pinterest, Instagram, YouTube, and Google+.
- Post positive messages on social networking sites to gain visibility.
- Keep profiles up to date.
- Add friends and patients consistently.

Sensory Analysis

This is the systematic evaluation of consumer products in terms of the use of human senses. That is, it is an evaluation of how the office's external and internal sensory cues affect the business.

The analysis begins from the time patients pull into the parking lot to the minute they leave the office. What will they see, smell, taste, hear, touch, and feel inside and outside? How can the practice become both inviting and crystal clear about the services provided? It is helpful to visit a number of offices in the local area to gather ideas about design in terms of sensory input and office flow. Beginning with the ending in mind, consider and rate the following items, asking what can be done to create an exceptional experience in each area, both inside and outside the office. Consider the following items:

- sights (colors, clutter, etc.)
- sounds (traffic noise, type of music, loud conversations)
- smell (body odor, aromatherapy, disinfectant; keep chemical sensitivities in mind)
- feel (furniture upholstery, regulation of heating and cooling)
- cleanliness
- décor

- doctors and staff (appearance, personal hygiene, etc.)
- landscaping
- parking lot
- signage
- lighting

Patients appreciate an office staff dedicated to providing a clean, friendly, and comfortable environment. It is not necessary to spend a large amount of money if one is observant and creative.

Summary

This chapter provided basic information and resources to contribute to the successful launching of a chiropractic practice. It can also be used by those more experienced in practice to return to the basics and reenergize their business. While this chapter represents a substantial starting point, there is much more to consider, and finding a mentor can help a new practitioner avoid the minefields of a new business start-up. If done right, a chiropractic practice brings the practitioner much joy in life, in addition to financial success. However, it takes work, vigilance, and well-thought-out strategies for growth.

References

1. Gerber M. *The E-Myth Revisited: Why Most Small Businesses Don't Work and What to Do About It.* New York: HarperCollins; 2004.

2. Senna MK, Machaly SA. Does maintained spinal manipulation therapy for chronic nonspecific low back pain result in better long-term outcome? *Spine (Phila Pa 1976).* 2011;36(18):1427–1437.

3. Cifuentes M, Willetts J, Wasiak R. Health maintenance care in work-related low back pain and its association with disability recurrence. *J Occup Environ Med.* 2011;53(4):396–404.

4. Globe G, Farabaugh RJ, Hawk C, et al. Clinical practice guideline: chiropractic care for low back pain. *J Manipulative Physiol Ther.* 2016;39(1):1–22.

5. Chou R, Huffman LH. Nonpharmacologic therapies for acute and chronic low back pain: a review of the evidence for an American Pain Society/American College of Physicians clinical practice guideline. *Ann Intern Med.* 2007;147(7):492–504.

6. Woolf S, Aron L. *U.S. Health in International Perspective: Shorter Lives, Poorer Health.* Washington, DC: National Academy of Sciences; 2013.

7. Kaptchuk TJ, Miller FG. Placebo effects in medicine. *N Engl J Med.* 2015;373(1):8–9.

CHAPTER NINE

Typical Chiropractic Practice

Marion W. Evans Jr., DC, PhD, MCHES; Cathryn S. Evans; Lyndon Amorin-Woods, BAppSci(Chiropractic), MPH; Christina Cunliffe, DC; and Jesse Politowski, DC

This chapter describes typical chiropractic practice in the United States, including aspects of starting a practice as well as day-to-day activities and skills and knowledge needed to successfully perform them. To provide additional perspective, it also includes a glimpse of typical chiropractic practice in Australia and Indonesia.

The Chiropractic Physician's Day-to-Day Activities

Before choosing a profession, it is helpful to have a good deal of information about what it is like to perform the tasks of that job on a daily basis. Many people have entered a field or profession not really knowing a lot about what happens day to day in the particular job they have selected. It is helpful to understand a typical day in the life of a doctor of chiropractic (DC) as well as the most common patients they see and tasks they perform. In many ways, a typical day in the chiropractic office is probably a lot like other small businesses or health care clinics. While patient care is the business, the same type of management is needed as one might see in any other shop or small business. Depending on whether the practice is a group practice shared with other professionals or a solo practice in which the doctor is the only practitioner in the office, someone has to oversee the operation. A DC must maintain the office from a business perspective and serve as the leader of the business or the "chief executive." In this respect, the DC is the president, the manager of all personnel, the head of marketing, the front public relations figure, and the doctor all in one. This can be a difficult role to become used to, and so the typical chiropractic education has courses that focus on practice management, or the business management aspects of health care operations. Some students will say that their college curriculum did not devote enough time to this particular part of how to set up a practice. However, there are also other ways to learn about small business management or clinical practice management, and much has been written about it as well.

Essentially, patient care is what the DC is going to focus on during most hours of the day. While in the early years of a new practice, a DC may have to manage some of the business operations alone, or with a limited staff, with time, typical offices will hire more than one staff person and task them with some of the supporting roles in the office. Answering the phones, scheduling appointments, following up with patients, record keeping, and routing people from the patient waiting area to treatment rooms can all be done by support staff once the clinic is making enough money to hire additional support. Chiropractic is hands-on. That is, practitioners apply manual therapies to a person's body. They touch people— literally! Potential chiropractors who have issues with this should rethink their career because this is a core part of what it is to be a DC. However, for those who enjoy helping others and being active during the day versus sitting down, and who like educating people about how to be healthy, this is a rewarding exchange. Some studies now show chiropractic practice to be among the most rewarding careers in the health care arena.[1]

The New Patient Begins a Doctor-Patient Relationship

Once DCs receive their degree, pass national and state board exams, and open their doors with approved business licenses and malpractice insurance, it is necessary to market the practice to get people to try their services. They need to generate patients through contact and referrals. (Ways to accomplish this will be discussed later in this chapter and were also detailed in the previous chapter.) Marketing will bring new patients in need of chiropractic care to the office. These will likely have spinal pain, since chiropractic does focus on the spine. In many cases, they will have other forms of musculoskeletal pain or even neurological pain. A typical doctor-patient relationship must start here. Acceptance of the new patient will depend on several things, and the new patient intake paperwork or computer-based intake will be among the first steps in determining this. There is no guarantee that people selecting chiropractic care are a good fit for this care, nor that the condition they have is going to respond to the care rendered. At times, only a short conversation is needed to understand that the potential patient might be better off in someone else's hands.

Intake, Staff Support, and Direction

Intake

Intake is the process of asking patients to fill out forms about their current condition, complaint, and overall health status. Some offices may do this with actual paperwork, where a patient will fill in the blanks with pen-and-paper forms. Others use an electronic intake with an iPad or tablet. Typically, some paperwork is required so that an electronic health record (EHR) can be established. Once the EHR is established, it becomes easier to track improvement, and in some cases, share information about care with other providers if the patient has formally given permission to do so. These forms are similar to ones used in most doctors' offices. They contain basic data about the patient, including age, sex, and "chief complaint" or what has brought her or him into the office that day; in some cases, the form will ask about tobacco use history and other significant health behaviors that may be addressed in the clinical encounter.

In addition to the intake paperwork, patients complete forms that record their insurance information, next of kin, and other important information and sign a right to medical privacy form, which is required by law. The forms might also include work history (important to know because some jobs have inherent health risks) and ask about patients' overall health goals. Do they simply want pain relief, or do they want to know more about what they can do to improve overall health? Questions like this can help busy practitioners determine if the client is a good fit for their type of practice. Patients will often have some understanding of what to expect in a chiropractic clinic, but this will not always be the case. Intake, patient history, and examination may indicate that the patient would be better off in another practice or in a different provider's office.

Staff Support

Should the office have staff, one task that may be handed over to them will be to interact with the patient in the early evaluation process—that is, providing the patient with forms to complete and entering information into the computer system. In many states, some training or certification is required by the state's licensing board in order for a staff person to be in charge of this information-gathering task. Patients' rights to privacy must be respected, and unique and sensitive information must be safely maintained. The DC is responsible for the actions of all staff working under him or her. The doctor should delegate the tasks that any staff person will do on a given day and make sure that patient confidentiality and rights are always preserved. However, managing the staff, directing them as to support duties around the office, is a part of what a DC must do on a daily basis.

Direction

Staff and front desk personnel are often the first impression of the practice, so they are very important. While staff can generate good ideas for the office and in many cases serve as a confidant to patients, they must be trained to tell the DC what they know about patient health, responses to treatment, and anything pertinent to the delivery of patient care in the office. The DC must play the chief executive role direction by directing office activity.

Interview or Review of Systems

Once the intake paperwork is completed, the doctor or the staff person that has been designated to assist in this area will take the patient back to a more private room where personal health history and a review of past medical conditions and the current situation can be discussed privately with the doctor. Patients will often tell the doctor many things, including things that the doctor may not want to know! However, for a good doctor-patient relationship to be established from the beginning, the DC must listen, not judge, and not blame people for their current situation, regardless of what they may have done to get them into it. Empathy is a key feature of a good health care practice. One has to be able to put him- or herself in that patient's situation and want to help restore the patient's desired level of health. The importance of respecting where people are as they arrive at the office and in their process of getting better, and the choices they make about their care, cannot be overemphasized. Patient autonomy is absolutely necessary. No provider should force a level of care on patients if they don't want it, no matter what the rationale.

In a typical review of systems, the doctor will review any past health issues and the affected systems of the body. To some degree, this is a part of the history-taking process. The doctor may also ask about old injuries and medical treatments and about the daily duties and specific demands of the patient's job. A review of the patient's various systems and organ function will help the DC determine an appropriate approach to treatment and how treatment outcomes may be affected. For example, if the patient has right-sided back pain that radiates to the right lower abdomen, it would be good to know if the patient still has an appendix. The doctor may want to ask more specific questions about past or current medical issues and what is being done about them. Next, the doctor will gather information about the patient's "history."

History

Most people have a history of some condition and perhaps a successful treatment. The review of systems established what shape the person is in and why, as it pertains to various systems of the body. The history elicits more detail on what happened in the past, what was done about it, and whether it was successful. It also records whether there were complications or limitations after the treatment or resolution of the condition. It will also ask about current treatment of the area of complaint and any conditions being treated currently, such as hypertension or diabetes. A good history, more than any other single aspect of intake, will often point the doctor toward the actual diagnosis. The doctor must listen carefully and pay attention to every detail in order to find out the essential facts in the patient's history. The patient is essentially telling a health "story," and the clues given in it provide the doctor with necessary detail on not only what is wrong but likely whether he or she can help the patient.

A good history will ask about the past: what has happened to them in the past, any previous treatments, and how the patient fared with those treatments. It may also ask about family history of various diseases, as some diseases have a tendency to show up in families. Even current medications or herbal and vitamin preparations that a person takes can be critical to know in order to make an accurate diagnosis and to render appropriate care in the current case. Therefore, a good history asks a lot of questions about patients' current complaint, other existing conditions, particularly chronic diseases, and how they are managed, including self-management strategies.

Examination

After the intake paperwork, review of systems, and history are complete, typically the next task a doctor will undertake is to examine the patient. This starts out with a physical evaluation, including vital signs: height, weight, temperature, blood pressure, and sometimes other basic measures, such as waist circumference. Measurement of the waist can be a predictor of cardiovascular disease, because a large waist size indicates the "apple shape" associated with increased risk of heart disease. While a staff member can also be designated to perform these basic vital sign measures, the doctor should always review them and discuss them with the patient, even if they are normal.

Once basic vital signs have been performed and there are no "red flags"—that is, signs or symptoms that signal something more serious, warranting referral to an emergency room or some other health care provider—the DC may proceed to the specific physical examination that the intake and history suggest is needed. For example, if the patient has upper back pain that radiates into the left arm, perhaps the problem is related to the back. However, cardiovascular problems, such as a heart attack, sometimes refer pain into this same pattern, so there could be a need for an immediate referral to the emergency room, or the doctor may need to focus on this pain and further evaluate it. Either way, the examination of the patient with hands-on care continues. Perhaps the doctor will press on an area where there is soreness or pain. If this causes further symptoms, and aligns with the patient's description of an injury to that area in his or her history, it could mean the DC has pinpointed the problem. While the physical exam often yields a clear-cut issue, supported by what was shown in the intake paperwork and history, sometimes further diagnostic tests are needed. For instance, it is common for a DC to order radiographs or X-ray, MRI, and ultrasound studies or to perform some of these in the office. These studies of the patient's area of injury or complaint may confirm a diagnosis or may be negative and so rule out suspected pathology. It will be up to the DC, and perhaps another specialist, such as a radiologist, to arrive at a conclusion on what these radiographic or special examinations mean.

Laboratory tests such as blood work and analysis of urine, skin, or other areas of the body may also be performed or ordered in a typical chiropractic practice. Depending on the patient's needs, the DC may want to evaluate his or her vitamin D or cholesterol levels. Since musculoskeletal conditions are common, and sometimes cancer spreads to bone, the DC might also order a bone scan done in a hospital environment. This would hopefully rule out cancer of bone, but in some cases, unfortunately, it rules it in. These findings, both positive and negative, must be shared with the patient. Patients want to know what can be done for their pain and suffering, and this is exactly what a doctor will cover in the report of findings.

Report of Findings

The report of findings is done after all available information has been gathered on the patient and the doctor has had time to evaluate that information and to think about what he or she can do to help. In some cases, the report may point to a condition the doctor can't help. At that point, it is appropriate to suggest another health care provider; with the patient's permission, the DC may call that doctor to inform him or her of the findings and set up the referral appointment. If the patient's health complaint is commonly treated successfully in the office, the doctor can share this with the patient in the report of findings.

Patients will want to know (1) what is wrong, (2) if the doctor can help them, (3) how long it will be before they have some relief, and (4) how much it will cost. They will also want to know what their insurance plan will and will not cover. DCs should discuss as much of this with the patient as they feel they know at the time. It is common to show findings or scans and radiographs at this time, if they show something that will help the patient understand his or her case. DCs should be careful not to alarm the patient about the condition unless this is truly warranted.

The report of findings is an appropriate time to recommend and describe a specific course of treatment, if one has been decided. Patients may ask, "Will the treatment hurt? How long will an appointment take? How many times must I come in for office visits?" Doctors should answer these questions as they outline the initial phase of care for the patient. As the patient's body responds to the early phases of treatment, the treatment plan will often change, and the patient should be kept in the loop. Since chiropractic care is hands-on, takes some time to render, and takes place over several visits, similar to physical therapy, there is plenty of opportunity to talk about the care, response to care, and various health education items that could improve the overall health status of the patient. These may be lifestyle-related behaviors. It is appropriate to discuss these with patients at the report of findings if they can speed recovery as well as during subsequent visits as the patient is beginning to feel better and may be more capable of making lifestyle changes. Self-care may be a valued part of the treatment plan. Dos and don'ts are also a part of the self-care plan. The DC will tell the patient which activities to avoid and which are acceptable (for example, that it is okay to work or to get gentle exercise each day).

Setting Up a Treatment Plan

Part of what every doctor must do is to establish a treatment plan that will get his or her patient better. The intake paperwork, history, exam, and any specialty exams all inform the DC as to what it may take to get the patient better. The actual estimate of what will be required as a treatment plan is based on the doctor's education and training. It is also important that the DC keep up with relevant scientific literature, so that the treatment plan reflects the best scientific evidence. In time, as doctors gain experience, the treatment plan will also reflect how patients under their care have responded in the past. The treatment plan may include manual manipulation performed by hand or with the assistance of an instrument, with the patient either seated or lying on a special chiropractic adjustment table. It may include applications of heat, ice, therapeutic ultrasound, and other treatment methods, such as specific exercises or home care. It may also include adopting a healthier diet to manage weight or stopping tobacco use. Those needed changes should be shared with the patient at the report of findings. DCs generally develop a treatment plan for the first week or two prior to the report of findings. While they may change, many of the hands-on procedures performed every day in chiropractic practice are very similar and are a standard part of chiropractic practice. Practitioners should also offer patients the opportunity to address some needed lifestyle changes that can add years to their life.

Following Up

After the first visit, some doctors want to call the patient and follow up, make sure they understand any side effects of the treatment, and are following home care or self-care instructions. While a staff person can also do this, it is a nice touch if the doctor is the one to make contact. The patient will appreciate it and know that the DC has his or her interests at heart. It is a good chance to remind patients that they need to apply ice, or soak in a hot bath, or do prescribed exercises. Communication is a critical skill to hone in any health care practice. A good rapport with patients is another key to a successful practice.

Use of Health Education and Health Promotion in Practice

While it seems like a given that health education would be provided in a health care practice, studies continue to show that the average health care provider only engages a minority of patients on the topic of health education and wellness. Lifestyle changes, when desperately needed, tend to go unaddressed, even when the patient has risk factors that could be changed with some guidance and support. On average, 35–40 percent of patients report that their health care provider engaged them on a needed topic of wellness or health promotion.[2] This ranges from advice on smoking cessation to needed changes in diet and exercise levels.

The most common causes of early death in developed countries continue to be tobacco use, poor dietary choices, lack of physical activity, and excessive use of alcohol. While all are behaviors that can be changed, most people have never been told by their doctor that these behaviors are a danger to their health. For the sake of the health of the public, this needs to change. The health care practice is full of opportunities to talk to patients about lifestyle change. In particular, DCs tend to have regular, prolonged contact with patients with treatment plans that often include multiple visits per week initially. The number of visits multiplies the opportunities to reinforce lifestyle messages—if only the DC will make this a part of routine clinical practice.

Various health promotion opportunities are noted in most patient charts. However, the opportunity passes when the doctor fails to discuss them when the patient is in the office. If the DC would address the four issues noted above—tobacco use, poor diet, lack of physical activity, and excessive use of alcohol—there would be measurable improvements in health for the practice and the community. Searight offers a look at simple screening tools and behavioral theories that can assist health care providers in this capacity.[3]

It is fairly easy to master some simple tools in advising and basic behavior theory and when to try and motivate the patient and when to leave well enough alone. If the clinic takes this attitude and can support patient self-efficacy, the outcomes are rewarding for doctor and patient. Self-efficacy is the patient's confidence that he or she can change a health behavior. DCs can help patients attain self-efficacy by working with them to set small, attainable goals, encouraging them, and putting resources clearly in their path.

The health belief model of health education suggests that patients have to perceive a significant risk to their health in order to consider changing a health habit. This theory has been tested many times and is one of the most prevalent models of health behavior. In addition to a perception of risk, patients need to know that the risk would have a significant negative effect on their health and that without change, that threat is imminent. Originally, this model was used to frame education programs to get people to make a single change, such as getting a flu shot. Other aspects of the model included having a key person "cue" one to take action. Over time, the health care provider or doctor has been seen as the single most powerful person to get someone to make a health behavior change. In the course of behavior change, people have to feel that they can be successful; this confidence in being able to make a needed change is called "self-efficacy." Having a person set small, obtainable goals is one way to build this confidence. It is important not to overstate risks in order to scare people into action. However, when there is a real threat to health, the doctor relaying that to the patient and asking him or her to consider making a change can be very powerful. This should be applied in every case where a patient has a modifiable risk factor.

The stages of change (the transtheoretical model) is a health behavior model that suggests that people move through five stages toward healthy behavior change: (1) precontemplation, in which the person has no desire or intention to make a behavior change in the next six months; (2) contemplation, in which the person is thinking about making a change within the next six months; (3) preparation, in which the person is planning concrete ways to start the process of a new behavior change; (4) action, in which the person actually begins to put the plan into effect, such as setting a date to stop smoking or starting to go to the local gym; and (5) maintenance, in which the person simply maintains the new behavior for at least six months, so that it feels well established.

When the doctor pays some attention to how a patient responds to "cues to action," he or she can often determine what stage of behavior change the patient is in. Major behavior changes are hard to accomplish. When a person does not feel well or is in pain, it can be even more difficult to make a change, and the process will be slower. Accepting people where they are and being supportive is the role of the doctor in this case. Slow progress is still progress. There are also great resources available for health care providers who want to advise patients on behavior change, and many of them have taken into account the person's stage. Directing patients toward behavior change in a manner that respects the stage they are currently in and gently moves them toward more progressive change is a skill that can be acquired and honed to make a very powerful tool in aiding patients in their wellness process. Staging the patient is a part of that process. For example, patients who have not considered a needed lifestyle change would be encouraged to think about it, whereas those who say they would try to make a change today if they only knew what to do next need to be given immediate resources to help them take action.

In any clinical practice today, the needs are likely to be the same. People will need guidance and opportunities to make changes, such as increasing levels of physical activity, eating a healthier diet, decreasing the amount of alcohol they drink, and quitting using tobacco of any kind. While each one represents a different challenge, each one also has established guidelines to best help patients. In the case of tobacco use, there are many free resources and cessation programs that health care providers can guide their patients toward. It is simply about choosing to have the practice focus on wellness and not simply treating pain or disease processes.

Assessing Risk

One way to ensure that wellness and health promotion is a central feature of the practice is to designate a staff member to be in charge of the resources the DC identifies as acceptable and ensure they are always readily available. It may be worthwhile to provide the designated resource person(s) with additional training in this area. It's easy to gather brochures, resources, and lists of low-cost or free supporting agencies or programs in the area. Partnering with other likeminded wellness professionals as a part of routine chiropractic practice is a great way for any future DC to start out on the right path. There is a growing need for clinical providers to assess not only the patient's "chief complaint" but also the state of his or her overall health. This is done with the intake and evaluation methods described above but with a focus on identification of modifiable behavioral risk factors.

Most generic health care forms available from office supply companies include questions about risks such as tobacco use, and most EHR systems have places to check these most fundamental risk factors. Adding questions to the history and completing appropriate vital signs and examinations will identify most risk behaviors. It's worth adding questions about how many days a week a person gets physical activity outside of the workplace and about dietary intake, including how many fruits and vegetables the patient typically consumes in a day.

When it comes to alcohol use, asking a single question about potential excessive use can reveal which patients might be consuming too much alcohol at one time or in general. The common question is "In the last year, how many times have you had more than five alcoholic drinks in one sitting?"[4] For women, the number is four drinks in one sitting. The answer can alert practitioners to delve further into a patient's consumption of alcohol and, where needed, prompt advice on reducing this risk. While having one too many at a major event at some point in the year, such as New Year's Eve, may not signify a drinking problem, if the patient consumes four or five drinks at a time three times a week, this denotes a problem and an opportunity to determine the patient's stage of readiness to make a change. With that comes an opportunity to assist in this process.

Promoting Health

The 2008 *Physical Activity Guidelines for Americans*[5] describe the needed levels of physical activity and strength training that will keep people healthy. For the most part, adults require a minimum of 150 minutes of physical activity per week. These minutes need not be attained all at once; it is the accumulation of the minutes of movement that is tracked. For added benefit, the recommendation is a total of 300 minutes. That means a vigorous walk three days a week, washing the car, tilling the garden, going to the gym, and playing with the kids all count toward the total. Basically, there appears to be no limit to how much benefit most people can gain from physical activity. Of course, in some cases it may be necessary to check with a patient's primary care doctor or do an evaluation taking into account the patient's medical history and current state to determine a safe level of exercise.

Patients enter health care practices in varying states of sickness or wellness. A person who is injured in a softball game playing in a summer league may not need advice on additional physical activity, whereas someone who has chronic back or neck pain and gets very little physical activity is likely to be a candidate for such advice. As a doctor, remember to accept people where they are and preserve autonomy and not attempt to coerce patients to take on an issue they do not wish to address. It can be frustrating when a doctor identifies a risk factor that can be changed only to find that the patient has no interest in this. However, this is a common situation with many patients, and future DCs should keep in mind that behavior change must be voluntary. Seatbelt laws, tobacco smoking ordinances, and child safety laws have enforced some behavior changes at the community level, but in general, in a health care practice, that is neither advisable nor possible.

Marketing the Practice

New DCs will face several obstacles in getting a practice started if they do so from the ground up. None of these obstacles are insurmountable, but it takes planning to market a new business of any kind, and a health care practice is no exception. The plan needs to brand the practice in a way that reflects what the practitioner sees as his or her purpose or focus. For example, a sports medicine focus might use branding that begins with the name of the clinic or practice itself. "North Side Chiropractic Sports Medicine" tells potential patients exactly what the practice is about. However, new DCs should consider that this might limit their patient base only to athletes and exclude many patients who might also benefit from chiropractic care. A way to avoid this limitation might be to brand the clinic as "spine and sports medicine."

When it comes to wellness and health promotion as a feature of the practice, the name of the clinic could also be a place to start. Everyone from the yoga studios to the pharmacy at the local grocery see themselves as in the "wellness" business; consequently, the term can be somewhat confusing to potential patients. It is certainly possible to brand one's clinic as one that promotes health and wellness without the name of the clinic bearing the overused word "wellness." Alternative descriptive names such as "lifestyle medicine," or "prevention-focused" may have more meaning to some patients. In any case, a doctor who wants to brand the practice as oriented toward wellness and health promotion must follow through and actually deliver on these in the practice.

A part of the process of getting to know the potential marketplace is to take the first several months to meet as many people as possible outside of the office. Someone needs to remain in the office to answer calls, or calls can be routed to the doctor's cell phone. New patients may not want to leave a message, so it is best to have a person answer the phone rather than calls going to voicemail. Speaking to the Rotary or Kiwanis Club, local garden club, or even the assisted living facility can establish the doctor's presence and what the practice does. This is part of how any health care practice is built. It's helpful to give talks to the local community on stress management, wellness, physical activity, fall prevention, and promotion of health and well-being as part of what the chiropractic practice is about in addition to explaining what chiropractic can do for typical musculoskeletal problems. Questions will come that will allow the doctor to show the community that he or she is a musculoskeletal specialist, but sharing tips on wellness and positive preventive measures is a much-needed and often unique service to the community. Many people use "wellness" in their signs or materials, but few really address behavior change in the areas just discussed in this chapter. This delivery of preventive care is needed and wanted in many communities.

Getting to know the local health care community, including practitioners at the local urgent care, dental, mental health, or podiatric clinics, is an effective way to promote a successful practice. While not every provider will refer patients, there will be many opportunities to cross-refer. Getting to know the best, most conservative family doctor is a great idea. Also, let the medical physicians know about the practice's emphasis on prevention and health promotion. Remember, family practice physicians are seeing many of the same patients for family medicine, so in many cases they are trying to get a patient to stop smoking, get more physical activity, or eat a healthier diet too. Finding a like-minded professional can result in referrals from those practitioners. Many patients will have chronic medical conditions. Some will want to change their behaviors, but for others it may be too late to reverse the changes poor health habits have set in place. When a new patient needs a family physician as well, the opportunity to share the patient with a good medical doctor can be the starting point for a collaborative arrangement that benefits both patients and the practices.

Health care practices can be marketed with ads on local television and in newspapers, pop-up ads on Google, and even an ad in a high school sports program. Choosing if and where to advertise is one of the responsibilities of the chief executive part of the job.

Some doctors are better at marketing than others; for some, it might be worth hiring a local marketing expert. When first starting out in practice, it may be a good idea to look at local colleges or small business institutes or other sources of free or low-cost assessments of the marketplace. Some resources are available for free. Regardless of which methods are selected, marketing has to be done in some capacity. It is a good idea in the beginning to simply ask new patients to refer people in need of chiropractic services if they are satisfied with care. They may not otherwise know that referrals will be appreciated and may be less likely to do so. Volunteering in the community or sponsoring a little league team are other ways to increase visibility. Sending a thank-you to people who refer patients is also a part of the business of practice. *Chapter 8 provides details of starting a successful practice.*

Insurance, Record Keeping, and Billing

Many insurance plans cover chiropractic care. Today, most companies are either self-insured or have a plan administrator that handles insurance benefits for employees. This is often combined with premiums they collect from employees. Many of these companies will only pay for care if the health care provider is on their plan administrator's panel of providers. To join a panel of providers of an insurance company will take time and effort, and the doctor must be proactive in applying—the insurance company does not seek out providers. This can take weeks to months once a license and proof of malpractice insurance is in hand. Medicare pays for some limited chiropractic services, but again, it is the responsibility of the doctor to apply to be an approved Medicare provider. This is often the first step in getting credentialed for other insurance plans as well.

Once a provider is listed on a few major insurance company panels as an expert in chiropractic, employees for companies that have their insurance plans administered by that insurance carrier can choose him or her. The doctor's fees will either be reimbursed, wholly or in part, to the employee or may be paid directly to the doctor on what is called "assignment of benefits" for services rendered. The patient will have to have a diagnosis and corresponding diagnostic code that is covered by the plan and a reasonable fee for the service that is negotiated in advance when the provider agrees to join the panel. That is, the insurance company sets the fee schedule and doctors who join the panel agree to abide by that schedule of payment. They may charge more, but they will only be reimbursed for the amount specified in the agreement. Each procedure has a specific procedural code. Knowing these codes and using them correctly can have a great impact on payment. Manuals are available and seminars are taught on how to appropriately code insurance forms. In addition, there are companies that specialize in coding, and practitioners may wish to pay that company a percentage of the fee so that their office does not have to handle billing and the filing of insurance forms. While most will be filed as a part of the EHR today, follow up is often required, and those billing and coding specialists can be helpful in that respect.

Record keeping is critical to patient care. First and foremost, it provides an accurate record of diagnostic procedures and what information was given to the patient. This is needed for patient care and also if an insurance carrier wants to see a record of the office visit and the treatment that was rendered in order to authorize payment. Having good, detailed records is a key to successful management of patients and getting paid. It can also serve as a defense if anyone ever questions what was done in an office visit or treatment session. Having the appropriate level of detail is important. A common saying in practice is "if it is not written, it did not happen." Having evidence of what was done, the rationale for why it was done, which procedures helped, and when a change in the treatment plan was needed can be important for patient care and critical for getting paid.

There will be occasions when an insurance company will ask for those records to compare what was billed with what the office record indicates was done for the patient. Having a good record is a part of everyday best practices in any health care setting. A staff member can fill in some of the daily notes for the doctor, but the doctor needs to know what is being entered and to have the opportunity to edit it because he or she is ultimately responsible for what appears in the record. EHR systems date and time stamp all office notes, so patient chart notes should be made as the visit occurs. When it comes to billings to the insurance provider or administrator, regardless of whether a third-party biller sends the charges in, it is the doctor who is responsible for what is billed. The patient record serves as an accurate reflection of what occurred on the visit as well as which services were billed. While the panel may list the provider as an approved member or preferred provider for the plan, the overall agreement for insurance coverage is between the patient, the company he or she works for, and/or the insurance carrier. A new doctor will spend some time with the patient record and will need to become well versed at accurate entry into the patient chart or record.

Other Aspects of a Successful Health Care Practice

Chiropractic practice is a very active health care business. It takes some physical conditioning; in successful practices, doctors will be on their feet a lot during the day. Since the practice is dependent on hands-on care, it is important not to risk injury to hands or limbs.

The demands of the job are such that, in order to be successful, one has to have a heavily science-based education, must past rigorous board examinations in order to become licensed, and must master many tasks in the small business world in addition to being a good doctor.

A typical day in the office is spent talking to patients, sometimes solving complex diagnostic puzzles, and working hard not to miss an uncommon diagnosis that occasionally appears in the chiropractic office. Those uncommon diagnoses may be putting a patient's life at risk. Occasionally, the report of findings will bring bad, sometimes even devastating, news. New practitioners should be prepared for this. For example, it is likely that within the first few years of practice, a young doctor will find a previously undiagnosed case of cancer or some other life-threatening disease in a patient who presented with what at first appeared to be a simple case of back pain. Becoming good at diagnosis is about listening to the patient;

this is how the uncommon condition is diagnosed in the office. History leads the way. When the report of findings brings bad news, it can be a very emotional time. When patients with whom the doctor and staff have established a warm relationship experience a life-threatening event, it can be depressing for the entire team and requires that the doctor comes to terms with it.

While a routine practice involves hands-on, physical care to patients, the job also requires personnel management and all of the problems that brings. A good doctor will have to be good at managing not only patients but also, eventually, the staff that supports him or her. While this can be a challenge, it's worth taking the time to find the right staff member—someone with a caring attitude, healthy, positive, and people oriented. He or she should also champion chiropractic care. At times, it can be difficult to juggle all of these variables in a small business setting. Having a front office business manager whom one can trust can be a major asset to practice. This should be a long-term goal of all practitioners.

Overall, a typical day in the chiropractic office can be fast paced, fun, challenging, and financially rewarding. As one prepares for any career, it is always a good idea to meet people who currently perform this job and are successful at it. The aspiring or new doctor should ask them what they have done to be successful, what mistakes they have made that might be avoided, and what makes the job rewarding for them. When possible, aspiring doctors would be wise to spend time in a practice in the area where they plan to locate their future practice. They should find out about insurance coverage in the state, the climate for growth in chiropractic in that area, and look for parts of the community where there is growth and need for a new doctor. With this type of preparation, there is a great chance to be successful and to join a community as a respected member of the health care team. If that can be accomplished, most will find a very rewarding career and be able to practice in nearly any city, state, or country that they choose. And nothing can be more rewarding than getting to live and work in an area of the world you have always wanted to be, while practicing a profession that has the potential to help so many people.

Chiropractic Practice in Australia: 2015

Australians consider this to be the "lucky country," one of the most livable countries on earth with a high life expectancy—over 80 years at birth. With a total health system expenditure at about 9 percent of GDP, Australia is about average compared with other OECD countries (e.g., United States spends 17 percent).[6]

Australia's health system is complex, best described as a web of services between providers, recipients, and organizational structures featuring a universal safety net called "Medicare" augmented by optional private insurance (this is not analogous to the United Sates' Medicare for seniors). A person does not usually need a referral for primary care, which includes services provided by general medical and dental practitioners and other allied health professionals, such as physiotherapists, dieticians, and chiropractors. While primary health care is delivered in a variety of settings, including general practices, Aboriginal and Community Controlled Health Services, community health centers, and private allied health services, at present chiropractors practice only in private practice settings. Private health insurance is not compulsory, and people who opt to buy private health insurance can mix and match the levels and type of coverage to suit their individual circumstances, thereby giving private health-fund-paying patients more control in choosing their provider. As of June 2013, 55 percent of Australians had some form of general coverage[7] with most private health insurers covering chiropractic care to some extent; however, reimbursements are limited, and there are invariably substantial gap fees payable by the patient.

To become a chiropractor prior to 1975 required Australians to travel overseas to study since the first jurisdictions to legislate chiropractic practice stipulated North American courses as the benchmark. While the first chiropractic program in Australia designed to be of international standard was located in Melbourne, Victoria, there are now other university-based chiropractic programs in the states of Western Australia, New South Wales, and Queensland. All of these courses closely reflect their international counterparts, and in the early years employed mainly non-Australian academic staff. This means firstly that a significant proportion of chiropractors practicing in Australia are overseas trained, and secondly, that local courses are based on internationally benchmarked, accredited curricula,[8] thus Australian chiropractors and their practices mirror their overseas cousins, and the therapeutic journey of chiropractic patients in Australia will invariably bear close resemblance to those overseas.

In common with other countries, in recent years Australia has seen a gradual shift in the dynamics of the wider health care landscape toward "patient-centered" or "holistic" care based on a biopsychosocial model, a model that resonates with chiropractors. Historically, Australian chiropractors have identified themselves strongly with a philosophy of health that espouses a "natural approach," including good diet, adequate rest and relaxation, physical activity, positive mental health and well-being, not smoking, not using drugs, and moderate alcohol consumption; in other words, chiropractors have occupied a "nonpharmacological, non-surgical spine care expert" health care space. However, to date they have effectively practiced in a "silo" alongside the mainstream health care system. As a result of this limited engagement, many other health care practitioners and health system administrators are likely to know little about the chiropractic profession, and this increases the possibility of attitudes and perceptions arising from stories found within the (sometimes negative) wider media, possibly explaining a widespread reticence to engage professionally with chiropractors. In an effort to address this gap, independent researchers in Australia have started collecting data from chiropractic practices at both national and regional levels by building a robust practice-based research network (PBRN) that will offer far greater insight into the current role and future potential for chiropractic in the Australian health care system. The initial PBRN uptake data reflects the strong engagement with professional associations where approximately 75 percent of the profession belong to at least one organization, the largest being the Chiropractors Association of Australia (CAA); around 35 percent of practitioners have also joined the PBRN.

In 2010, with the advent of the Australian Health Practitioners Regulation Agency (AHPRA), chiropractic in Australia transitioned from state legislatures and became a nationally regulated profession alongside medicine, physiotherapy, dentistry, and various other professions. Chiropractic is thus equally represented in the legislation as a self-regulating profession. However, the role of chiropractic in the broader health care system remains somewhat unclear; the profession has the same responsibilities but fewer rights than other regulated professions. Australian chiropractors essentially have no other employment options as chiropractors other than private practice with limited referral rights or academia/research.

This contrasts, for instance, with physiotherapists, who may work in hospitals, workplaces (as consultants), sports and community centers, women's health centers, rehabilitation centers, aged care facilities, mental health centers, chronic disease management centers, the private sector, schools, and education and research facilities. Consequently, the profession is currently working hard to expand the role of chiropractors in the Australian health care system via participation in various multidisciplinary task forces and working parties.[9] Notwithstanding, the average number of services provided by chiropractors is approximately two-and-a-half times that of physiotherapists.[10]

In Australia, as in other countries, government-generated models of care for musculoskeletal health care provision, which includes spinal pain, have increasingly focused on shifting services from hospital to community-based settings and improving access to multidisciplinary care. This shift is aimed at improving outcomes for patients, containing health care costs, and making use of the available, appropriately trained workforce. For example, the Western Australia Department of Health Musculoskeletal Health Network has produced a Spinal Pain Model of Care[11] and the Framework for Persistent Pain (to be published in 2016), in which guidelines for multidisciplinary care, service navigation, and the patient care journey are described. These models of care and frameworks contain numerous potential opportunities[9] and roles for chiropractors in the context of multidisciplinary care, particularly in the area of musculoskeletal/spinal health.[12]

Existing data on chiropractic practice or patients are primarily from the United States, Canada, and Europe, with relatively few studies of satisfactory quality providing insight into chiropractic practice in Australia. Studies[13–17] indicate that, as in other countries, the vast majority of people in Australia consult chiropractors for spinal pain and related musculoskeletal disorders, they are predominantly referred by word of mouth (family, friends, and acquaintances), and they pay for their care out of pocket along with receiving private insurance rebates; around 16 percent of Australians visit chiropractors annually. The level of direct referral to chiropractors by medical practitioners is very low; however, the federal government–funded universal health system (Medicare) provides coverage for chiropractic referral for a limited number of musculoskeletal imaging item numbers (plain film X-ray) and a limited number of patient visits under a "Chronic Disease Management" initiative as well as coverage by the Department of Veterans Affairs (DVA) for service personnel. There is also coverage for chiropractic services delivered under workers' compensation and traffic accident claims; however, the referral protocols and fee rebates paid to practitioners vary significantly by state.

Typical Chiropractic Practice in the U.K.

A clinical practice in the U.K. will look and feel very similar to one in other established jurisdictions around the world, but there are some differences worth highlighting.

The practice of chiropractic in the United Kingdom is regulated by the General Chiropractic Council (GCC), which is an independent statutory body established by Parliament and is responsible for setting and maintaining the standards required for safe and competent practice. The GCC's primary purpose is to ensure the safety of the public; their code, which includes a code of practice and standard of proficiency, lays down what is expected from chiropractors to ensure the quality of patient care.[18]

Chiropractors must follow the code in order to maintain their registration, as the right to be called a chiropractor is linked to registration with the GCC. However, the code is broad based and does not limit or prescribe the way chiropractors practice, as long as they can demonstrate that they are following these guidelines and working safely in the best interests of patients. The GCC has produced a helpful booklet for potential patients that outlines what they can expect from a chiropractor, including what happens in the clinical encounter, how many sessions might be needed, and how they might respond to chiropractic care.[19]

As chiropractic is recognized as a primary care profession, chiropractors are able to refer their patients to a wide range of other health care providers within the U.K., including general practitioners (GPs), who are generally regarded as the principal gatekeepers to the National Health Service (NHS) in the U.K. Increasingly, GPs are referring patients with musculoskeletal complaints to chiropractors, and in general the relationship between chiropractic and the medical profession is positive and respectful.

Chiropractors are required to take a holistic, patient-centered approach to their practice and to consider patients' general health needs, including their physical, psychological, and social well-being. They will therefore take an integrated approach to the health needs of their patients, considering not only their presenting physical condition but also their lifestyle (such as sleep, diet, stress levels, work/life balance) and social factors, including how much support they have at home. As well as helping with pain management, injuries, and rehabilitation, chiropractors will commonly offer advice on self-help, exercise, nutrition, and how to modify lifestyle in order to get the patient to understand the role that they themselves play in maintaining their health.

The types of chiropractic intervention used will be dictated to a large extent by the presenting complaint, and one of the first tasks will be to take a full clinical case history, followed by a physical examination, including neurological and orthopedic tests if needed and referral for any further diagnostic tests. The vast majority of chiropractors in the U.K. do not have their own X-ray equipment and will routinely refer into the NHS if a patient needs any sort of imaging for diagnostic purposes. Under U.K.'s regulations, images, including X-rays, must only be taken for clinical reasons. This means that certain chiropractic techniques that routinely require X-rays as part of their diagnostic procedures could potentially cause problems. With that exception, a very wide range of adjusting techniques are in common use.

Although the majority of chiropractors will have a musculoskeletal focus, many choose to work in preventive and wellness care, which proves popular with the population. Open-plan adjusting is not common in the U.K., though chiropractors do use this style of practice while keeping within the GCC's code.

Chiropractors in the U.K. provide care for patients of all ages who present with a range of acute (short-term) and chronic (longer-term) conditions. Roughly 55 percent of patients will present with back pain, 25 percent with neck or shoulder pain, 10 percent with headaches, and 10 percent with extremity problems, or any combination of those. Some chiropractors will choose to focus their practice on, for example, older people or athletes, and there is no restriction on chiropractors working with children as long as they can demonstrate that they are properly trained and qualified to do so.

Virtually all chiropractors work in private practice, and patients pay cash direct to the practice for their chiropractic care, most usually immediately after the treatment session. Some practices do operate an advance payment plan system, though care needs to be taken on how this is operated, following the relevant guidance issued by professional associations. A wide range of other useful guidance can be found on the GCC website.[20]

All U.K. private medical insurance (PMI) companies recognize chiropractic, and reimbursement is made to the chiropractor on receipt of an invoice for each patient care session. The majority simply require the chiropractor to register with them and the full cost of treatment will be reimbursed, but an increasing trend is to limit the number of sessions that can be reimbursed and, in the case of one PMI, to fix the price that the chiropractor can charge. Relatively few chiropractors have a contract to provide chiropractic services under the NHS, but anyone interested in this type of practice will need to become recognized as an appropriate provider by demonstrating how they meet a wide range of clinical governance guidelines.[21]

In order to maintain their registration, all chiropractors need to complete 30 hours of continuing professional development (CPD) each year, of which half must be learning with others. Chiropractors generally attend conferences, seminars, and training courses to complete their CPD, but they may also choose to undertake independent reading or research as long as this can be linked to the improvement of patient care.[22]

Chiropractic Practice in Indonesia

In terms of patient care, Indonesian chiropractic practice is very similar to practicing in the United States. Chiropractors do the typical consultation, examination, and report. However, an important part of a typical report in Indonesia is education about chiropractic. Many patients have never heard of chiropractic prior to their visit. Therefore, the doctor of chiropractic (DC) must explain what chiropractic is and what he or she will do prior to any therapy. He or she should be prepared to answer the patients' questions about chiropractic in general. Most foreign DCs will require a translator during patient interactions, as many Indonesians do not speak fluent English. Most commonly, the translator will double as a chiropractic assistant.

Indonesian patients are similar to "typical" chiropractic patients in the United States in terms of their presenting complaints, which are often back pain, neck pain, or headaches. However, personal relationships and sharing of their culture are very important to Indonesian patients. They expect a much closer doctor-patient experience and appreciate spending more time with the doctor, both in and out of the office. The DC will receive many lunch invitations, frequent dishes of local cuisine, and the occasional gift. DCs need to understand this and be willing to interact more closely with their patients and show simple cultural gestures, such as wearing a traditional "batik" shirt to work or learning the national language, Bahasa Indonesia. This will go a long way to enhance patient retention and referrals.

The office staff (aka chiropractic assistants [CAs]) serve many roles in the office. They work as translators, front desk staff, collections, schedulers, and more. Because of the language barrier for most foreign DCs, they must rely heavily on the office CA to run the office smoothly. As is true with the patients, building relationships is even more important with the DC's staff. Spending time with the staff, in and out of the office, will go a long way to maintain good office morale and motivation. The staff will teach the DC the language and culture. They will be the doctor's biggest advocates and promote him or her to many prospective patients.

In general, Indonesians are very open to the idea of natural health care options. They are willing to try conservative options before using medicine or surgery. Other natural health care options in Indonesia include traditional Chinese medicine, acupuncture, reflexology, and Kerokan, a type of traditional Indonesian medicine in which a coin is rubbed across the back. These can be forms of competition, but most people are willing to try different therapies together.

Most practices in Indonesia are cash-based practices. Some of the international workers' insurance covers chiropractic, but most Indonesian insurance does not, as it is not completely understood or completely licensed yet. Unfortunately, because of this situation, only the affluent middle or upper class can afford chiropractic care.

Most practices are owned privately, either independently or as small groups of clinics. Any business in Indonesia must have an Indonesian as majority owner, so many chiropractic offices are owned by a local Indonesian business partner who partners with a foreign chiropractor.

Patients will either pay the clinic for services at the completion of each visit or buy packages of treatment visits. Compensation to the DC tends to be on a commission basis. That is, the DC is often paid a percentage of the services or patient visits for that month. Another common compensation option is a base salary plus bonuses based on services provided. The clinic owner then keeps whatever is collected, minus the DC commission and overhead. Most commonly, the chiropractor is paid in Indonesian rupiah, the local currency, the value of which is frequently lower than that of the U.S. dollar. This is something DCs must consider if they have financial obligations in the United States, such as student loans, which must be paid in U.S. dollars.

There is currently no national chiropractic law or licensure in Indonesia. As far as legality goes, practicing in Indonesia is essentially one big gray area. This means that it is neither legal nor illegal to practice chiropractic. Therefore, enforcement is not consistent, and it is particularly important that DCs make sure they have all appropriate work permits and visas. The health department or immigration agency may make individual decisions to apprehend and deport a foreign DC, which can happen even if one chiropractic practice reports on another one to the health department. This will continue to be possible until a national chiropractic law is signed.

There are approximately 100 chiropractors practicing in Indonesia. Most of these are foreign, with only about one-fifth being Indonesian. Most Indonesian chiropractors are medical doctors who have taken a conversion course in chiropractic. Roughly only 30 Indonesian chiropractors have completed the conversion course. With Indonesia holding the fourth-largest population in the world, there is much potential for success in chiropractic.

Note: Dr. Amorin-Woods would like to acknowledge Dr. Andrew Vincent and Dr. Gregory Parkin-Smith for reviewing the section about practice in Australia.

References

1. United States Department of Labor. Occupational Outlook Handbook. Chiropractic. http://www.bls.gov/ooh/healthcare/chiropractors.htm#tab-6. Published December 15, 2015. Accessed April 10, 2016.

2. Evans MW, Ndetan H, Singh KP. Primary prevention: what are we missing in primary care? *Am J Heal Stud.* 2012;27(2):82–96.

3. Searight HR. Realistic approaches to counseling in the office setting. *Am Fam Physician.* 2009;79(4):277–284.

4. American Public Health Association. Alcohol Screening and Brief Intervention. http://www.integration.samhsa.gov/clinical-practice/alcohol_screening_and_brief_interventions_a_guide_for_public_health_practitioners.pdf. Accessed April 10, 2016.

5. U.S. Department of Health and Human Services. Physical Activity Guidelines for Americans. Washington, DC: USDHHS; 2008.

6. Worldbank. Health Expenditure, Total (percent of GDP) by Country. http://data.worldbank.org/indicator/SH.XPD.TOTL.ZS. Accessed January 10, 2015.

7. Australia Institute of Health and Welfare. Australia's Health System. http://www.aihw.gov.au/australias-health/2014/health-system/. Accessed December 21, 2015.

8. Council on Chiropractic Education Australasia Inc. Standards for Standardisation Programs in Chiropractic. 2004. http://www.ccea.com.au/Documents creditation/Standardisation%20Programs%201011.pdf. Accessed January 7, 2016.

9. Amorin-Woods LG, Parkin-Smith GF, Saboe V, Rosner AL. Recommendations to the Musculoskeletal Health Network, Health Department of Western Australia related to the spinal pain model of care made on behalf of the Chiropractors Association of Australia (Western Australian Branch). *Top Integrative Health Care.* 2014 Jun 30;5(2):ID: 5.2002.

10. Engel RM, Brown BT, Swain MS, Lystad RP. The provision of chiropractic, physiotherapy and osteopathic services within the Australian private healthcare system: a report of recent trends. *Chiropr Man Therap.* 2014;22(1):1–7.

11. Department of Health WA. Spinal Pain Model of Care. Perth: Health Networks Branch, Department of Health, Western Australia; 2009. http://www.healthnetworks.health.wa.gov.au/modelsofcare/docs/Spinal_Pain_Model_of_Care.pdf. Accessed June 27, 2015.

12. Parkin-Smith G, Amorin-Woods L, Davies S, Losco B, Adams J. Spinal pain: current understanding, trends, and the future of care. *J Pain Res.* 2015;8:741–752.

13. Ebrall P. A descriptive report of the case-mix within Australian chiropractic practice. *Chiropr J Aust.* 1993;23:92–97.

14. Xue C, Zhang A, Lin V, Myers R, Polus B, Story D. Acupuncture, chiropractic and osteopathy use in Australia: a national population survey. *BMC Public Health.* 2008;8(1):105.

15. Brown BT, Bonello R, Fernandez-Caamano R, Eaton S, Graham PL, Green H. Consumer characteristics and perceptions of chiropractic and chiropractic services in Australia: results from a cross-sectional survey. *J Manip Physiol Ther.* 2012;37(4):219–229.

16. French S, Charity M, Forsdike K, et al. Chiropractic Observation and Analysis Study (COAST): providing an understanding of current chiropractic practice. *Med J Aust.* 2013;199(10):687–691.

17. French S, Densley K, Charity M, Gunn J. Who uses Australian chiropractic services? *Chiropr Man Therap.* 2013;21(1):31.

18. General Chiropractic Council. *Code of Practice and Standard of Proficiency.* London: General Chiropractic Council; 2010.

19. General Chiropractic Council. What Can I Expect When I See a Chiropractor. http://www.gcc-uk.org/publications/publications-for-chiropractors. Accessed May 2, 2016.

20. GCC Publications. The Code: Standards of Conduct, Performance and Ethics for Chiropractors http://www.gcc-uk.org/publications/publications-for-chiropractors. Accessed May 2, 2016.

21. Society of Radiographers. Any Qualified Provider AQP/New NHS Structure (England). http://www.sor.org/career-progression/managers/any-qualified-provider. Accessed May 2, 2016.

22. General Chiropractic Council. Continuing Professional Development (CPD) Mandatory Requirements. London: General Chiropractic Council; 2004.

CHAPTER TEN

Chiropractic Specialization Career Paths

Stefanie Krupp, DC, MS; and
Clinton Daniels, DC, MS, DAAPM

Within the chiropractic profession, practitioners may specialize in a particular population, technique, or philosophical or integrative approach. According to the National Board of Chiropractic Examiners' *Practice Analysis of Chiropractic 2015*, 34 percent of chiropractors have worked toward and/or achieved certification in a clinical specialty area.[1] Chiropractors may gain expertise over time through practice experience and professional development but may also seek additional credentials or authority through graduate programs, residencies, or other postgraduate training. This chapter examines the specialty opportunities for doctors of chiropractic, including training, typical practice requirements or equipment, patient base, and value-added services, and will indicate in some instances how a specialty may impact or be affected by scope of practice. Some states may not acknowledge or allow recognition or marketing of some or all of these chiropractic specialties.

You might notice some overlap among many of these specialties; however, each specialty is defined based on added credentials, the focus of the practice (whether more narrow or more broad), and the patient base. The following practice specializations are covered in this chapter:

- manipulative (adjustive) techniques
- soft tissue techniques
- acupuncture
- sports chiropractic
- rehabilitation
- integrative pain management
- personal injury (PI)
- radiology
- neurology
- orthopedics
- nutrition
- functional medicine (FM)
- diagnosis and internal disorders (DID)
- primary care
- special populations (pediatrics, geriatrics, women's health)
- military medicine
- manipulation under anesthesia (MUA)
- occupational health and ergonomics
- forensics
- animal chiropractic
- nonclinical career specialties

Individual interests, needs of a local or niche population, and/or mentorship can motivate a chiropractic physician to pursue additional training or expertise. Specialty practices and added credentials through certifications, graduate degrees, and/or diplomates give chiropractors added authority in their local region as well as on a national or international scale. With added authority, other general practice chiropractors and other local health care providers may refer patients to them for their specialty services. It is also a way for a chiropractor to create added value to their services or gain confidence in providing services beyond more routine chiropractic care.

Manipulative (Adjustive) Techniques

Within the chiropractic profession, manipulation of the spinal and other joints is usually referred to as "adjustment." Thus, these techniques can be called "manipulative" or "adjustive." Though most chiropractors use a variety of techniques for patient care, some focus their practice on a single adjustive technique or protocol.[1] Commonly known treatment techniques include Cox Flexion Distraction, Gonstead, Activator, sacro-occipital technique (SOT), upper cervical, applied kinesiology (AK), and Thompson (also known as "drop," "drop table," or "Thompson drop"). These techniques often require special equipment, such as table design or features and tools (instruments, upholstered blocks). A 2005 study found that after the generic adjusting technique known as "diversified," the most common techniques used by North American chiropractors were flexion distraction (39%), Gonstead (36%), and Activator (35%).[2]

Diversified technique is the most common technique taught in chiropractic programs, so it is not considered a specialty technique. There are a variety of reasons why chiropractors may deviate away from diversified adjusting when they go into practice. Diversified adjusting is a high-velocity, low-amplitude manual force applied to joints to restore proper motion and can be considered a very physically demanding adjusting approach. Doctors may choose to specialize in one or a few particular techniques because of a preference to treat a certain patient population, like children or elderly patients, to protect the doctor's body mechanics, or to accommodate a doctor's injury or other condition.

Low-force techniques are commonly added to or substituted for diversified adjusting, which may include using drop tables, flexion distraction tables, adjusting instruments, or pelvic blocking. The choice to use a low-force technique may be based on certain patient characteristics or presentations: those with history of cancer, osteoporosis, or other cause for bone fragility; very young or very old patients; or those who may be fearful or anxious of a more forceful adjusting style or of hearing the joint cavitation noise from manual adjusting. There may also be a benefit to doctors using low-force techniques since they are considered to cause less wear and tear on the doctor's body. Therefore, some doctors opt to exclusively use a low-force method for adjusting.

Those who specialize in chiropractic techniques or protocols often start in chiropractic college by joining clubs, taking elective offerings, and attending continuing education courses offered on and off campus. Chiropractic students learn about techniques and protocols through the curriculum as well as through practicing doctors. Many new chiropractors are mentored by experienced doctors as they start in practice.

Most of the widely known techniques taught through continuing education courses to doctors of chiropractic provide certifications or diplomates, including Cox flexion distraction, Activator Methods, Gonstead, and applied kinesiology. Training is also offered through companies that sell specialized equipment, such as instrument adjusting tools and tables. Certifications and diplomates often require completing a minimum number of course hours and passing an examination but are not acknowledged by the American Chiropractic Association or state boards as specialties. The International College of Applied Kinesiology (ICAK) offers a diplomate called the diplomate of the International Board of Applied Kinesiology (DIBAK). The Gonstead Clinical Studies Society (GCSS) offers both diplomate (DGCSS) and fellow (FGCSS) programs. The Council on Upper Cervical Care of the International Chiropractic Association offers the diplomate in chiropractic upper cervical procedures (DCUCP). Techniques that provide certification or diplomate status may require ongoing continuing education courses to maintain active status or to be listed in the provider directory on the certifying body's website.

Some insurance companies recognize technique specialties for reimbursement, although some technique specialties may not qualify as approved treatment approaches depending on the amount of research supporting their use. Activator, flexion distraction, and drop table are often approved as treatment approaches but require the appropriate documentation and paperwork according to the insurance company contracted provider requirements. Technique specialties follow the same scope of practice as a typical doctor of chiropractic in each state.

Soft Tissue Techniques

Chiropractic physicians commonly use soft tissue techniques in combination with or in lieu of manipulative therapy. Soft tissue techniques are typically aimed at lengthening tight or shortened muscles, releasing fascial restrictions, reducing trigger points (sites of taut muscle fibers), and/or increasing range of motion. Some of the more commonly used soft tissue therapies include Nimmo, Post-Isometric Relaxation (PIR)/Proprioceptive Neuromuscular Facilitation (PNF), Active Release Techniques (ART), and Graston Technique/Instrument-Assisted Soft Tissue Mobilization (IASTM). A survey of Australian chiropractors revealed that practitioners with 10 or more years of experience were more likely to apply soft tissue or low-force techniques instead of high-velocity, low-amplitude manipulation.[3] Practitioners often select soft tissue techniques based on their practice style, flow, and patient population.

Nimmo technique was developed around the theory that physiopathologic reflexes cause increased muscle tonus, trigger points, and ultimately painful conditions. Nimmo-trained chiropractors evaluate for trigger points through manual palpation. Upon detection of trigger points, mild manual pressure is applied to the trigger point for five to seven seconds in sequence for several cycles until the trigger point releases.[4] Treatment with Nimmo technique prior to joint manipulation can conceivably reduce the amount of force necessary for manipulative thrust.

Post-isometric relaxation and proprioceptive neuromuscular facilitation are low-force muscle energy procedures that serve as joint mobilization and muscle relaxation. Each of these practices is commonly taught as a standard part of chiropractic school curriculum, but providers may also seek out continuing education specific to these treatments. PIR involves the practitioner placing the muscle of interest in a stretched position until he or she reaches a "barrier" of tension. Next the patient is instructed to isometrically resist further stretch for 5 to 10 seconds and then relax. After the patient relaxes the involved muscle, the provider passively lengthens the muscle to the next "barrier," and the whole process is repeated as necessary until desired length is reached. Incorporation of inhalation/exhalation and/or eye movements can further facilitate muscle relaxation. The primary difference between PIR and PNF is the amount of resistance exerted by the patient. With PNF the procedure is the same, except patient resistance to stretch is much stronger (i.e., up to 100 percent of their maximum strength), and stretch by the practitioner during the relaxation phase is more aggressive.[5]

Active Release Techniques is a patented hands-on soft tissue system–based massage technique that treats dysfunctions of muscles, tendons, ligaments, fascia, and nerves. The technique was founded on the principle of recognizing and treating cumulative-injury disorders or overuse injuries. ART protocols involve shortening the tissue of interest, applying a contact tension, and then lengthening the tissue so that it slides relative to adjacent tissues. The protocol is generally recommended to be repeated three to five times or until the clinician subjectively determines the tissue is functioning properly. ART offers one- to four-day seminar courses on the diagnosis and treatment of musculoskeletal conditions related to the spine, extremities, and other musculoskeletal topics.

Instrument-assisted soft tissue mobilization (IASTM) techniques, such as Graston Technique and Gua Sha, use tools to mechanically mobilize scar tissue, increasing its elasticity and loosening it from surrounding tissues. Available tools range substantially in price and material. Common materials include stainless steel, porcelain, buffalo horn, jade, and plastic. It is hypothesized that through scar tissue mobilization, IASTM introduces a controlled amount of microtrauma in order to reinitiate the inflammatory process of healing. This is believed to trigger a rush of blood, nutrients, and metabolic processes, which facilitate healing of the injured tissue. Graston Technique offers basic and advanced training in a weekend seminar format.

Despite the expense of specialized IASTM tools, many chiropractors use these tools to reduce stressors that may result from hands-on approaches.

Acupuncture and Oriental Medicine

Advanced training in acupuncture and/or Oriental medicine allows chiropractors to offer expanded treatment options, particularly for patients who may not have responded to traditional chiropractic care. With this added specialty, a chiropractor may have the opportunity to work in integrative settings, such as hospitals, that may have otherwise excluded chiropractic. The demand for acupuncture and Oriental medicine has been steadily rising due to increased evidence supporting the relatively low risk to treatment. Licensure requirements vary by state; some states allow chiropractors to perform acupuncture under their chiropractic license while others require a separate license. Certification in acupuncture is optional but can be a requirement for licensure depending on the state. Most health insurance companies also require licensure to cover acupuncture services. *Advanced training and licensure options for acupuncture and Oriental medicine are covered in Chapter 7.*

Acupuncture incorporates some similar evaluation approaches to chiropractic but also uses its own distinctive assessment and treatment techniques. Acupuncture may be incorporated in a chiropractic practice with a traditional approach, using ultrafine needles inserted into specific meridian points on the body, but may also be more progressive with electroacupuncture, acupressure, or "dry needling." Dry needling uses acupuncture needles for myofascial pain control, locally placed in muscle and fascia and not using meridians. This technique can be learned from continuing education seminars offered to musculoskeletal specialists like chiropractors and physical therapists but may not be allowed in all states depending on the limitations of scope of practice. Acupressure, which uses pressure instead of needles, is an alternative application of acupuncture concepts when needles are outside the scope of practice. Other acupuncture treatment approaches, such as moxibustion, cupping, tui na, exercise, and breathing techniques, may also be incorporated.

Patients seeking care from chiropractors who also offer acupuncture services may want treatment options that complement or reduce the use of high-velocity, low-amplitude adjusting in helping with pain management or treatment of muscle tightness and spasm. Additionally, a chiropractor who specializes in acupuncture and Oriental medicine may offer more comprehensive health and wellness services beyond the typical musculoskeletal practice, which can be considered primary care or family practice as well.

Sports Chiropractic

Chiropractors interested in working with athletes have numerous paths to pursue. Many chiropractic offices focus on managing athletic injuries in their local community, working with local high school athletes and weekend warriors. Other practitioners serve as official team chiropractors for college sports teams, professional sports teams, and Olympic and Paralympic events. Doctors of chiropractic can work in a purely chiropractic capacity by providing manipulation and soft tissue services, or they can administer pregame athletic taping, on-field emergency care, and sideline injury care, and prescribe rehabilitative exercise. In some states, chiropractors are permitted to perform preparticipation physicals as well. Chiropractors can serve as part of an interdisciplinary team with athletic trainers, physical therapists, and medical doctors, or as the chief medical officer guiding all athletic care.

The American Board of Chiropractic Sports Physicians offers postgraduate training and credentialing as certified chiropractic sports physicians (CCSP) and diplomates of American Chiropractic Board of Sports Physicians (DACBSP). Several chiropractic colleges offer master's degree programs in sports medicine. To date, credentialed DACBSP chiropractors have served as the chief medical officer of the Pan American Games, USA Archery, USA Fencing, and as managing director of sports medicine for the United States Olympic Committee.

All National Football League (NFL) and Major League Baseball (MLB) and most National Basketball Association (NBA) teams now have official team chiropractors. The men's and women's professional golf tours have chiropractors available for players at all of their tournaments. The Professional Football Chiropractic Society was formed in 2001 with a mission of education and communication to enhance the perception of chiropractic in sports and ultimately with the general public. They now provide annual continuing education on professional sports chiropractic topics in Indianapolis during the NFL scouting combine. The Professional Baseball Chiropractic Association followed suit in 2008. *Chapter 13 discusses sports chiropractic in depth.*

Rehabilitation

Physical rehabilitation has become a mainstay of chiropractic care. There are many forms of rehabilitation, ranging from educating patients on low-tech therapeutic and corrective exercises to applying passive physical modalities, such as ultrasound, electric stimulation, and lasers.

Some practices even use high-tech gym-based or decompression offices with lots of expensive equipment.

Recent years have seen a surge in popularity of the low-tech and minimalist type of rehabilitation programs. These frequently involve a progression from isometric holds to increasingly dynamic and functional movements centered on concepts of developmental kinesiology. Low-tech rehabilitation commonly incorporates basic equipment, such as foam rolls, resistance bands, balance boards, and kettlebells. There is a large overlap in the rehabilitation world between injury treatment and personal training. Chiropractic rehabilitation specialists commonly partner with CrossFit and other gyms to help keep their clients healthy and guide the transition from injury to return to activity.

The American Chiropractic Rehabilitation Board (ACRB) offers diplomate board certification as a chiropractic rehabilitation specialist. In addition, there are several national organizations that offer advanced postgraduate seminars and training in rehabilitation. Some of the leading organizations include Rehab 2 Perform; Prague School of Rehabilitation; Rehabilitation Institute of Chicago; McKenzie Institute, USA; and Functional Movement Systems. Physical rehabilitation is also embedded in sports chiropractic seminars and training, so many chiropractors with a strong rehabilitation focus may also have expertise or credentials in sports chiropractic.

Integrative Pain Management

Working in an integrated environment can be very appealing for chiropractic physicians. These positions allow providers to manage complex and challenging cases, learn from and teach allied health care professionals, and practice in a hospital-based environment, and they open up opportunities in clinical research. In some capacity, almost all chiropractic clinicians are involved in the prevention, treatment, or management of pain. Acute and subacute pain are typically related to some sort of tissue injury and resulting inflammatory process. Acute and subacute pain are typically successfully managed with provider intervention or can be self-resolving. However, chronic pain is a much more complex issue that may result from persistent nervous system sensitization/pain amplification, movement dysfunction, lack of physical activity, poor dietary lifestyle, history of physical or emotional trauma, cultural perceptions, and most commonly a combination of these. The complex nature of chronic conditions does not typically respond to narcotic medications, surgical intervention, or any individual method of treatment and frequently requires a team-based integrative approach.

The American Academy of Pain Management defines integrative pain management as an evidence-based, patient-centered, holistic model of care that emphasizes lifestyle changes as a first-line treatment and is inclusive of all appropriate health care members in a team approach. A 2012 study on integrative medicine practices in the United States found that 38 percent of integrated centers included chiropractic physicians.[6] Integrative rehabilitation programs commonly center on mindfulness meditation, cognitive behavioral training, physical activity, nutrition, sleep hygiene, pain medication management, and physical rehabilitation.

Personal Injury

Personal injury (PI) is an area of specialty that primarily involves treating patients injured in motor vehicle accidents or at work (workers' compensation). It may also include injuries sustained in other ways. This practice specialty benefits from diplomates and certifications in forensics, occupational health, and pain management. These practices often work closely with lawyers and medical doctors; and PI chiropractors may find themselves providing testimony on the patient's behalf in court in support of the significance of an injury (or injuries). Patients may be comanaged with pain clinics since the presenting injuries may cause substantial pain that can be alleviated by pharmaceuticals. Appropriate use of pharmaceuticals can allow chiropractors to perform treatment on a patient who may otherwise be too sensitive to treat with a manual approach. These practices may also provide second-opinion exams or independent medical exams.

The typical patient population for a PI practice includes a mix of patients presenting either with an acute (new) injury or with a chronic (long-term) injury that requires ongoing care. Often the injury resulted from a slip and fall or collision, so strains, sprains, disc bulges, and herniations with potential neurological symptoms are common. The typical treatment approaches will include manual therapy, such as adjustments and soft tissue treatments (massage), and may even include rehabilitation. Some practices work closely with massage therapists and physical therapists so that the chiropractor can focus on one aspect of the treatment. Some of the injuries may be fairly complex and require multiple approaches to gain medical improvement and successfully manage the overall condition.

Often the marketing for a personal injury practice is not geared at patients but at referral sources, such as lawyers and medical doctors. An interesting aspect of these referral sources is that PI practices then see patients who may not otherwise have sought care from a chiropractor. This expands the demographic to include a greater volume of patients in varying socioeconomic levels, from a multitude of cultural backgrounds, and with preexisting conditions. These patients often continue care even after their injury case has been resolved, which ultimately offers PI practices a very diverse population base.

Working with motor vehicle insurance companies, lawyers, and/or workers' compensation benefits to cover the patient's treatments can require a substantial amount of knowledge as to what needs to be documented or written into narrative form and how to submit and track billing statements and payments (claims). Often payments can be delayed until clear fault or injury has been established, or the total amount paid for treatment may be reduced based on settled amounts, which deters some chiropractors from focusing on this patient population. Having a well-trained support staff can alleviate some of the difficulty with this aspect of practice.

Many recent graduates find themselves initially exploring personal injury practices as associates and learning the ropes from experienced doctors. Because these practices often focus on injuries that garner higher frequency of visits in short periods of time (over a few weeks or months), they provide new grads with the opportunity to get their hands on a high volume of patients. There is much to gain from working in this type of environment, since good documentation and appropriate billing practices are crucial to success in this specialty area. Additionally, recent graduates find they can significantly improve their routine treatment skills for musculoskeletal injuries. However, the pace of this practice environment may send some recent graduates into more wellness-focused or family practices, which can provide long-term holistic patient relationships and less intensity.

Radiology

Chiropractors who pursue postgraduate residencies and the diplomate (DACBR) in radiology function as imaging specialists called chiropractic radiologists. Advanced training in radiology and diagnostic imaging encompasses plain films (radiographs), fluoroscopy, computed tomography (CT), magnetic resonance imaging (MRI), and diagnostic ultrasound, as well as other options for advanced imaging. Chiropractic radiology as a practice specialty is typically referral based, providing consultation services at the request of other qualified doctors associated with private practices, hospitals, and teaching institutions. Chiropractic radiologists have expertise in the diagnosis of pathologies and contraindications to manipulative therapy. They are able to provide interpretation of routine radiographic studies as well as consultation for complex imaging procedures. Their training enables them to assist referring physicians in the necessity and appropriateness of radiology services and then in the use of diagnostic findings to support clinical decision making.

This is a competitive specialty because limited slots are available in diagnostic imaging residency programs at chiropractic institutions and not all institutions offer programs. *See Chapter 7 for more details on graduate and diplomate information.* Chiropractic radiologists must gain recertification every five years by performing certain educational activities, such as publishing scientific papers and attending annual symposia, or retaking and passing an ACBR certification examination.

Diagnostic imaging specialists may also have their own chiropractic practice where they treat musculoskeletal injuries and other conditions similar to any other typical chiropractic office. Some chiropractors find that they want to be the authority in their area and incorporate radiographic analysis into their practice, in which case the DACBR is an appealing credential. In rural areas, a chiropractor may be the closest imaging option for the local population. There are also chiropractors who have combined another specialty with diagnostic imaging for an even more unique specialty, such as imaging indications and analysis specific to sports injuries. This specialty and associated credentials also provide opportunities to serve as an adjunct instructor, lecturer, seminar speaker, or administrator for chiropractic institutions and other associations.

Neurology

A chiropractic neurologist uses the musculoskeletal system and the sensory systems as they interact with the neurological system to improve quality of life. They incorporate a variety of treatment modalities, including manipulation as well as other sensory-based modalities to facilitate improvements in health. Reasons patients might seek out a chiropractic neurologist include movement disorders, dystonia, poststroke rehabilitation, and radiculopathy or nerve entrapment. Patients may also seek care from a chiropractic neurologist for chronic pain or recurrent musculoskeletal conditions that may have a neurologic component. Chiropractic neurologist programs provide advanced training to expand on training in chiropractic school, including topics in neuroanatomy, neurology, and neurologic conditions. They may also incorporate nutrition and functional medicine concepts and treatment approaches, so some chiropractors who pursue the diplomate in neurology may further specialize in both neurology and functional medicine.

Multiple groups have organized postgraduate educational curriculums and certifications in chiropractic neurology. The American Chiropractic Association recognizes diplomate training from the American Chiropractic Neurology Board (DACNB); the DACNB is accredited by the National Commission for Certifying Agencies (NCCA); and the International Board of Chiropractic Neurology offers diplomate training.

Orthopedics

Chiropractic orthopedics is a subspecialty of chiropractic that incorporates the nonsurgical evaluation and management of spinal and extremity conditions. Diagnosis and treatment of orthopedic conditions is a standard part of chiropractic-school curriculum, but more in-depth training and networking and mentoring opportunities are provided through the Academy of Chiropractic Orthopedists. Chiropractic orthopedic specialists have completed advanced postdoctoral training in nonsurgical orthopedic, neurologic, and pain evaluation and management, as well as diagnostic imaging and neurodiagnostics. Training concludes with a specialty examination demonstrating proficiency in evaluation and nonoperative management of conditions of the neuromusculoskeletal system. This specialty and certification affords practitioners an evidence-based, patient-centered integrative medicine model that prepares them to work in community health center settings and gain additional authority with orthopedic presentations and management.

The Academy of Chiropractic Orthopedists provides organization and education for chiropractors interested in advanced orthopedic training. Practitioners with diplomate certification who are in good standing with the academy are titled Fellows of the Academy of Chiropractic Orthopedists (FACO). To maintain clinical competency, the academy maintains recertification on a three-year cycle. In addition, the academy publishes the peer-reviewed and indexed *Journal of the Academy of Chiropractic Orthopedists* (*JACO*).

Nutrition

Though chiropractic programs have coursework in nutrition, advanced courses and expanded practice options in nutrition and functional medicine are a great way to offer patients added holistic services that complement chiropractic care. Since a patient's diet provides the building blocks for healing and repair of the tissues in their musculoskeletal system, improved nutrition can have a positive impact on patient outcomes. Though it is easy to provide a few quick diet recommendations to patients as they are receiving chiropractic adjustments or adjunctive therapies, some chiropractors incorporate more in-depth analysis and recommendations to their patients. Even if nutrition was not a strong interest as a student, many doctors find themselves learning more while in practice because patients ask questions or because supplement companies offer free trainings and samples.

As with many other specialties, advanced training in nutrition can start as early as chiropractic college. Quite a few chiropractic institutions offer advanced nutrition electives or master's degrees in nutrition. Additionally, nutrition is a common continuing education topic offered at chiropractic schools and state association conferences and through supplement companies. Nutrition courses and webinars are readily available on the Internet, with some being more recognized than others. Due to many fad diets, publicity in the media, and food and supplement company claims, nutrition is one area where it is of utmost importance to use the research and information literacy skills gained from chiropractic programs and select training and information sources that are highly reputable and supported by research.

Advanced training in nutrition at the postgraduate level often covers reviews of biochemical pathways and mediators; symptom surveys and nutrition-related outcomes assessments; in-depth review of systems and history taking; review or addition of specific laboratory tests, including blood, saliva, and stool testing, genetic testing, and immune reactivity and allergy testing; diet protocols, such as elimination diets, gut repair protocols, and detoxes; and a wide variety of supplement protocols and the mechanisms of action for the ingredients. Also important is covering drug-induced nutrient depletion and nutrient-herb-drug interactions.

There are a number of professional organizations related to nutrition that a chiropractor can get involved with for networking and educational opportunities. Nutrition is one of the recognized specialties of the American Chiropractic Association, which has a Nutrition Council. Additionally, the American Public Health Association has a Food and Nutrition Section. There are also several national organizations, including the National Association of Nutrition Professionals, the American Nutrition Association, and the American Society for Nutrition, which offers the monthly journal *The Journal of Clinical Nutrition*. Professional memberships and affiliations in nutrition can also be beneficial in building other business opportunities and expertise, such as guest lecturing, workshops, webinars, and other speaking engagements.

Though many certifications in nutrition and wellness topics can be gained from postgraduate seminars from a variety of sources, there are a few that are recognized more broadly. As mentioned in Chapter 7, graduate work in nutrition fulfills the educational requirements to sit for the national certification exams to be credentialed as a certified nutrition specialist (CNS) or a certified clinical nutritionist (CCN) through the Clinical Nutrition Certification Board (CNCB). There is also a certification through the International Society of Sports Nutrition (ISSN) for a credential as a certified sports nutritionist (CISSN). Lastly, there are two diplomate options, including the diplomate of the American Clinical Board of Nutrition (DACBN) and the diplomate of Chiropractic Board of Clinical Nutrition (DCBCN). The American Clinical Board of Nutrition offers the diplomate to all health care professionals whereas the Chiropractic Board of Clinical Nutrition diplomate is specific to chiropractors.

Chiropractors offering nutritional counseling or nutrition recommendations without these additional credentials do not typically satisfy the requirements to bill insurance providers for nutritional counseling. Even with nutritionist credentials, insurance providers may only authorize payment for nutritional counseling for specific nutrition-related disorders, like diabetes, or insurance companies may only allow registered dieticians to provide nutritional counseling. Both the provider and the patient should review the patient's insurance coverage to determine if coverage exists. However, because of the rapport that chiropractors build with their patients and the level and type of care they offer, many patients opt to pay for nutritional counseling out of their own pockets and do not worry about insurance coverage.

When providing nutritional recommendations, chiropractors must be clear that they are not diagnosing, treating, or curing organic diseases outside the scope of practice in their state, or outside the legal claims that can be made by supplement companies. Most chiropractors avoid this by carefully documenting the patient's signs and symptoms and offering recommendations for symptoms, such as white spots on nails, which can indicate a zinc deficiency, or bumps on the arms, which may be indicative of a fatty acid deficiency. For those who offer nutritional counseling in their practice, regular research and continuing education supplies emerging data on nutritional interventions, minimizing adverse effects, inappropriate advice, and outdated recommendations. It is also important to carefully check the scope of practice for each state where the chiropractor is licensed to determine to what degree nutritional advice is within scope.

Nutritional counseling helps patients who are overwhelmed with food choices, who recognize they are making poor food choices, who have a recent diagnosis or chronic disease that would benefit from nutritional interventions, or who may just want to improve their overall quality of life or lose weight. Patients may have restricted diets either by choice or due to a health condition or want guidance in selecting foods that will help them achieve their health and wellness goals. Patients may be at a particular stage in life, like pregnancy, or have a milestone or event that is motivating them to get in shape and manage their weight. Though a typical chiropractor has enough education to offer recommendations, advanced training in nutrition helps provide long-term treatment strategies for these patients.

Chiropractors who want to use a nutrition specialty to expand their career options may find job opportunities in industry or the private sector, including nutrition and health communication, consulting, corporate wellness programs, nutrition-related business ventures, research, public health, school systems, health clubs, nursing homes, and food companies, depending on educational background, credentials, and professional experience. Graduate degrees in nutrition also open doors to teach courses in nutrition and biology in higher education.

Functional Medicine

Functional medicine is a specialty that incorporates nutrition as well as lifestyle recommendations and strategies to improve the health and well-being of patients. Many chiropractors who have a nutrition focus also incorporate functional medicine training and approaches in their practice. Though at times the difference between nutrition and functional medicine may seem to be semantic, functional medicine practitioners often have more in-depth evaluation and patient-intake procedures with a more intense treatment protocol. They look for root causes of disease and dysfunction through a variety of assessment methods, which can include extensive patient history, environmental exposure, diet throughout the life of the patient starting from childbirth, family history, medication and supplement history, symptoms surveys and systems reviews, and laboratory testing. They may incorporate physical examinations that look at indicators for nutrient deficiencies, assess a multitude of biometric and health parameters, and establish a baseline for overall system function.

In addition to nutrition, some practitioners find other avenues into functional medicine through specialties like neurology, internal disorders, primary care, pediatrics, sports chiropractic, or Oriental medicine. All types of health care providers may specialize in functional medicine, ranging from medical doctors to acupuncturists to nutritionists and naturopaths. Some may pursue training through a master's degree in nutrition offered by one of the chiropractic institutions mentioned in Chapter 7. Additionally, continuing education opportunities are offered through webinars, weekend seminars, conferences, certification programs, supplement companies, and laboratory companies. Certifications are not necessarily broadly recognized, but one of the most well known is through the Institute for Functional Medicine (IFM). The IFM has speakers who are featured at the national level on lecture circuits for conferences and also on news and popular media.

Functional medicine practitioners do not typically bill insurance for their services because this type of care may actually be considered more of a luxury. Patients who seek the care of functional medicine practitioners often expect to pay out of pocket and want more from their doctor than what is offered under their insurance benefits. Some of the examination and treatment procedures may also be considered experimental or not well-established and proven treatment methods, which can be another reason insurance companies will not provide coverage. Because patients are seeking a higher level of care and often paying more for services, they expect more attention and explanation from a functional medicine practitioner than other mainstream providers. Patients also pay out of pocket for the special tests, supplements, and dietary items that are recommended by their functional medicine provider.

Additional training in functional medicine does not expand scope of practice. Chiropractors who specialize in functional medicine must be very careful how they offer treatment recommendations and manage patients on medications. The natural approaches they use with patients may decrease the need for prescription management of chronic conditions, but chiropractors cannot manage a patient's prescription medication so the patient must be referred back to the prescribing physician. For this reason, some chiropractors either comanage patients with a holistic medical doctor or obtain additional degrees to practice as a nurse practitioner or medical doctor.

Functional medicine practitioners may provide conservative holistic care for all types of chronic conditions, but some opt to specialize further by focusing on one type or group of conditions. A functional medicine practitioner may only treat patients in one of the following subspecialty areas: hormone or thyroid disorders (diabetes, Hashimoto's, Grave's), autoimmunity (including multiple sclerosis, rheumatoid arthritis, etc.), or gut disorders like irritable bowel syndrome, small intestine bacterial overgrowth, Crohn's, and ulcerative colitis, among others. Some practitioners may focus on a special population like pediatrics cases or women's health and infertility. Chiropractors who become functional medicine specialists may even no longer manually adjust their patients and primarily provide care only through diet, supplement, and lifestyle management recommendations.

Diagnosis and Internal Disorders

Another specialty recognized by the American Chiropractic Association with its own council and diplomate is called "Diagnosis and Internal Disorders." This specialty may use nutrition and functional medicine approaches but also provides primary care to a broader patient base. Doctors practicing in this specialty often employ a broader variety of evaluation procedures, such as electrocardiograms, vascular Doppler ultrasound, spirometry, DEXA bone density testing, and other diagnostic tools. Treatment approaches include diet and supplement recommendations, botanical medicine, homeopathics, manipulation, soft tissue work, and other conservative treatment approaches. Training in diagnosis and internal disorders for the diplomate involves a 300-hour postdoctoral course along with passing a certification test and maintaining at least 12 hours of continuing education in related coursework each year. The American Board of Chiropractic Internists (ABCI) is the certifying body for the diplomate (DABCI).

This type of specialty does not expand scope of practice, and depending on the state, there may be limitations on the breadth of diagnostic and treatment services that a chiropractor with advanced training in diagnosis and internal disorders may offer. The practice population encompasses patients who want holistic and natural management of a variety of conditions or maintenance of a healthy lifestyle. These types of patients may also consider or use other complementary and alternative medicine (CAM) providers, such as naturopaths, acupuncturists, and functional medicine practitioners. A specialist in diagnosis and internal disorders may opt to no longer provide chiropractic manual procedures and instead cotreat with other chiropractors.

Primary Care

Though all chiropractic programs prepare graduates to function as portal-of-entry providers, many chiropractors focus the majority of their practice on musculoskeletal conditions and refer patients for comanagement with other health care providers for other conditions or for annual health screenings. However, chiropractors have the ability to diagnose and manage a variety of nonmusculoskeletal presentations, depending on the scope of practice in their state and patient base. In some states, chiropractors can perform blood draws and other types of laboratory procedures in their office. The patient population is similar to those who seek care from a DABCI, but depending on the practice setting may include a broader patient base if the provider is functioning as the primary care facility for a rural town. In a more urban setting, it may depend on the region and city culture, local market, and expertise of the provider whether he or she caters to a niche population or maintains a broad patient base. For patients who do not want prescriptions or more invasive treatment, chiropractors are uniquely poised to offer holistic family care with a conservative approach.

In order to specialize in primary care and family practice, the DABCI is one option for additional training and certification. Other postdoctoral training options include continuing education seminars offered through a variety of institutions, such as naturopathic and medical universities and integrative medicine conferences. Chiropractors may also decide to pursue additional degrees and credentials related to the practice of medicine, including an MD, DO, NP, or ND. Another avenue to this specialty may be advanced training in Oriental medicine.

Special Populations (Pediatrics, Women's Health, Geriatrics)

Chiropractors learn the fundamentals in managing special patient populations, such as pediatrics and geriatrics, during their chiropractic training. Additionally, chiropractic students are exposed to lab procedures for gynecology and proctology and have a good understanding of the components of women's health, such as normal and abnormal hormone and reproductive system function. Chiropractors can handle the more common presentations of conditions for these populations and know when to refer for more advanced or specialty care. However, some chiropractors may decide to specialize in one of these areas through postdoctoral training, typically diplomate programs and/or associateships.

Pediatrics is a specialty with diplomate certification for chiropractors offered either by the International Chiropractic Association Council on Chiropractic Pediatrics (ICACCP) or the International Chiropractic Pediatric Association (ICPA). These programs provide in-depth training in the holistic evaluation and care of children and women before, during, and after pregnancy. The curriculum covers diagnostic and assessment procedures as well as manual treatment skills for different stages of development and a variety of conditions. Modules include radiology, nutrition, functional medicine and immunology, sports injuries, orthopedics, neurology, and special needs. Some chiropractors may obtain the diplomate training to support a family practice model.

Pediatric chiropractors commonly manage asthma, birth trauma, colic, constipation, ear infections, head or chest colds, and upper respiratory infections as well as neck, back, and extremity pain.[7] They typically incorporate more technique styles beyond diversified, including instrument-assisted adjusting, other low-force manual techniques, and craniosacral work as well as the use of specialized tables made for pediatric patients who may have a unique shape, size, or function.

Women's health is a specialty area that may incorporate fertility, hormone balance, stress reduction, gynecology, pregnancy, nutrition, and weight management. Chiropractors who want to specialize in women's health may seek postdoctoral training through women's health seminars and conferences, integrative and functional medicine seminars, supplement companies, and institutions. Additionally, diplomates in pediatrics, diagnosis and internal disorders, and nutrition are also complementary certifications. Women's health specialists may also include or further focus on female athletes. Not every state will allow chiropractors to perform gynecological exams or other adjunctive assessment procedures, but those services can easily be comanaged and provided by other local providers.

With the baby boomer population advancing in age and increasing average human lifespan, *geriatrics* is a growing specialty that provides care directed at the elderly population, or those over 60–65 years of age. Musculoskeletal conditions, particularly back pain, still play a large role in this specialty, but the treatment approaches start to vary since bone fragility and decreased flexibility may make it more difficult to use certain manual adjustment approaches. Additionally, prescription medication side effects, lack of physical activity, balance issues, and a lifetime of accumulated macro and micro-trauma make the evaluation of a geriatric patient potentially more challenging. Training in geriatrics can come from technique seminars (particularly low-force techniques, such as instrument adjusting, flexion distraction, and drop table), and postdoctoral courses or certifications in orthopedics, rehabilitation, and neurology. Chiropractors are well equipped to manage a broad array of typical and even atypical neuromusculoskeletal complaints of the geriatric population, in addition to offering guidance in fall prevention and improving overall function.[8] They may gain expertise over their professional career, or they may join a practice that already specializes in or has a large geriatric patient base or practice in an area known for having a large population of retirees, as many Southern states in the United States, including Florida, Arizona, and Arkansas.

Military Medicine

Chiropractors interested in serving active duty soldiers or military veterans can seek federal employment with the Department of Defense (DoD) or the Veterans Health Administration (VHA). Openings for positions with the DoD and VHA are posted on usajobs.gov and are extremely competitive. In addition to clinical competencies, an evidence-based approach, and a background in academics, research and publishing can better position doctors for these positions.

Chiropractic physicians have been integrated into the military health care system since 1995 and into the Department of Veterans Affairs since 2004. Chiropractic care is now available at 65 military treatment facilities and at 51 Veterans Affairs facilities.[9,10] Presently, training opportunities in military medicine include a competitive one-year VA residency and clinical externships within the VHA and DoD at sites across the United States.

Within military and veterans' facilities, chiropractic care is treated as a specialty, and care requires direct referral from a primary care physician or another health care provider. While back and neck pain comprise the bulk of VHA chiropractic consultations, practitioners in these systems must be prepared to manage complex patients with lots of comorbidities, posttraumatic stress disorder, amputees, and victims of traumatic brain injuries related to improvised explosive device blasts.[11] Patient satisfaction with chiropractic care is high, and preliminary findings show that chiropractic management of common conditions shows significant improvement.[12]

Manipulation Under Anesthesia

Manipulation under anesthesia (MUA) of the spine and surrounding soft tissues has been proposed to disrupt or stretch adhesions and allow for restored joint mechanics. It is theorized that adding anesthesia to manipulative procedures eliminates pain-inhibiting reflexes and allows for relaxation of muscles, thus increasing treatment efficacy.[13] The application of MUA is generally reserved for patients who have received conservative care for six to eight weeks without substantial improvement and without contraindications to mobilization/manipulation or the use of anesthetics. The generally accepted phases of MUA treatment are (1) sedation, (2) manipulative procedures, (3) additional stretching/traction procedures, and (4) follow-up in-office care without sedation. There is no established standardization of MUA or follow-up care.

To determine procedure candidacy, the MUA physician typically evaluates the patient. Ideal patients present with segmental joint and/or global motion restrictions thought to be the result of fibrosis and have failed conservative therapy, such as in-office manipulation. When appropriate, the patient is then examined by the anesthesiologist to determine suitability of anesthesia care. From a chiropractic standpoint, MUA carries the same risk as traditional manipulation; therefore, additional specialized tests are not required, except as necessary for diagnosis. Candidates for MUA include:

- intractable nonsurgical joint pain, muscle spasms, decreased range of motion
- nonsurgical nerve entrapment syndrome
- disc protrusions/extrusions
- failed back surgery syndrome
- chronic cervicogenic headaches
- complex regional pain syndrome
- postsurgical adhesions
- adhesive capsulitis

Patients with osteoporosis or bone-softening diseases, acute fracture/dislocation, malignancy, heart disease, uncontrolled diabetes, and any contraindication to anesthesia would not be candidates for MUA.

Anesthesia is provided under the direct supervision of a board-certified anesthesiologist or appropriately licensed and certified physician. The anesthesiologist selects the anesthesia based on the patient's medical condition and is responsible for all medical decisions. The chiropractic physician does not administer any medications or make any anesthesia-related decisions. The involvement of a doctor of chiropractic in MUA is limited to local state scope of practice. A certified MUA physician must carry the appropriate malpractice insurance to perform MUA.[14]

Occupational Health and Ergonomics

Chiropractors interested in applying biomechanical, ergonomic, and chiropractic principles to avoidance of workplace injuries and improving productivity and quality of life for workers may want to specialize in occupational health. There are many businesses that would benefit from chiropractic services related to occupational health, including trucking and vehicle operators, manufacturing and warehouses, material handlers, nursing homes and health care facilities, and other businesses that involve prolonged sitting or repetitive motions.

There are growing opportunities for chiropractors to work with businesses to provide an array of services supporting workplace safety and employee health promotion. Chiropractors often provide care to injured workers, but they can also positively impact associated absenteeism, lost time from work, and future injury prevention. Postdoctoral training equips chiropractors with skills to communicate, interact, and strategize with employers for accident and injury prevention, ergonomics, and identification of work-injury problems related to back pain and other musculoskeletal conditions. Chiropractors may gain proficiency in offering supportive services, such as substance-use testing, preplacement examinations, certified medical examiner physical examinations, "return to work," independent medical examinations, employee education, and wellness services. These services are highly marketable because they ultimately support the company's bottom line.

For this particular specialty, it is beneficial to engage in postdoctoral training and gain certifications in order to increase credibility, service delivery, and competitiveness with other professionals in the industry. Diplomate training is offered through Northwestern University of Health Sciences and the American Chiropractic Board on Occupational Health in occupational health and applied ergonomics, resulting in the credential of diplomate of the American Chiropractic Board of Occupational Health (DACBOH). Other advantageous certifications include the certified health education specialist (CHES) through the National Commission for Health Education and the certified wellness practitioner (CWP) through the National Wellness Institute. Chiropractors with this specialty may do independent consulting part time or full time and may also find full-time career opportunities with large corporations.

Forensics

Chiropractic forensic specialists have training in the application of medical and scientific facts to legal issues, most commonly related to injury and disability cases. They serve as expert witnesses to courts and medical facilities and provide independent medical exams for insurance companies. They have organized, systematic approaches to conducting analyses, investigations, inquiries, tests, inspections, and examinations for gaining facts to make expert opinions that are objective, logical, unbiased, and understandable by the requesting agency.

Forensic chiropractors have training in disability determination systems and programs, impairment rating systems, independent medical examinations, functional capacity and physical assessment systems, return-to-work and fitness-for-duty assessment (such as those for the Department of Transportation), fraud and abuse investigation, maximum medical improvement determination, and causation. This training affords chiropractors the focused awareness of injury and disability evaluation, data and records analysis, written reporting skills, and expertise to testify on forensic conclusions. Forensic professionals do not provide treatment as part of these evaluation and consulting services.

The Council on Forensic Sciences (CFS) of the American Chiropractic Association provides education, advocacy, and networking opportunities for chiropractors interested in learning more about medicolegal issues. Diplomate certification as a forensic examiner (DABFP) is offered through the American Board of Forensic Professionals. They also provide national certification in impairment rating based on the AMA Guides to Impairment. A related credential is the certified medical examiner (CME) for the Department of Transportation, which is required to be listed in the National Registry of Certified Medical Examiners (National Registry) by the Federal Motor Carrier Safety Administration (FMCSA). Another useful certification may be the certified independent chiropractic examiner (CICE[SM]) offered through the American Board of Independent Medical Examiners (ABIME). Chiropractors can still provide many of these examination and consulting services without additional credentials, but for providing expert testimony, it is very beneficial to gain the additional knowledge and authority that comes with the diplomate or related certifications.

Animal Chiropractic

Chiropractors who love animals may pursue additional training in anatomy, physiology, and assessment and treatment approaches for household pets or farm and competition animals, such as horses. Animal chiropractic, or veterinary chiropractic, training includes manual adjusting, instrument-assisted adjusting and adjunctive therapies such as light therapy, myofascial work, botanical and homeopathic therapies, and nutritional advice. Conditions treated by chiropractors or veterinarians with expertise in animal chiropractic include neck, back, leg, and tail pain and injuries such as disc and joint problems; muscle and nervous system conditions, including seizures; and organic symptoms, such as vomiting, respiratory or urinary infections, diarrhea, or constipation.

Parker University is the only chiropractic institution offering training in animal chiropractic, but other programs exist in the United States. Parker's program focuses on the equine and the canine but also covers cats, birds, cows, pigs, and other small house pets. The instructors review the vertebral structure for a variety of species and the unique consider-ations in the treatment of animals, such as restraint. The program includes hands-on live animal experience. Certification is offered from the Animal Chiropractic Certification Commission (ACCC) of the American Veteri-nary Chiropractic Association (AVCA). Both veterinarians and chiroprac-tors may seek certification, which is valid for three years and requires 30 hours of approved continuing education every three years to maintain certification.

Chiropractors who gain certification to treat animals may still have a traditional practice and offer services with animals on the side through local veterinarians. This may be out of scope for a chiropractor depending on the state—it may be that only veterinarians can provide chiropractic treatment to animals. Before pursuing training or performing treatment on animals, chiropractors should check their state's chiropractic-related laws and regulations and should contact the state board if it is unclear whether it is within their scope to treat animals.

Nonclinical Career Specialties

For chiropractors who want to use their education as a stepping-stone to other private and public sectors, obtaining training, certifications, and graduate degrees can be beneficial in bridging their knowledge, doctoral training, and experience with the appropriate background to pursue other professional opportunities. There are a variety of reasons why chi-ropractors may not practice clinically, including injuries, expanding interests, or prior professional experience. Chiropractors may find them-selves experts because of their practice experience in billing and coding, practice management, human resource management, and employee train-ing, particularly for chiropractic assistants. They may find opportunities as claims adjusters or working in the health care insurance industry as medical advisers. The electronic health records or electronic medical records industry is ripe with opportunity in medical informatics, research, training, and consulting on design and implementation. Often these other career pathways require some additional training, beneficial credentials, or industry contacts for a smooth transition from clinical practice into another career.

Chiropractors who have successfully built their own practices may find a niche in marketing, communications, and practice management consulting, helping other practices become just as successful. Some chiropractors no longer practice themselves but oversee chains of chiropractic practices or create franchises. Business degrees or advanced training provide added authority, knowledge, and principles for this type of career path.

Chiropractors who have gotten very involved in their local communities or with local or national advocacy groups for chiropractic may find careers in politics at a local, state, or national level. Additionally, service-oriented and policy-minded individuals may be drawn to public health or public policy, eventually obtaining training or degrees such as a master's in public health (MPH), professional doctorate in public health (DrPH), or doctoral degrees in community health, health promotion, and public health (PhD). Lastly, as covered in more depth in other chapters, careers in education and research are options both within and outside of chiropractic that can be alternatives to or in addition to a clinical practice.

References

1. Christensen M, Hyland J, Goertz C, Kollasch M. *Practice Analysis of Chiropractic*, 2015. Greeley, CO: National Board of Chiropractic Examiners; 2015.

2. Coulter ID, Shekelle PG: Chiropractic in North America: a descriptive analysis. *J Manipulative Physiol Ther.* 2005;28(2):83–89.

3. Clijsters M, Fronzoni F, Jenkens H. Chiropractic treatment approaches for spinal musculoskeletal conditions: a cross-sectional survey. *Chiropr Man Therap.* 2014;22:33.

4. Koo TK, Cohen JH, Zheng Y. Immediate effect of Nimmo receptor tonus technique on muscle elasticity, pain perception, and disability in subjects with chronic low back pain. *J Manipulative Physiol Ther.* 2012;35(1):45–53.

5. Emary P. Use of post-isometric relaxation in the chiropractic management of a 55-year-old man with cervical radiculopathy. *J Can Chiropr Assoc.* 2012;56(1):9–17.

6. Horrigan B, Lewis S, Abrams D, Pechura C. *Integrative Medicine in America: How Integrative Medicine Is Being Practiced in Clinical Centers across the United States.* Minneapolis, MN: The Bravewell Collaborative; 2012.

7. Pohlman KA, Hondras MA, Long CR, Haan AG. Practice patterns of doctors of chiropractic with a pediatric diplomate: a cross-sectional survey. *BMC Complement Altern Med.* 2010;10:26.

8. Dougherty PE, Hawk C, Weiner DK, Gleberzon B, Andrew K, Killinger L. The role of chiropractic care in older adults. *Chiropr Man Ther.* 2012;20:3.

9. Department of Veterans Affairs. Department of Veterans Affairs Health Care Programs Enhancement Act of 2001, Pub. L. 107-135. http://www.gpo.gov /fdsys/pkg/PLAW-107publ135/pdf/PLAW-106publ117/html/PLAW-106publ117 .htm. Accessed November 27, 2015.

10. Lisi AJ, Khorsan R, Smith MM, Mittman BS. Variations in the implementation and characteristics of chiropractic services in VA. *Med Care.* 2014;52(12 suppl 5):S97–S104.

11. Lisi AJ, Goertz C, Lawrence DJ, Satyanarayana P. Characteristics of Veterans Health Administration chiropractors and chiropractic clinics. *J Rehabil Res Dev.* 2009;46:997–1002.

12. Green BN, Johnson CD, Daniels CJ, Napuli JG, Gliedt JA, Paris DJ. Integration of chiropractic services in military and veteran health care facilities: a systematic review of the literature. *J Evid Based Complementary Altern Med.* 2015 [epub ahead of print].

13. Digiorgi D. Spinal manipulation under anesthesia: a narrative review of the literature and commentary. *Chiropr Man Therap.* 2013;21(1):14.

14. Gordon R, Cremata E, Hawk C. Guidelines for the practice and performance of manipulation under anesthesia. *Chiropr Man Therap.* 2014;22:7.

CHAPTER ELEVEN

Academic Careers in Chiropractic

Phillip Ebrall, BAppSci(Chiropractic), PhD

"I think teaching is one of the highest callings and a great privilege."[1]

A successful teacher within a chiropractic program is one who, apart from knowing the content, knows how to deliver it and understands students and how they learn. This means there are two core dimensions: a specialized knowledge of a field that must be taught and a specialized knowledge about how to effectively achieve learning outcomes.

The result is a gulf unappreciated by most field practitioners but embraced by those who have chosen to follow the academic pathway. The gulf is straightforward: the four to seven years spent earning one's qualification to allow registration and associated entitlement as a doctor of chiropractic does nothing to confer any right to stand in a learning space and teach chiropractic. This gulf is not ameliorated by years of practice nor by a desire to earn external income while building one's own practice, nor least of all by an altruistic desire to give something back as one enters the eve of retirement from practice.

There are occasions where any of the above may fit with certain activities of an institution, and these are explored below. However, the key point is that in a way similar to a professional chiropractic qualification being two degrees (typically a bachelor's plus a DC in the United States, or a double bachelor's in some countries, or a bachelor's/master's in others), to become a chiropractic academic requires additional qualification in learning and teaching, ranging from a graduate certificate through to an MEd or a doctorate (PhD or EdD).

Licensed chiropractors without such formal qualification in education may be considered for the role of tutor, a member of the academic team who reinforces the core learning presented by the qualified academic in accord with the approved curriculum. They may also be considered for appointment as clinical educators, if they have five to seven years of equivalent full-time practice, and to act as clinicians to supervise patient care in an institution's outpatient clinics.

A Very Brief Historical Overview

D. D. Palmer determined to teach his newly developing art and science two years after he gave the first chiropractic adjustment.[1] This was about 1897, and the school followed two years later, opening in 1899.[1] It is reasonable to see this as the commencement of opportunities for one to become a chiropractic academic, albeit still within that which historian Gibbons considers the Tutorial Period (1897–1905)[2] of the chiropractic educational establishment. The majority of the first chiropractic academics were graduates of Palmer's School of Magnetic Cure (incorporated under the laws of the state of Iowa), which by 1903 had become known as the Chiropractic School and Cure and offered diplomas.[1]

The next serious institution to commence teaching chiropractic was the National College of Chiropractic in Chicago, which began late in 1906 in Davenport, Iowa, before relocating to Chicago in 1908. It was founded by John Howard. The National College of Chiropractic evolved into the National University of Health Sciences and now offers a chiropractic degree program alongside a doctor of naturopathic medicine in the College of Professional Studies in suburban Chicago and also through a relationship in Florida. Palmer University delivers from three campuses and keeps a passionate commitment to the chiropractic paradigm.

Over the ensuing years, a number of new colleges were formed and a need started to develop for competent chiropractic academics. Canada was the second country to create opportunities, and while its earliest attempts were poorly organized, a stronger sense of structure and direction was instituted in 1945 with the establishment of the Canadian Memorial Chiropractic College.[3] This institution was the first to introduce what became the standardized curriculum, designed by John Nugent in 1942.

In broad terms, Canada was followed by England in 1965 and Australia in 1975. Before Australia commenced program delivery with a government-funded institution in 1975, it had provided a number of short programs in multidisciplinary environments (usually osteopathy and naturopathy and, in at least one case, the same program leading to awards in both chiropractic and osteopathy) for a number of years beforehand, largely in the southeastern states. These smaller establishments were absorbed either into Phillip Institute or the Sydney College of Chiropractic.[4] The Sydney College of Chiropractic became Macquarie University, and the program at Phillip Institute became Royal Melbourne Institute of Technology (RMIT) University. They were the first two chiropractic programs in the world to achieve full standing in a government university system.

The first chiropractic program in 1906 in the United States was about nine months in duration and the educators were mainly graduates. This is not a negative observation, as it reflected health professional education at that time. It was around 1910 that Flexner made radical changes to the manner in which medical education was delivered. He did not do so as a medical physician but as a secondary school teacher and principal.[5] It was not until the year 2000 that "A Systematic Review of Faculty Development Initiatives Designed to Improve Teaching Effectiveness in Medical Education" was published[6] and a little later that an academy of medical educators was established.[7] Structured activities to improve global medical academics continue.[8]

Historians have a predilection for categorizing activities as "periods,"[2,9] and it may well be an effective approach to help understand the development of global events. However, chiropractic education, and hence chiropractic academia, was sporadic in its commencement across various countries, and each took different approaches. It is not possible to uniformly apply a "one size fits all" classification by period.

Each country had its own groups of academics who felt their way was superior to others' and formed their own institutions, not always exclusively chiropractic but including such offshoots as spondylotherapy.[10] Chapman-Smith and Cleveland III point out the complexities of the international chiropractic environment.[11] Chiropractic academics are now served by an international, peer-reviewed journal (*Journal of Manipulative and Physiological Therapeutics*) that came into existence in the mid-1980s, dedicated to publishing research and scholarly articles pertaining to education theory, pedagogy, methodologies, practice, and other content relevant to chiropractic's academe.

Japan, which has recognized practicing chiropractors since 1916, commenced a formal educational program, now accredited, in 1995. Today there are some 47 chiropractic educational programs worldwide and most are university based or affiliated. The vast majority are fully accredited by one of the Councils on Chiropractic Education, which each serve various regions of the world; others are in development/establishment mode.

A critical component of institutional and programmatic assessment is evaluation of the variety and quality of the chiropractic academics. External accreditors look for source diversity to avoid an institution's perpetuation of its own views. This ensures a variant of being "fit for purpose" to ensure academics are teaching within areas of their competence and overall qualification without an institution becoming incestuous. The predominant academic paradigm of chiropractic programs is that put forward by Gatterman, the patient-centered paradigm.[12]

Terminology

Chiropractic academics work with two very different sets of terminology. The first has to do with their activity and the second, their environment.

Enlightened educational institutions have moved beyond "teaching" and speak of "learning." The difference is that the act of teaching developed several hundred years ago and is variously referred to as "the sage on the stage" or "talking head" or by some other pejorative term. The act of teaching implies a transfer of knowledge as opposed to fostering learning and understanding.

The contemporary view is more one of reaching a shared understanding, demonstrated at early levels of study as competency, then rising to capability during the clinical learning years, and attaining professional knowledge at the time of graduation. Biggs, a noted educator, expresses this through a knowledge hierarchy.[13] In this hierarchy, declarative knowledge (being able to describe factual matters) and procedural knowledge (being able to know what to do) form the foundation. Functioning knowledge (knowing "why" and "how") and conditional knowledge (knowing when to act) then lead to professional knowledge, the top level.

Current trends in education indicate that the term "learner" is preferred to "student." A related trend is to see academics as "learners" as well. "Teachers" would then more appropriately be called "learning leaders." The reasons for a chiropractic academic to be considered a learner are given a little later in this chapter.

The contemporary chiropractic classroom consists of small groups participating in shared discovery and learning with the support of a learning leader. Any institution in the 21st century that continues to pretend it can deliver a "class" as a 50-minute lecture to a flat floor or tiered theater is kidding itself. The main driver of change from this significantly outdated approach to learning relates to the millennial students, considered as "Gen Wi-Fi" learners, now commencing their chiropractic education. The change away from "50-minute blocks of boredom" is facilitated by an educational process called "chunking" (see below) and e-delivery.

The above terminology is universal. However, the second set of terminology, that relevant to academic progression as opposed to content, is country specific. As an overview, there are two general systems, the Germanic/British and that of the United States.

One form equates titles such as "professor" with proven attainment in a specific academic field. This is the same system adopted in Australia and most other British-derived cultures, which means a person with the title "professor of chiropractic" has met extensive and detailed criteria, reviewed by peer panels and the university's academic board, before being accorded the title. The key point to note is the earned title is accompanied by a named rank.

On the other hand, the American system is seen as being opposite in that advancement by rank carries a title. There are times a certain position of academic rank, perhaps as simple as being tenured, may be termed "professor." On the other hand, criteria may be used that are similar to those in the British/Germanic system, which is very long established from as far back as the Heidelberg University in 1386.

What this means is that in countries following the British/Germanic system, a lecturer is a lecturer as specifically appointed to that position on the basis of qualifications. Within the United States, a tenured lecturer may be called a "professor" by his or her students, whether or not the academic has the qualifications that would support professorial appointment under another system.

The Australian government structural system for academics, a scheme to which all tertiary institutions in that country subscribe, presents five levels of academic appointment based on what is termed "academic merit." This essentially means the intellectual, academic, and behavioral characteristics define where one fits on this ranking scale. The Australian system parallels those used in other countries that have a common source for their educational system titles and may also be loosely equated to the typical U.S. structure. Within the structure below, sessional, fractional, part-time, or casual appointments are acceptable for levels A and B, but from Level C one is reasonably expected to be committed to the academic career path within a full-time contract or tenured appointment.

Level A—Tutor/associate lecturer (most junior); in the United States, this is instructor.

Level B—Lecturer; in the United States, there is no equivalent of this level.

Level C—Senior lecturer; in the United States, this is assistant professor.

Level D—Reader/associate professor; in the United States, this is also associate professor.

Level E—Professor (most senior); in the United States, this is also professor.

Beyond this, an academic enters the "executive ranks" of the university where terms start with dean then, generally, pro-vice-chancellor (PVC), deputy-vice-chancellor (DVC), and then vice-chancellor (VC). An interchangeable term for a PVC or DVC is "provost." U.S. colleges usually run only with "dean" but may add a provost to provide a buffer between the president and the student body.

At the senior level, the VC is essentially the chief operating officer, answerable to a board of directors known as a council, a group created to facilitate close engagement with the broad communities in which the university operates. Colleges in the United States have lower levels of government funding and a greater reliance on private donors, tuition fees, and unique fund-raising events, so must rely heavily on their president as CEO to represent and promote the institution externally.

Both senior leadership roles require internal academic management to be in the office of the dean of academic affairs in the United States or the office of the DVC (learning and teaching, or academic) in Australia. European and other structures may not be quite as clear.

The above observations show the sheer complexity of operating a successful chiropractic educational institution. In reality, while chiropractic academics may represent a relatively small group, one institution represents a coalition of very complex businesses, engaging ground staff, cooks, librarians, security, and many, many more.

The one thing chiropractic academics must know is that their performance can only be as good as those who work together let it be. This is another imperative for chiropractic academics to sublimate their ego and concentrate as hard as possible on the prime task of creating new chiropractors.

While it is expected that a noted chiropractic educator will rise to become academic dean in a U.S. college, such pathways are not as likely in other countries. It is not common for a chiropractic academic to proceed beyond being an expert in his or her discipline field, with the positions of dean, PVC, or DVC currently essentially unobtainable. The reasons may vary but often begin with the fact that a chiropractic program in a true multidiscipline tertiary institution is a comparatively small program, and to start on a management track that could lead to a dean or PVC role, one needs to serve with merit in lower-level management roles, such as associate dean. Chiropractors generally seem to lack the background and education to earn such positions.

Academic Enhancement Activities

Once the academic ranking system is understood as it applies to any particular institution, the potential chiropractic academic must then determine both an entry point and a stream of academic activity.

The initial decision is to make the time to review the options, which are binary, either a part-time (or sessional) or a full-time appointment. This decision requires one to understand one's strengths and desired future direction. If the prime choice is to maintain practice and contribute as a chiropractic academic when possible, one may choose to consider tutorial positions or clinical supervision positions.

It must be stated that while roles such as these are critically important within every well-rounded chiropractic program, every applicant/appointee will still be required to gain educational qualifications (Box 11.1). Such roles are not about "doing it my way" or the "copy and paste" method, which is sometimes mistaken for learning attainment. They are about contributing to the greater goal of the program and institution (one road of induction) while learning how to be a valuable learning leader (the second journey). A position such as a tutor or duty clinician should never be seen as inferior; neither should it ever be trumpeted to boost the ego of the incumbent. Such roles are cogs that happen to be critical components of the educational gearbox, regardless of their size, as long as the slant of the thread totally meshes.

It is this latter comment that will be addressed shortly. No gearbox will operate smoothly and produce the maximum power to the driving wheels in the absence of every piece being interconnected.

When one becomes sufficiently bold to apply for a full-time or ongoing appointment, the first point of consideration is the field of expertise. This may be basic science, social science, diagnostic science, clinical supervision and management, or, of course, chiropractic science. One should only consider an area in which one already holds, or is working toward, a doctorate and has appropriate experience.

The myths that must be dispelled are those that suggest years one and two of any program can be taught by a fairly low-level academic, while more senior years must be taught by the elite academics. The reality is the

---

Box 11.1

The Learning Achievement Required for a Career as a Full-Time, Tenure-Track Chiropractic Academic

1. A professional qualification in chiropractic from an accredited chiropractic institution.

2. Registration in good standing with the licensing body responsible for the jurisdiction in which one resides or practices.

3. Items 1 and 2 may qualify an applicant for an interview regarding an academic vacancy. Recognition and priority will be granted to practitioners who have a publication record. Typically, somewhere between 5 and 20 peer-reviewed papers in the indexed literature, along with positive responses to items 1 and 2 should guarantee an interview.

4. Either hold a doctorate in an area relevant to chiropractic education or be enrolled in one and making good progress.

5. Either hold some qualification in tertiary learning and teaching or be prepared to enroll in and undertake the program of that nature offered by the institution.

6. Listing of recent publications.

7. Demonstration of ability to convey concepts of critical thinking, scholarship, and research to learners.

---

reverse, and this author argues strongly that an institution's most qualified and gifted chiropractic academics belong in the beginning years. After all, the basic science subjects are delivered by academics with a PhD in anatomy, physics, chemistry, or other basic science fields. So, what sense is there in putting a chiropractic novice educator within that mix? Should it not also be a chiropractor with a relevant PhD qualification?

At this formative level, a chiropractic academic with a PhD will infuse the research and critical enquiry environment that is so essential to commencing learners to provide a base for their future individual growth. When this is added to qualification in education that facilitates communication and support, the institution may feel very comfortable. The effective leading of learning in all of the various fields presents quite a wall of challenge to any person who selects chiropractic academic as a career path.

Qualifications

The distinctions made to this point are the choice between (1) a part-time or sessional engagement and (2) a full-time career as a chiropractic academic. The reader may have also concluded that terminology about positions is not really that important, as it tends to only reflect the environment in which the institution operates.

Therefore, regardless of the names on the rungs of the ladder one must climb, we need now to look at those things that give one the ability to climb, from tutor (lecturer, instructor, assistant professor, depending on institutional conventions) to being a full professor based on merit, which in turn reflects knowledge and respected academic status.

The bottom line is quite straightforward and breaks with the traditions set by learned chiropractors acting as teachers and tutors during the profession's first century. Now, becoming a chiropractic academic is a career path in its own right.

This is the point where it becomes difficult to commit to an academic chiropractic career. As previously stated, the knowledge hierarchy outlines the pathway to professional knowledge.[13] Not only must one have impeccable declarative and procedural knowledge, it is also necessary to be able to apply it appropriately.

This hierarchy of knowledge illustrates that becoming a chiropractic academic requires more effort than being a practicing chiropractor. The starting point has to be an educational qualification equivalent to academic peers and appropriate for the profession. Thus follows the need for qualifications to (1) demonstrate that the skills in the professional area are at a sufficiently high level and (2) there is an ability to impart them. The former is demonstrated by doctoral-level studies, either completed or in process, and the latter by educational studies, again either completed, in progress, or ready to be undertaken with the institution to which one has applied.

Continuous Learning (Professional Development)

If we presume one has spent seven or more years gaining professional qualification, then commenced doctoral studies in addition to publishing a handful of case reports or some other scholarly work, we may reasonably expect a respectable institution would consider the applicant worthy of appointment.

Yet there is a plethora of other considerations. To this author, who has established five or more new or revised programs across seven campuses in four countries in three languages, these additional matters fall into two groups. The first is the academic's own academic path of research and scholarship. Second, there is the ongoing learning that is needed in order to remain contemporary as an educator. While licensing bodies or registration boards remain unclear as to what constitutes continuing professional development (CPD) for academics, the fact remains that quality universities and tertiary institutions provide an abundance of CPD for their staff. So, in addition to an appointed chiropractic academic holding the additional qualifications to confer validity in that position, one must undertake a program of professional development. The main reason is that registration bodies see chiropractic education as a field of practice and apply the same principles as they do to clinical practice to ensure its practitioners retain safety and currency.

At times, these offerings by educational institutions may appear of low relevance. Sometimes there may be gems, but regardless of the expectations, an academic must participate to be seen as a good citizen within the institution's academic community. And, quite frankly, the more that chiropractic academics participate, the more influential becomes their position within their academic peer groups.

Academic Freedom

There are two ways to consider the concept of "academic freedom." The first is to appreciate that in today's commercially driven tertiary education environment, the more important duty is academic *coherence*. When one is employed as an academic, one has the usual contractual responsibilities to one's employer. This equates to a uniform endorsement of the institution's position.

This level of pro and anti ideas must never be mistaken for academic freedom. It is simply the traditional basis of how workplaces operated in 19th-century society. Naive chiropractic appointees might believe their word is the definitive expression of chiropractic, no matter whether or not it is even vaguely contemporary. This is not academic freedom; it is academic immaturity.

One person's opinion does not equate to freedom. In fact, the term "academic freedom" is better considered as "academic responsibility." This requires the academic to develop evidenced-based and innovative arguments. The "freedom" relates to the fact the argument may extend to areas not yet considered plausible, which in turn releases and recruits other minds to bring their perspective to the question.

The greatest abuse of academic coherence in this sense is seen in those people appointed to casual academic duties as tutors or clinical supervisors and who act as if they know everything. This can only be seen as a reflection of their simplistic attitude toward the richness of academic tradition. The saddest abuse of academic coherence comes from those with a tenured appointment who decide they do not wish to follow the institution's position on chiropractic. This is a very touchy topic in contemporary chiropractic education.

Those trained in education know the disconnect for the learner occurs within successive chiropractic classes where one learning leader will put forth one idea and concept, then another learning leader will contradict it. The initial reaction of the academics is "we are showing the student how to think differently about a common topic." However, this statement is made in ignorance of the reality that students all want to pass, so they "learn" the best answer that will please a particular examiner.

This illustrates the difference between a "student" and a "learner." The latter will be "right" no matter the answer they offer, because it will be an answer that has been thought about, developed, and hopefully expressed coherently.

The underlying principle is that when the surroundings are safe, an individual's expression may be greatest. This is the principle underpinning, for example, Japanese society. There are societal rules, such as respect for elders and other people's property, that produce an inherently safe and stable environment that allows individual expression, which in the Shinto tradition causes no harm. This principle should define the environment in which chiropractic academics practice their profession.

The first and most important act is to create a unified sense of purpose for the particular chiropractic program. Potential students in the United States and Canada sometimes select a college based on its philosophical stance. This level of independent distinction is lost when a chiropractic program exists within the setting of a large university. The chiropractic program is only one program in a suite of perhaps 100 or so programs that compete for the same resources, such as space and related facilities, and often, the same students.

Basic Premise

Every applicant for a position as a chiropractic academic must become very familiar with the manner in which the institution presents itself. This means that applicants should declare their concordance with the institute's views and their desire to not only abide with them but refine them as needed through appropriate processes.

Every responsible tertiary institution will have statements representing a vision (Sidebar 11.1) and mission (Sidebar 11.2). It will also have a statement of values; an example of this is provided below.

Sidebar 11.1

An Example of a Vision Statement for a Chiropractic Institution

[Institution name] will be the destination of choice for the individual, regardless of socioeconomic background, wanting to graduate as a highly skilled chiropractor who is practice-ready and capable of engaging with the community as a leader and productive practitioner within tomorrow's health care team.

It is expected that every chiropractic academic will work to support and enact this vision.

Sidebar 11.2

An Example of a Mission Statement for a Chiropractic Institution

The chiropractic program at [institution] will meet our students' aspirations by providing the highest-quality, innovation-based education, characterized by inclusiveness in our scholarship and learning activities and openness in our assessment processes. We will emphasize exemplary engagement with the community and demonstrate leadership by personal example and positive attitude. Our practice of chiropractic will be enjoyable, ethical, and compassionate.

It is expected that every chiropractic academic will work to support and enact this mission.

Values for a Chiropractic Program within a Large, Multidisciplinary University

Each of the following values is a revision of one of the larger institution's values, in order to maximize alignment:

- We value the capability to formulate and communicate views requisite to academic argument as a chiropractor and the ability to communicate using appropriate language, level, and style.
- We value the capacity to locate and identify resources appropriate to chiropractic and to apply, interpret, and analyze information to address specific tasks and needs.

- We value the ability to act as a cooperative, productive individual within a team, taking responsibility for developing, setting, and achieving group goals while evaluating one's own strengths and weaknesses as a leader, team member, and/or an autonomous worker in a team context.
- We value information technology competence.
- We value problem solving and the ability to develop solutions to given situations and/or questions and to formulate strategies to identify, define, and solve problems including, as necessary, global perspectives.
- We value critical thinking, including reflective self-evaluation with the capability to think creatively within the context of health care in general, and specifically, chiropractic.
- We value cross-cultural competence and a respect for cultural diversity that allows the relative merits of ideas and actions to be discussed from different cultural perspectives and for a chiropractor to operate effectively within a socially diverse global environment.
- We value ethical practice where a chiropractor demonstrates an understanding of the legal and moral fundamentals of best practice, makes reasoned judgments on the value of particular actions, and articulates an appropriate personal value system in terms of social behavior and civic responsibility.

It is expected that every chiropractic academic will ensure each value is represented in the guide to the course/subject they deliver. There is no point in expressing values unless they are embedded in the chiropractic program's day-to-day activity.

In addition to a statement of values, there should follow an expression relating that institution's teaching style to ensure concordance among academics (see below). It is at this point that the concept of academic responsibility becomes active, in which faculty accept their allegiance to the institution's mission, vision, and values.

The Need for Concordance in Chiropractic Academia on the Use of the Term "Subluxation"

Overview

Chiropractic education and practice should be influenced by evidence, sourcing and weighing all available evidence, including the literature, the practitioner's experience, and individual patients' preferences and locus of understanding with regard to their health and well-being.

The discipline and its educators embrace an identity of chiropractic informed by the World Federation of Chiropractic and consider the whole patient within a continuum from pain and dysfunction to health and well-being.

Academics have an abiding responsibility to work to understand and explain the core tenets of chiropractic. They have the duty to use their academic abilities to explore and explain in the tradition of true science.

Key Tenets

- Chiropractors use the term "subluxation" to describe a collection of clinical findings indicative of therapeutic or prophylactic intervention by a chiropractor. In this sense, subluxation is a clinical framework for structuring evidence.[12]

- Chiropractic students must have competencies in diagnosis and basic spinal adjusting, grounded in clinical and basic sciences, contextualized in terms of the chiropractic profession and its history. Chiropractic academics must teach these competencies.

- In this sense, "basic spinal adjusting" is a collection of specialist techniques that address a form of clinical dysfunction evident within any altered structure and function of the spine.

- Learners will progress through tiered clinical practice courses, commencing with close clinical supervision and concluding with an intern year of minimally supervised practice that parallels an associate-type practice.

- There are additional terms of learning where students may follow their clinical interest, be it a style of practice (for example, rural health) or a style of technique. Should the student seek additional formal learning in these fields, it will be at the student's expense and arrangement with the knowledge and support of the institution.

- Flexible learning is a feature of each year of the program. Clinical skills classes and clinical practice require mandatory attendance, and all classes must be supported by high-level online learning and assessment.

Campuses have long outlived the 1960s concept that universities are the key to understanding the meaning of life. The responsibility now is for every chiropractic academic to be a model corporate citizen for his or her institution and to lead learning journeys using the best available methodologies while representing the institution as a businessperson should. For example, every time academics travel, representing the institution that employs them, the dress code should be business attire. Academia has a strong parallel with successful real-world activity.

Other Key Issues in Chiropractic Academics

The other little-known fact about being a chiropractic academic is that it is not a nine-to-five proposition. It is a total life immersion. Quite frankly, should readers hold a dream of becoming successful academics, they must realize it means writing on their MacBook over breakfast in the airport lounge in one city, adding another paragraph while flying in the back row of economy, then another while transiting through the lounge in a second city, then finishing it at destination at two o'clock in the morning. This may well be about 30 minutes before an on-site residential student knocks on their door seeking counseling and one's pastoral care role takes over (a real-life scenario of this writer).

This type of work is all-encompassing and occupies the pure space for learning that should be owned by a learning leader. It is into this clear space that every learning leader must take every learner, kindly, gently, and safely. Every chiropractic academic must have certification that he or she is cleared to work with children, even though college students are technically adults—they are still impressionable young people. Although even within Australia there are varying ways of certifying this—one state calls it a "blue card" while another calls it a "red card"—what it means is that the holder is acknowledged by the government as being a person with no record of dubious behavior with young people. Why is this relevant to being a chiropractic academic?

There are several reasons. The first is that every clinical tutor must carry such a card to ensure he or she is registered and enabled to work with young people and children. The next is to ensure classroom teachers (instructors/learning leaders) are beyond reproach when working in practical situations where students are in underwear. The simple fact is that a chiropractic academic deals with the human body. The earlier in the program, the more important it is for this intimate style of learning to be conducted with a level of dignity that embraces and respects privacy and imbues trust in the learner.

Should such questions raise issues, it may suggest the learning leader with such issues is not an appropriate person to work in that environment, which may in turn suggest he or she is not appropriate for appointment to the team of chiropractic educators.

Chiropractic academics must remain current with contemporary developments in education theory and practice. To this end, one must be prepared to invest a considerable number of hours, often at inconvenient times, to participate in "how-to" sessions. Regrettably, many such sessions are delivered by fellow academics who may know less of the topic than expected, which means a great deal of patience is required. However, attendance at such sessions must be recorded for two purposes. The first is to create one's personal record of aligning with the institution, while the second is to provide evidence of CPD for one's professional registration/licensing body.

It is also to be expected that academics will make significant investment in their own technology. It matters not whether this is tax deductible; what does matter is that an academic's productivity must be continuous and seamless.

The Contemporary Curriculum

Today's applicant for the position of a chiropractic academic will have made the initial choice between sessional or part-time employment and full-time or potential tenure-track employment. Reliance on past interpretation of these roles, based perhaps on one's own personal experiences as a student, suggests one role, that of clinical supervisor, for example, is more likely a one-on-one experience between the supervising academic and the learning clinician about a patient. The skills that must be brought to bear are those that convert such a privileged encounter into an enriching learning experience.

This is where "evidence-influenced" and innovative practice may be properly realized. The learning leader is reasonably expected to have a broad knowledge of any particular case a learning clinician may bring to her or him. Every health care record (patient file) should include copies (electronic or paper) of articles relevant to the case from the current literature. The learning clinicians will thus have built a compendium of current evidence relevant to the cases they have managed.

Another preconceived idea is that a lecture takes 50 minutes of the academic's time as a "talking head" to an often-half-empty classroom. The fact that most learners no longer attend "lectures" in turn may drive academics to employ devious tricks to enforce attendance. However, it has to be accepted by every chiropractic academic that today's world is no longer yesterday's world—and it is the academic who has to change. There should not be a chiropractic institution in the world that continues to schedule 50-minute lectures. These belong to the dinosaur age. The lesson is to bulldoze the lecture halls and build spaces for small group learning (similar to Apple stores). This means that established chiropractic academics need to relearn how to lead learning. Any chiropractic academic who is not using contemporary learning approaches and the appropriate supportive technology should stand down and retire.

Today's learning environment requires the following:

- Breaking a 50-minute lecture into bite-size pieces, called "chunking." This is a genuine academic term and means that the academic will present a learning element, with evidence, in less than 10 minutes.
- Recording and making the chunks available online.
- Enabling the learners to assemble the chunks like Lego blocks to make something of relevance to them.
- Embracing the concept of anywhere, anytime learning, where learners may pull up a chunk on their platform in any location and learn at their own pace.

The next step is radical as it means no more lectures: use small-group learning. This means fracturing the timetable and making chiropractic academics accountable for a wide range of learning content, any pinch of which may be offered at any particular time.

Up to this point, this chapter has been somewhat positive about chiropractic academia as a career path, albeit one that may never be populated globally by a large number of people. Therefore, it is time for a reality check. The following outlines the expectations for academic faculty in chiropractic institutions in the future:

- Hold a professional qualification in the discipline of chiropractic and be of good standing with licensing or registration authorities.
- Hold or obtain a PhD on a topic relevant to the field of teaching.
- Enthusiastically engage in the institution's CPD activities.
- Embark on a formal academic qualification in learning and teaching.
- Write and publish regularly in the peer-reviewed, indexed literature.
- Know every learner by his or her first name, and use it.
- Be sufficiently mentally flexible to function in a collective of small groups where each group may be playing with the learning dimensions around one individual project at a different year level at the same time in the same learning space.

Chiropractic education can be a brilliant experience, and a wonderful career may be crafted within that domain. How can this occur? The entire thrust of this chapter is that becoming an academic is a learned skill. Some brief comments follow that may be of assistance.

Shift to Capability

Many observers, including accreditors, fail to differentiate between competency and capability. In short, anyone can teach a clinical act, such as how to take a blood pressure reading. The "capability" lies in knowing when it is indicated. Competency is simply doing something reasonably well, while capability is knowing when and why to do it and then interpreting it within the context of the patient.

The move from competency to capability in health education is one of the major challenges at this time.

Social Media

When social media are mentioned, first thoughts turn to bevies of students using Facebook, Instagram, Weibo, Mixi, and others. The most valuable advice to an academic is to not get engaged. Leave the Facebook page to the experts in the institution.

When the unsubstantiated website claims of chiropractic colleges in Canada and the United States were explored by Sikorski and Grod in 2003,[14] they found "more than half of the chiropractic colleges in Canada and the United States made unsubstantiated claims for clinical theories or methods on their websites."[14] The investigators concluded this behavior likely reflected what was taught in the schools.

Chiropractic's quest for greater legitimacy and cultural authority is delayed by this tendency. The learning outcomes from today's prolific use of social media, indeed including by institutions to self-promote in addition to providing a forum for learners, points strongly to a significant responsibility of chiropractic academics, which includes setting the highest possible example if and when a decision is made to use social media.

Millennial students see email as dated and social media sites as being straightforward and easy to access. They are useful for rapid communication among a group (for example, an announcement about a delay in the commencement of a particular class), but they generally lack permanency and privacy. The question of permanency presents a conundrum as every social media expression becomes a perpetual representation of the individual. The lack of permanency referred to within the context of intraclass communication is more along the lines of "You posted it when? Yesterday? I don't do 'yesterday.'"

Anywhere, Anytime Learning

In contrast, the concept of "anywhere, anytime" learning is one that must be embraced by instructors and academics with regard to course or subject content. Learners already have this attitude when it comes to the use of libraries. Interestingly, some of the heaviest users of library content may never actually set foot in the physical building. Academics must always remember that librarians are their best friends.

In the way that libraries have become curated collections of electronic pathways, academic courseware is becoming a curated collection of learning chunks. The instructor or academic is the curator, so it goes without saying she or he must be both current and capable with an institution's electronic learning platforms.

Every academic will have negative stories to relate about these "distributed learning systems" and various versions of electronic systems that require learners to locate a particular site then try to find their particular place in their learning journey and then eventually pull the content to their device.

The next generation of such distribution systems will reverse the technology and instead push the content to the learner. The benefit is obvious. The learners proceed at their pace on their pathway through the learning chunks. As soon as one task is completed, the next and most relevant learning object appears on the learner's device.

Packages such as iBooks by Apple have amazing utility to gather and order content and distribute the learning chunks in manageable sizes. Quizzes, embedded objects, interactive videos, and so on have been delivered in this and antecedent formats by this author since about 2005. The options are straightforward. Today's academics either embrace technology and make it work for them and their learning groups or end their career with acetate overheads, dry-erase markers, and whiteboards.

Anywhere, Anytime Clinical Assessment

The concept of cramming 80 to 120 students into a classroom is so outdated it is difficult to imagine any chiropractic institution taking this approach in the 21st century. Of course, they will be urged to for its cost-effectiveness, another phrase for which is "price gouging." Every academic is familiar with the bell curve of results from tests and assessments, clinical or otherwise. It is a statistical anomaly that any one group of, for example, 100 learners, will have most scoring in the middle hump, which may be cleverly set by the academic to produce a class median grade of a certain value, perhaps 60 percent.

The bell curve naturally tapers off at either end so a few score the high distinctions and a few fail. This approach to assessment is outdated and reflects the weakness of using multiple-choice questions. which themselves produce their own mini bell curves. Rather than allow any real measure of individual performance in a group environment, this approach is not only flawed in a standard classroom setting, it is next to meaningless when it comes to assessing clinical capability.

Imagine the lowest score you could ever award clinical learners based on their observed interaction with a patient. If the clinician notes "hopeless," then the institution is liable to be challenged as to how such an incompetent learner "made it that far" to actually put hands on a patient. Further, clinician learners may have a valid case against institutions to which they have paid good money in order to bring them to a point where they are safe to work with patients, but have not.

The problem quickly becomes complex, and most clinician assessments end up as an ego-driven exercise by a handful of chiropractic clinicians who may have failed in practice and are now failing in education. The clinical learner must receive a grade that is legally protective of the institution, which means every clinical student has to be ranked as "passing" or "close to passing."

Therefore, there have to be very clear markers of capability before a learner engages with patients. As noted earlier, capability is a superior measure to competency as it requires the learner to process a variety of incoming data and formulate evidence-based decisions relevant to a unique situation. As time goes by, these decisions and outcomes should come closer to the core tenets of the institution.

The assessment processes need to come to measure the decision-making capability of the clinical learner. A good place to start is with case reports and copies of other literature that closely align with the presenting signs and symptoms of the patient. Hence the term "anywhere, anytime clinical assessment" requires full engagement by learners so they may make cogent, evidenced-based arguments to whichever clinical supervisor happens to be on duty and demonstrate that not only do they have the capability to make such argument, they have the capability to continue a trial of therapeutic intervention while measuring patient outcomes.

Suddenly, with just one or two very simple steps, a senior student's clinical learning and associated practice becomes empowered.

Fields of Research and Scholarship

Appointment as a chiropractic academic across all aspects of the spectrum, from sessional clinical supervisor to research chair, demands a steady output of academic papers. A typical output from a full-time academic would be three or four papers per year in the reputable peer-reviewed, indexed literature. Various countries require researchers to identify a field of research.

As a chiropractic academic, one must find a way to be involved in scholarship. It helps to think of "research" as being inquisitive work while scholarship is more a process of critical reflection and review. One may elect to write about one's teaching approach or some other innovation being developed, so in general scholarship may be thought of more as qualitative work while research is often more a quantitative methodology.

This is a simplistic suggestion. The real point to understand is that earning appointment as an academic is just the beginning of a long and complex career path. It is not so much the hackneyed idea to "publish or perish," as that concept now serves little purpose. Academics will write and publish because it is "what academics do." And not only will they perform in this way for their own reputation and career trajectory, they will do so for the specific benefit of their learning group. Below is an example of one DC's pathway to an academic career.

Academic Careers: Mentoring Faculty in Teaching and Scholarly Activity

Dana Lawrence, DC, MMedEd, MA, is a professor and head of the Center for Teaching and Learning at Palmer College of Chiropractic in Davenport, Iowa. He was also the editor of the *Journal of Manipulative and Physiological Therapeutics* (*JMPT*) for many years. He has devoted his career to chiropractic teaching, learning, and scholarly activity. Below, he discusses his experience.

How did you get into the academic side of chiropractic?
"I applied for a teaching position at National College of Chiropractic (now National University of Health Sciences) within eight months of my graduation in 1979. I had already worked as a teaching assistant in both the physiology and technique departments, and I counted many faculty members as friends. And I came from a home where my mom was a teacher, so I really found I enjoyed academic pursuits much more than I did clinical ones. I was hired to teach, and within a year had begun to work behind the scenes with the *JMPT*. The rest, as they say, is history."

How did you become a journal editor? Any particularly striking events or impressions you can share about JMPT, *especially in its early development?*
"I volunteered to help the *JMPT* editor, Dr. Roy Hildebrandt. I knew very little about journal management, but under Dr. Hildebrandt's tutelage I began to gain skills related to editing, layout, and scientific writing. I spent

eight years working with him before I took over as editor. I think in the early days of the journal I was struck by how this little publication seemed to be holding its own against much bigger journals, how it was helping to provide a solid foundation for chiropractic science. And I also began to meet people within the profession, people who were instrumental in its growth."

What are the most fulfilling/inspiring things about being involved in chiropractic education?

"Contributing to the future growth of the profession in every way I can—by training students, by working with faculty, by helping to add to our knowledge base."

A minority of chiropractic academics enter research as a full-time career, with teaching being a secondary part of their work. Following are interviews with three chiropractors whose career path, although closely aligned with academics, is focused on research.

Research as a Career Path in Chiropractic

"Being a researcher is like climbing a mountain whose cloud covered summit I don't really expect to reach, but it's a good hike."

—*James Whedon, DC, MS*

Research has become increasingly important in the era of evidence-based practice. Chiropractic educational institutions, like those of all other health professions, are now teaching the principles of evidence-based practice and include research in the job description for faculty. Also, an increasing number of chiropractic practitioners and faculty are seeking advanced training in research and joining the faculty of conventional universities, to pursue clinical, health services, and basic science research, most often within departments of rehabilitation. However, most faculty doing chiropractic research at this time are employed by chiropractic universities within a division or department of research.

Jerrilyn Cambron, DC, MPH, PhD, is currently a professor in the Department of Research at the National University of Health Sciences (NUHS) in Lombard, Illinois. NUHS was the first chiropractic college to become a full-fledged university, training multiple health professions rather than just one. It was also one of the first chiropractic colleges to build a strong research component into the institution.

How did you get into research?

"Great question! I was a research assistant as a chiropractic student, but I expected to practice once I graduated. But soon after starting a practice, I found that it just wasn't for me. Just then, I received a call from a faculty member in the research department saying she was planning on leaving and thought I would be a great fit. I applied and got the job. My plan was to be there for a year or two, but it has been over 20 years now! This path unexpectedly opened up and it was absolutely the right one for me."

What type of background/training did you have when you began your career in research?

"I was a research assistant for two years before I became faculty in the research department. Once in the position, I realized I needed more research training so completed an MPH in public health (epidemiology/biostatistics) while working full time. Grad school was such a good fit and I enjoyed it so much that I stayed to get a PhD as well. These degrees helped me become an independent researcher."

What do you find most interesting, fulfilling, inspiring?

"Even though answering research questions through clinical trials is interesting and fun, I am most fulfilled by helping people with research literacy and study design. Teaching others how to search on PubMed, read an article, incorporate the information into their practice (or not!), and even design small studies helps our entire profession grow."

What is your advice for other DCs who would like to become involved in research?

"First, read as many articles as you can. Then, consider starting by submitting a case report to a scientific journal. Going through the peer-review process with a journal is a big part of research, so doing that early will help an individual determine if they are cut out for it. If peer review doesn't scare you away from getting involved, then consider getting an advanced degree. Chiropractors are not trained to do research, but you can learn these skills in grad school. Finally, consider collaborating with other researchers especially in the beginning in order to learn from them."

Michael Schneider, DC, PhD, is currently an associate professor in the School of Health and Rehabilitation Sciences and associate professor, Clinical and Translational Science Institute, at the University of Pittsburgh. He works full time in research after being in private chiropractic practice for over 25 years.

How did you get into research?

"I was always interested in scholarly activity, published case reports, etc. while in practice." As a practitioner, it always bothered him that he felt like he was experimenting all the time, with not much real evidence to support what he was doing. "I pursued a PhD on a part-time basis. I could do this because my practice was close to the university, and my partner could cover for me. But because I needed to support my family, I didn't consider research as a full-time career until our kids went to college."

What do you find most fulfilling or inspiring about a research career?
"Clinical practice is great, but you can only help one person at a time. With research the impact is so much greater—you can affect people even globally. When you publish high-quality research, and serve on scientific advisory panels, it helps the whole profession. This is how the profession advances."

James Whedon, DC, MS, is currently director of health services research at Southern California University of Health Sciences. Before this, he was the recipient of a National Institutes of Health Career Development grant at Dartmouth College.

How did you get into research?
"Until I applied for my first grant relatively late in my career as a chiropractic practitioner, I had not planned to get into research. After about 12 years practicing chiropractic in Massachusetts, I worked at the teaching hospital for Dartmouth Medical School, where I was responsible for administering the trauma registry. I could see that the trauma registry offered untapped potential as a source of research data, and in collaboration with attending physicians at Dartmouth, I published the results of several small trauma-related projects. One of the papers was a case report of an adverse event following spinal manipulation, which sparked a research interest in chiropractic safety. I read a journal article about opportunities for complementary health care providers to obtain NIH grant funding for research training. Without really knowing what I was getting into, I obtained the support of my department to apply for an NIH grant, and I also had the good fortune to be mentored through the application process by several very experienced researchers. I was awarded a five-year research career development grant, which funded my training at Dartmouth and afforded ample protected time for me to conduct my first major research project."

What do you find most interesting, fulfilling, or inspiring?
"I am interested in pursuing research that promises to support a vision of *health care justice.* All people should have the right to access health care services that they need and want, regardless of their background, circumstances, socioeconomic status, or where they live."

What is your advice for other DCs who would like to become involved in research?
"Find a mentor! (Even better, two or three mentors.) Your mentor must be an experienced and publicly funded researcher. They should be someone whom you respect, and who respects you and is able and willing to take

the time to help. It's fine if they come from a different field, but there should be some common area of interest."

Peer Review

Academic faculty are aware of peer review. However, they usually place it more in the context of submitting articles for publication in journals. Peer review within the area of scientific publication has received negative publicity lately, with biased reviews seemingly common, along with other unsavory and unethical practices.[15,16]

Peer review in the context of forging a career as a chiropractic educator is a vastly different process. It requires an enlightened education institution and a high degree of trust and support among the chiropractic teaching team.

It becomes the role of the manager of the academic unit to guide this, and it may be as small increments that start with sharing a group's work in a safe forum. This writer has seen this function brilliantly in an East Asian university of high global repute, where the relevant chiropractic academics sat down together in one room and worked through every question and answer they and their peers had written for an exam series.

On the other hand, as successful as that was, another institution used a process where each academic provided her or his bank of questions for a particular major clinical assessment. Issues came to the fore when the request was made for the model answers, and it was discovered that in one particular topic a full third of the basic content for that topic was never delivered, let alone assessed. The academic had chosen to drop it from the curriculum.

If the manager of that assessment structure had not persisted with an open and transparent process, there is no other possible outcome than the creation of class after class of half-taught clinicians.

Every chiropractic institution is urged to immediately implement an open-door teaching-space policy and ensure its academics are on the same page. Formative feedback is an important part of this process.

The Evolving Environment

A critical part of our evolving environment is the development of mature accreditation processes. There is no doubt that institutional and programmatic accreditation has played a vital role in conferring the level of respectability now globally enjoyed by chiropractic programs.

However, there is room for improvement, and it is richly rewarding to see the Council on Chiropractic Education Australasia take the old processes, turn them upside-down to shake the coins out of the pockets, and rebuild to create something that has the promise of being enlightened, mature, and equitable.

While this is a strong, positive step forward, we still see global pockets of ignorance and biased academics with political agendas. It is interesting to confront this issue and attempt to determine why some outcomes of the accreditation processes in Europe should be so different to the thoughtful processes evident, for example, in the United States, where institutional missions are respected.

It is at this point that the environment must be revisited to determine whether there is really any wisdom in putting chiropractic students, who learn a health and wellness paradigm, in the same classes as medical students, who learn the best technologically and pharmaceutically supported ways to reverse disease processes and put broken bodies back together.

This is not a criticism of chiropractic versus medicine; it is a simple question about how we may better serve our respective academic paradigms and the nature of the contemporary learning journey that could best facilitate this.

A creative futurist would say the stronger each paradigm is, the healthier our society. And that is simply what constitutes a chiropractic academic: a person who develops leaders in a paradigm of health and wellness.

Conclusion

An utterly useless task is to try to determine the custodians of chiropractic. There would be 40-plus college presidents, thousands of chiropractic academics and students, plus a heap of people on the fringes of academia, and each group feels that they are the custodian. However, what if we come to the realization that we are each custodians in our own way? The beauty of this volume is that it sets out many ways to protect and develop the future of the profession. Valid career paths for every eccentric have been presented. This writer just happens to be a bit of a chalkie, and after 30 years or so has some sense of the space academics must fill within various cultures.

References

1. Peters RE, Chance MA. Chiropractic education: the beginning. *Chiropr J Aust.* 1997;27:51–63.

2. Gibbons RW. The rise of the chiropractic educational establishment: 1897–1980. In: Scheiner S, Schwartz L, eds. *Who's Who in Chiropractic International.*

2nd ed. Littleton, CO: Who's Who in Chiropractic International Publishing Co.; 1980: 339–352.

3. Biggs L. Chiropractic education: a struggle for survival. *J Manip Physiol Ther.* 1991;14(1):22–28.

4. Devereaux EP, Cice J, O'Reilly BK. History of the Sydney College of Chiropractic. *Chiropr J Aust.* 2006;36(1):17–32.

5. Flexner A. Medical education in the United States and Canada. Bulletin Number Four, 1910. *Bull World Health Organ.* 2002;80(7):594–602.

6. Steinert Y, Mann K, Centeno A, et al. A systematic review of faculty development initiatives designed to improve teaching effectiveness in medical education. *Med Teach.* 2006 Sep;28(6):497–526.

7. Cooke M, Irby DM, Debas HT. The UCSF Academy of Medical Educators. *Acad Med.* 2003 Jul;78(7):666–672.

8. Berman JR, Aizer J, Bass AR, et al. Creating an academy of medical educators: how and where to start. *HSS J.* 2012 Jul;8(2):165–168.

9. Bolton SP. A retrospective view of historical periods in Australian chiropractic history. *Chiropr J Aust.* 2006 Mar;36(1):9–16.

10. Waldwell W. *Chiropractic: History and Evolution of a New Profession.* St. Louis, MO: Mosby Year Book; 1992: 86–103.

11. Chapman-Smith DA, Cleveland III CS. International status, standards, and education of the chiropractic profession. In: Haldeman S, ed. *Principles and Practice of Chiropractic.* New York: McGraw-Hill; 1992: 111–134.

12. Gatterman MI. A patient-centered paradigm: a model for chiropractic education and research *J Alt Comp Med.* 1995;1(4):371–386. doi:10.1089/acm.1995.1.371. http://online.liebertpub.com/doi/abs/10.1089/acm.1995.1.371. Accessed September 8, 2015.

13. Biggs J. *Teaching for Quality Learning at University.* 2nd ed. Berkshire, UK: Open University Press; 2003.

14. Sikorski DM, Grod JP. The unsubstantiated website claims of chiropractic colleges in Canada and the United States. *J Chiropr Edu.* 2003;17(2):113–119.

15. Vyas D, Hozain AE. Clinical peer review in the United States: history, legal development and subsequent abuse. *World J Gastroenterol.* 2014 Jun 7;20(21): 6357–6363. doi:10.3748/wjg.v20.i21.6357. http://www.ncbi.nlm.nih.gov/pmc/articles/PMC4047321/. Published June 7, 2014. Accessed September 14, 2015.

16. Triggle CR, Triggle DJ. What is the future of peer review? *Vasc Health Risk Manag.* 2007 Feb;3(1):39–53. http://www.ncbi.nlm.nih.gov/pmc/articles/PMC1994041/. Accessed September 14, 2015.

CHAPTER TWELVE

Opportunities for Multidisciplinary Practice

Jordan A. Gliedt, DC; and Cheryl Hawk, DC, PhD, CHES

Over the last several decades, the prevalence of chronic disease and its impact on patients, society, and the health care system has been of significant public health concern. Recent analyses have shown that about half of the adults in the United States—approximately 117 million people—suffer from at least one chronic health condition (CHC), and one in every four adults suffers from two or more CHCs.[1] Between the years 2002 to 2009, the number of adults with two or more CHCs increased from approximately 23.4 million to 30.9 million.[2] The rise in CHCs has come at a great expense to the health care system, with an estimated 86 percent of all health care spending in 2010 being attributed to the management of CHCs.[3] This translates into about 71 cents of every health care dollar spent in the United States being expended on treating people with CHCs.[3]

Chronic musculoskeletal disorders are one of the most common categories of CHCs to cause disability, with spine-related disorders as its greatest contributor.[4] It is estimated that effectively 100 percent of the adult population is affected by back or neck pain at some time in life, with about 85 percent experiencing low back pain alone at some point in their lifetime and up to 37 percent of the population being affected from low back pain at any given time.[5,6] As CHCs have gained a heightened level of attention, health care has experienced a significant transformation in ideology in hopes to more effectively manage these problems with an emphasis on team-based care and interdisciplinary collaboration. The shift to team-based care is epitomized by the development of accountable care organizations (ACOs) and patient-centered medical homes (PCMHs) in which outcome-based care and cost containment are emphasized with patient engagement, shared decision making, and interdisciplinary collaboration.

Particularly with the growing rate of chronic spine-related disorders, the integration of chiropractic care into health care delivery systems is naturally increasing. Chiropractic care is now a covered benefit in most major health insurance plans throughout the United States. The occurrence of chiropractors serving as part of a multidisciplinary team is ever growing. It is estimated that approximately 7–8 percent of chiropractors currently practice in an integrated health care facility. Some prominent examples of multidisciplinary care settings that offer chiropractic care are Brigham & Women's Hospital's Osher Center for Integrative Medicine, Medical College of Wisconsin & Froedtert Hospital Spine Care Clinics, University of Maryland School of Medicine Center for Integrative Medicine, and the Veterans Affairs (VA) Health Care System.

The introduction and growth of chiropractic in the VA Health Care System is the most notable and successful example of chiropractic inclusion on a large scale in integrated medical settings in the United States. The VA operates the largest integrated health care system in the United States, which includes 144 hospitals, more than 1,400 other associated health care facilities, and more than 326,000 employees.[7] Approximately 7 million veterans are provided with health care services each year with more than 86 million outpatient visits to the VA.[7] Chiropractic care was first introduced into the standard medical benefits at the VA in 2001, and VA facilities began delivering on-site chiropractic care in 2004.[7] In Box 12.1, Reed Phillips, DC, PhD, the chair of the Chiropractic Committee to the VA, gives an insider's view into how this initiative started. Since that time, the rate of chiropractic use, workforce, and academic endeavors has grown considerably. Chiropractic use grew quickly within the VA. Patients seen in VA chiropractic clinics increased in the first year by approximately 112 percent and by approximately 18 percent each subsequent year through 2015.[7] Between the years 2005 and 2015, VA chiropractic clinics experienced a total 821 percent increase in patients seen.[7]

With such a marked increase in chiropractic use, the demand for an increase in the VA chiropractic workforce grew as well. In 2005, a total of 13 chiropractic physicians were employed full time at the VA.[7] Each year thereafter showed an increase in numbers of full-time chiropractic

---

Box 12.1

History of Chiropractic in the U.S. Department of Veterans Affairs

In 2001, Public Law 107-135 went into effect, requiring the VA to provide chiropractic care to all veterans. Reed Phillips, DC, PhD, was chair of the Chiropractic Committee to the VA. This committee made the recommendations that made this historic action possible.

Our charge was to make recommendations to the secretary of the VA regarding the inclusion of chiropractic services in the VA Health Care System. As a federal advisory committee, membership had to include all interested parties. Thus, the committee included two medical physicians, an osteopathic physician, a physical therapist, a physician assistant, and six chiropractors representing various chiropractic organizations. At the outset, the committee was labeled as one destined to fail because people believed there was no way any agreement could be reached with such a diversity of backgrounds. Three years later, 69 recommendations were put forward with only two lacking unanimous agreement. And the disagreement was only among the chiropractors, not between the medical and chiropractic contingents. Now, chiropractic is an integral part of the VA system.

---

employees, and a total of 86 chiropractors were employed full time in 2015.[7] In addition to on-site chiropractic care, off-site chiropractic care provided for eligible veterans through VA benefits has shown significant growth. In 2015, the VA had granted a total of 159,533 off-site chiropractic visits, compared to 8,244 in 2005.[7] To date, more than 10 VA medical centers have an academic affiliation with numerous chiropractic colleges, allowing chiropractic students to gain valuable experience in multidisciplinary care as student clerks during a several-week rotation.

In 2014, the VA initiated an inaugural year-long chiropractic residency training program in integrated clinical practice. The continued growth of chiropractic within the VA in the last decade has exemplified the value of chiropractic inclusion in clinically integrated medical settings, and it is estimated that growth will continue.

Chiropractic opportunities in multidisciplinary settings have seen growth in various fields and are not limited to traditional clinical environments alone. Chiropractic inclusion in sports medicine settings has also seen noteworthy expansion and is now commonplace. Though sports medicine settings may be different from traditional outpatient medical facilities, team-based care remains essential. Usual members on a sports medicine team may also include athletic trainers, physical therapists, orthopedic surgeons, and primary care physicians. Essentially every franchise in the National Basketball Association and National Football League has an official team chiropractic physician associated with the sports medicine team. Other major professional sports venues regularly use on-site chiropractic services alongside other health care approaches, including those in Major League Baseball, Minor League Baseball, the National Hockey League, and the PGA Tour. Chiropractors have additionally gained noticeable inclusion into the United States Olympic Committee (USOC) sports medicine staff. Chiropractors are an integral part of the sports medicine program within USOC. Along with physical therapists and athletic trainers, multiple chiropractors have been appointed staff privileges, director-of-care responsibilities, and represent part of the sports medicine staff at Summer and Winter Olympic Games. *Chapter 13 discusses sports chiropractic in greater detail.*

Traditionally, chiropractors have operated in independent practices, providing individualized chiropractic care. However, recent trends are directing a shift in the model and delivery of health care across all specialties. This has created an array of new opportunities for chiropractors to practice in multidisciplinary settings and participate in interprofessional collaborative team-based care. Although opportunities in integrated primary care and sports medicine settings appear to be the most typical environments at this time, integrated opportunities exist in other specialties as well, such as chronic pain management, geriatrics, and pediatrics.

This trend promises to not only provide better patient care but is also an exciting opportunity for new doctors of chiropractic (DCs) to consider. This chapter will present insights from five DCs practicing in multidisciplinary settings to help others who are interested in pursuing this opportunity.

Chiropractic in a Rehabilitation Practice

Rehabilitation practices, providing care for patients with chronic pain or recovering from injuries, are a good fit for chiropractic. However, perhaps because chiropractic evolved outside the health care mainstream, it can still be challenging for DCs to join a multidisciplinary rehab practice. Dr. Eric Roseen, DC, has successfully done so and has also accomplished an even less common feat in becoming a National Institutes of Health–funded research fellow at an academic university. Dr. Roseen shares his experience and insights on his journey below.

Dr. Eric J. Roseen, DC, currently practices at Joint Ventures Physical Therapy and Fitness, a multidisciplinary clinic in Boston, Massachusetts. He also has the rare distinction of serving as a research fellow in the Program for Integrative Medicine and Health Care Disparities in the Department of Family Medicine at Boston Medical Center and Boston University.

Dr. Roseen says, "I was always interested in multidisciplinary practice. As a high school wrestler, I had a good experience with my chiropractor and really felt like a clinical career as a sports chiropractor was a good fit for me. As a college student-athlete, this desire really solidified; many of my closest college friends were going into other health care careers. It always made sense to me that I would work alongside them." He felt that it was natural to collaborate and integrate with other health care providers to provide the best patient care possible.

The Route to Multidisciplinary Practice: Barriers and Facilitators

When he entered chiropractic college, Dr. Roseen found that there were very few opportunities to practice in "mainstream" health care settings. He had to find out about integrative practices on his own initiative by researching what was available and then determining whether he could serve his internship in one of them. Eventually he was able to arrange his internship in a hospital-based spine care center. His experience in this setting helped pave the way to his current position in a multidisciplinary clinic that includes chiropractic, physical therapy, personal training, massage, and acupuncture.

How could his self-motivated efforts have been facilitated? "I wish there would have been more in the curriculum about the logistics of multidisciplinary practice. For example: What does onboarding look like? What should a chiropractor in this setting get paid? How to triage patients? How to comanage patients? Which patients should receive my care, and who would do better with PT, massage, or acupuncture? Or clear guidance for use of more aggressive treatments like an injection, or surgery? How to communicate this decision-making process to other health care professionals? How to bill in these settings?"

Because chiropractic college academic and clinical coursework and experience provided limited training in this area, Dr. Roseen attended professional conferences at which he was able to meet and network with other DCs who were in such settings. "Conversations with these individuals really shaped how I think about chiropractic care and spine care in general. They were very helpful in understanding why DCs should be integrated into the mainstream, what this could look like, and why it often is very challenging." Now, some of these professional conferences, such as the Association of Chiropractic Colleges–Research Agenda Conference, have organized special sessions and even annual conference themes focusing on interdisciplinary and multidisciplinary practice and schedule breakfasts and other meetings for DCs in such settings where they can compare experiences and network.

Dr. Roseen's current research fellowship at Boston University has also been an invaluable experience. How did he obtain this coveted and highly competitive National Institutes of Health (NIH) training opportunity? "I wrote a grant to NIH with the help of my mentor (Rob Saper, MD, MPH) to gain research experience while assisting him with a large randomized controlled trial of yoga versus physical therapy versus education for chronic low back pain. I found we had a lot in common with how we thought about back pain, and [I] have really enjoyed my time at Boston University working with Dr. Saper's team." Motivated DCs or even chiropractic students should learn about current NIH training opportunities and be sure they have excellent knowledge of current clinical research and research methods. In the new era of evidence-based practice, research knowledge, and even better, research experience, are not just helpful but in many cases essential for joining a multidisciplinary practice.

What do you find most fulfilling or inspiring about multidisciplinary practice?
"When I get to comanage a patient. I've had patients who haven't responded to my care over a couple of weeks and they get one acupuncture treatment and are significantly better. Or a primary care provider refers someone with acute back pain for chiropractic care and they see firsthand a surprisingly quick recovery. It goes both ways and it's incredibly exciting and informative each time."

Can you give an example that epitomizes your experience in multidisciplinary practice?
"One of my first patients in practice presented with chest pain. He thought he may be having a heart attack. He was a really busy, stressed-out, high-profile businessman about to leave for a much-needed vacation. His primary care provider brought him down the hall to me after he had gone through a series of tests that showed that he had noncardiac chest pain. I was able to find a trigger point in his shoulder girdle that re-created the chest pain. One treatment significantly reduced his symptoms and he was well reassured and able to enjoy his vacation. This shows the value of

multidisciplinary practice: instead of being shuttled from one office to another, or, even worse, being told there was 'nothing wrong,' this patient was able to have his problem diagnosed and treated in a timely and economical manner, thanks to practitioners from different fields being located in one setting and being able to understand what one another does and being willing to work together." (Note: details about the patient have been changed to protect the patient's identity.)

What is your advice for other DCs who would like to become involved in this type of practice?

"Read. Write. Present. Publish. Be familiar with literature on the conditions you will see the most. This is most likely back and neck pain. It has always surprised me how little primary care providers and other health care professionals know about the care I provide—and about practice guidelines for common musculoskeletal conditions. It's okay; they have to know a lot about other things (my wife is a primary care provider in training). In fact, it's a great opportunity to educate them. For example, a broad basic education on best practices in managing low back pain (identifying red flags, when to image, nonpharmacologic treatment options, clinical practice guidelines) is incredibly helpful for primary care providers. Other health care providers are often surprised to learn that there is a large evidence base, including many high-quality randomized controlled trials, for spinal manipulation. Getting comfortable with presenting and discussing this type of information is really important. If your own 'self-study' can build into a literature review, case report, or case series, you may have the opportunity to publish. Preparing a manuscript for publication, although challenging, is an important experience for those interested in multidisciplinary practice and clinical research."

Chiropractic for Children with Special Needs

Sharon Vallone, DC, has an interdisciplinary pediatric practice, Kidspace, working with children with special needs in South Windsor, Connecticut. The philosophy at Kidspace is that children with challenges should be given every opportunity to thrive in a safe and nurturing multidisciplinary health care environment.

When asked how she got into this very unique practice setting, Dr. Vallone explains, "I've been associated with Kentuckiana Children's Center in Louisville, Kentucky, in one way or another since I was in chiropractic college, having met Dr. Lorraine M. Golden during a fundraiser run by our college's president, Ernest Napolitano, a classmate of hers at Palmer College. Dr. Golden had envisioned and founded a multidisciplinary facility in Louisville, Kentucky, in 1956 to provide chiropractic and other important health care opportunities for children with special needs.

"My story isn't quite as exciting but was definitely motivated by her incredible passion and mission. In 2002, my grandson was born with microcephaly. In 2008, in talking with my friend, who was also one of my grandson's therapists, we realized we needed a Kentuckiana in Connecticut to serve Ethan and all the children we had met on our journey with him and during my career as a chiropractor primarily working with families, many with children with physical, behavioral, and developmental challenges. So together, we founded Kidspace Adaptive Play and Wellness."

Their goal was to form a collaborative with professionals who also cared deeply for children and their families and understood their needs and financial burdens. Their perspective must be that the child comes first, and the environment must be safe and welcoming at all times. The professionals at Kidspace do not sit at a desk or wear a white coat; they join the children in their play to begin each therapeutic session.

Currently, in additional to chiropractic, recreational therapy, and qi gong, they have added other dedicated, loving health professionals: two naturopathic physicians (NDs) who specialize in children with neurological impairments, another chiropractor, a craniosacral therapist, a massage therapist, and a family counselor. There is also a consulting speech therapist and art therapist (who also uses animals in the healing process).

It is especially important for students reading this to know that both their new DC and NDs came to join Kidspace by first "hanging out" and then interning at Kidspace while they were still in professional school. Dr. Vallone explains, "They both spent every spare minute they had during school to 'hang out' and 'help out,' while completing their rigorous education, which showed us their dedication."

How did you prepare to develop a multidisciplinary facility like Kidspace?
"I learned about this type of practice at Kentuckiana, which is the model for Kidspace. First I worked as a volunteer, and then as a temporary director, and later serving on the board of directors at Kentuckiana. A veritable hands-on classroom!"

Since you learned through an apprenticeship model, were there aspects of running this type of enterprise that you wish you had but had to catch up on later?
"Grant writing! How a board runs (Roberts Rules of Order)! How to do research!"

What do you find most fulfilling or inspiring working in this interdisciplinary setting?
"It's still the one-on-one clinical experience with my patients, their cuddles, their laughter, and their tears and their amazing journey, successes and failures, and indomitable spirits." She explains that each child is

unique, and so their approach to each child is also unique, individual-ized to best fit his or her needs. So it is always interesting!

Is there a particular experience that you feel sums up or somehow captures the essence of this practice?

"Colton is one of our Kidspace kids. Colton has Down syndrome and was referred by an early development agency for large motor develop-ment." The play therapist started Colton on the "magic gym" and real-ized, in observing his movements, that he had structural restrictions that required chiropractic care to correct. His mom was at first skeptical, but, after Dr. Vallone explained what she would do, she agreed to treat-ment. "Within a short period of time Colton became mobile, and he made rapid progress." Dr. Vallone felt he would also benefit from nutri-tional advice, so she brought in the ND for consultation. Colton responded well and continued to improve and is still doing well even after the family moved away from Connecticut. "Colton is thriving and has become more and more active—he has even joined a gymnastics team," Dr. Vallone said. "Our population is growing daily, and our hall-ways are bustling with the sounds of happy children. We have played with hundreds of children and have seen so much progress over these past two years. It is such a joyful experience to work with these children and their families!"

What is your advice for other DCs who would like to become involved in this type of practice?

"Mine might be more of a unique specialty practice because of our client base. But whatever your passion, whomever your client base, a collaborative practice is one of the most fulfilling ways to practice as we can turn to each other for support when we may be at a dead end or need a second set of eyes to see with!

"It provides a stronger foundation for patient care and gives the patient a sense of security that they have a team working in their best interest and have a broader knowledge base to draw from. In our case, our parents know we understand their particular circumstances because of our own personal experiences with family members who are considered 'differently abled.' We are a community within a community."

Chiropractic within the Veterans Administration

Jordan Gliedt, DC, is currently one of the select group of chiropractors who provide care in the U.S. Veterans Administration. Competition for these positions is fierce, and the salary and job security are only the smallest portion of why these positions are coveted: the clinicians in the VA know that it is an honor to serve the nation's veterans, and it is excit-ing and fulfilling to work with the best-of-the-best health care providers to manage the complex needs of VA patients. Dr. Gliedt, who worked in a multidisciplinary practice prior to joining the VA, shares his journey:

How did you get into interdisciplinary practice?
"I entered chiropractic school with the assumption that all health care professions, including chiropractors, inherently worked together as a team specifically designed for the benefit of the patient. So, in many ways, I always carried an expectation and desire to work in an interdisciplinary medical setting.

"While in chiropractic school, I had the great fortune of completing a brief student rotation within the local VA Medical Center. At that time, the chiropractic school I attended had a relationship with the local VA so that those entering their final term with an interest in interdisciplinary practice, who also met recommended GPA requirements, could apply for and potentially be selected for voluntary clerkship under the direction of the local VA chiropractor. Unfortunately, beyond this limited experience, there were very few offerings available during my chiropractic training to gain experience in this type of environment.

"Soon after graduation, I opened a private practice within a physical therapy clinic, which was housed in a large orthopedic and sports medicine facility. I made it a point to seek many neighboring physicians of multiple spine/musculoskeletal specialties in order to interact and gain as much understanding of their disciplines as I could. During this time, I was graciously granted opportunities to shadow several physicians in outpatient clinic environments and also as a surgical guest observing a variety of surgical procedures. I subsequently had the fortune of making acquaintance with a local orthopedic surgeon and was invited to volunteer several hours per week participating side by side in day-to-day training activities with residency-trained physicians who were completing orthopedic/sports medicine fellowship training.

"Throughout these encounters, I was able to gain valuable interaction and recognize the various approaches, strengths, and limitations of both chiropractic and nonchiropractic management strategies. It was these interactions which also allowed other disciplines to become familiar with the benefits of chiropractic care, and this opened additional opportunities to further explore potential positive outcomes of chiropractic inclusion in interdisciplinary settings."

What type of preparation did you wish you had but had to catch up on later?
"In hindsight, I can see that the greatest gap in my understanding was how the entire breadth of the patient encounter was managed, outside of traditional chiropractic treatments. I wasn't adequately prepared to discuss options of care outside of a chiropractor's scope of practice. I had very little appreciation for general procedural mechanisms, indications and contraindications of nonchiropractic treatment approaches, as well as when it may be appropriate or inappropriate to provide chiropractic treatments for patients receiving different forms of concurrent care outside of chiropractic."

What do you find most interesting, fulfilling, and inspiring, and do you have an experience that somehow sums up or captures the essence of this practice?

"The opportunity to be a highly valued member of a team providing multidimensional treatment options and strategies to help people suffering from chronic spine pain is very rewarding. Chronic pain appears to be exceedingly complex and multifactorial, and the ability to have meaningful contributions as part of a team to offer individualized diverse strategies to these complex issues and see patients respond is quite satisfying.

"Being on a team of multidisciplinary providers creates a daily atmosphere of continual learning opportunities and improvement in patient care. Consistent review and collaboration allows for prompt and appropriate treatments, enrichment of individual management approaches, and greater individualization to comprehensive patient care."

What is your advice for other DCs who would like to become involved in this type of practice?

"I think the most important habits one must commit to in order to become involved in interdisciplinary medicine settings are (1) learn and stay abreast on the latest scientific literature and best practice concepts; (2) become and remain involved in local medical community interaction opportunities. These practices allow one to appreciate the benefits and limitations of individual and multimodal approaches to patient-centered care. This also can produce a pathway of trust and relationship building with other members on the patient's health care team, which is the first step to a strong interdisciplinary cooperation."

Another Perspective on Practice within the Veterans Administration

Pamela Wakefield, DC, has worked in the St. Louis, Missouri, VA since 2006. Originally, Logan University, where she is a faculty member, created an affiliation with the St. Louis VA. Logan provided equipment and a DC, and the VA provided space. She was the second DC to work at this VA, and the first woman.

What type of preparation did you have for this position?

"Although I observed the previous DC before I transitioned in as the primary chiropractor, I had no specialized training in caring for veteran patients. But I had many years of experience as a practicing chiropractor and was a clinical faculty member at Logan."

What type of preparation do you wish you had and had to catch up on later?

"A list of abbreviations and acronyms would have been helpful, and a map of the facilities. I feel I learned most of the computer records system along the way—even now after 10 years I learn something new about the software every now and then! In retrospect, it would have been helpful if I had generally been more well read, and specifically if I had a better understanding of the strong influences of disability, disability payments, and substance abuse in the VA patient population. It would have really helped if I had been more familiar with multidisciplinary care—what was being done in other places; what worked, what didn't work: successes, barriers, pitfalls."

What do you find most interesting, fulfilling, inspiring?

"Being part of the Interdisciplinary Pain Program is the most interesting. The patients have complex chronic pain with a heavy psychosocial overlay. I've learned a lot about pain psychology and pain medication. I tell friends it has given me a true understanding of the parable of the lost sheep. If you can help one chronic pain patient, it's a great joy! Overall, this has been a great experience for me, and hopefully for all stakeholders. The patients we see enjoy having chiropractic and acupuncture offered. The providers who refer to us appreciate our collaboration.

"Most fulfilling, however, has been my association with my VA peers. Since 2007 I have had an opportunity to meet with other VA chiropractors at least 10 times and the experience is always uplifting. We openly share information and coordinate with each other for the betterment of chiropractic care within VA. We have no competition with each other, no opposing agenda—we work together to make chiropractic successful and available for as many VA patients as possible.

"Most inspiring has been treating the older veterans, especially WWII veterans, some of whom have received care from VA all or most of their lives and so have never seen a chiropractor before!"

Do you have an experience that you feel sums up or somehow captures the essence of this practice?

"After we moved to the building that housed the Spinal Cord Injury Unit, one of the physicians came down the hall to tell me he had just seen a veteran, who was paraplegic, and who asked if he could see the chiropractor for his low back pain. This is something that could never have happened without different practitioners working together under the same roof."

What is your advice for other DCs who would like to become involved in this type of practice?

"Securing a chiropractic position in a multidisciplinary setting is very competitive. Be smart: your grades, your résumé, your activities, your posts on social media—all these matter when you are being considered. Write well, constantly read the journals, and stay up to date."

Integrative Medicine Clinic

Interdisciplinary care is a specific type of multidisciplinary practice in which the providers on the team collaborate on patient care plans rather than simply coexist in the same facility. "Interdisciplinary team work is a complex process in which different types of staff work together to share expertise, knowledge, and skills to impact on patient care."[8] Integrative medicine, in which conventional and complementary health care professions are brought together, is inherently inclined toward interdisciplinary collaboration. Dr. Brian Morrison is director of Chiropractic Services, Center for Integrative Medicine, University of Maryland School of Medicine. He describes his work there and how he came to join the center in this interview.

How did you get into this practice?
"The University of Maryland School of Medicine has had an integrative medicine clinic since 1991. The clinical program of the Center for Integrative Health and Healing, called the Center for Integrative Medicine, is on the campus of the University of Maryland Rehabilitation and Orthopedic Institute. Located on the west side of Baltimore, it is approximately 10 miles from my private office location.

"I have always developed excellent relationships with local physicians. This began when I was fortunate to enter the Chiropractic Family Practice Residency at Lindell Hospital in 1987 in St. Louis. This innovative program gave me my start in learning the skills required to collaborate in patient care with medical practitioners. One of my mentors, Norman Kettner, DC, was instrumental in developing this program, which was based on a podiatric medicine residency.

"In 2003, the director of CIM developed an ankle problem and she decided to seek alternative care. She was referred to me by other medical colleagues. She was impressed by our evidence-based approach that used manual therapy and rehabilitation to quickly resolve her condition. She became curious about chiropractic and manual therapy, spending a good portion of her visit time discussing these topics. She invited me to spend some time at the center, and after a short while I was offered the opportunity to become an independent practitioner at the center, which meant renting a space and seeing referred patients. I was responsible for my own billing and documentation. Shortly thereafter an integrative medicine elective was created. This program was an introduction to integrative medicine modalities for fourth-year medical students. I was asked to present a program to the director and other instructors. Other DCs were invited to present programs as well. Thankfully, my presentation was chosen, and I began teaching a three-hour introduction to chiropractic and manual therapies for physicians. I was then asked to create a manual medicine program for second-year students as part of their pain and analgesia module. The fourth-year elective was sparsely attended until Dr. Delia Chiaramonte took it over in 2010. She created a dynamic program, complete with shadow experience in outside clinics, and opened it up to residents in family, internal, and preventive medicine. Now there are two full sections each spring semester. My course has expanded to six hours with a three-hour practicum, and I teach a three-hour course on pain science. This came about in 2012 after I was asked to present a program entitled "Change Your Brain, Change Your Pain" for the Center's Annual Health and Wellness Conference. I have been a regular speaker since then. In 2014, I was offered an official position as clinical faculty with the University of Maryland. In 2016, I was named director of Chiropractic Services for the CIM and was asked to bring on a second DC."

What type of preparation did you have?

"As mentioned, the Lindell Hospital Chiropractic Family Practice program under the direction of the late Dr. Russell Forbes was instrumental for me in learning how to participate as a member of a health care team in a hospital inpatient and outpatient setting."

What type of preparation did you wish you had but had to catch up on later?

"Formal training in the educational field would have been very helpful."

What do you find most fulfilling or inspiring?

"Teaching medical colleagues requires that one stay abreast of health care trends and current literature. I find sharing this information to be very fulfilling. Treating patients in conjunction with medical and other integrative practitioners causes you to consider all the social, behavioral, and medical factors that impact the patient suffering from any disorder."

Do you have an experience that you feel sums up or somehow captures the essence of this practice?

"A current patient suffered a head trauma two years ago with an associated cervical sprain injury. He then went on to develop shingles affecting the injured scalp area and subsequent severe postherpetic neuralgia. His family dynamics changed radically as a result of his condition. Clearly he has complex health care needs! In order to meet them, we collaborate as a team that includes trauma surgeons, plastic surgeons, neurologists, psychologists, psychotherapists, a chiropractor, massage therapists, acupuncturist, and an integrative medicine physician. Each provider has a role, and we communicate our observations and treatment ideas to one another.

"Currently I am guiding him through pain education and graded motor imagery, along with manual therapy as required while he continues with integrative medicine and psychotherapy. He is coming along, experiencing only brief periods of pain, improved function, and has developed excellent coping skills. He is tapering from his opioid pain medication. I am convinced that in a nonintegrative setting he would be languishing in pain management and likely be dependent on opioids."

What is your advice for other DCs who would like to become involved in this type of practice?

"Never stop learning! Don't be afraid to speak to physicians, particularly primary care. Managing musculoskeletal problems is not their specialty, and you can position yourself as an ally. Become involved with your local hospital by attending grand rounds. Perhaps even present a case!"

References

1. Ward BW, Schiller JS, Goodman RA. Multiple chronic conditions among US adults: a 2012 update. *Prev Chronic Dis.* 2014;11:E62.

2. Ford ES, Croft JB, Posner SF, Goodman RA, Giles WH. Co-occurrence of leading lifestyle-related chronic conditions among adults in the United States, 2002–2009. *Prev Chronic Dis.* 2013;10:E60.

3. Gerteis J, Izrael D, Deitz D, et al. Multiple chronic conditions chartbook. AHRQ Publications No. Q14-0038. Rockville, MD: Agency for Healthcare Research and Quality; April 2014.

4. Vos T, Flaxman AD, Naghavi M, et al. Years lived with disability (YLDs) for 1160 sequelae of 289 diseases and injuries 1990–2010: a systematic analysis for the Global Burden of Disease Study 2010. *Lancet.* 2012 Dec 15;380(9859):2163–2196.

5. Schmidt CO, Raspe H, Pfingsten M, et al. Back pain in the German adult population: prevalence, severity, and sociodemographic correlates in a multiregional survey. *Spine.* (Phila Pa 1976) 2007;32(18):2005–2011.

6. Cassidy JD, Carroll LJ, Cote P. The Saskatchewan health and back pain survey. The prevalence of low back pain and related disability in Saskatchewan adults. *Spine.* (Phila Pa 1976) 1998;23(17):1860–1866.

7. Lisi AJ, Brandt CA. Trends in the use and characteristics of chiropractic services in the Department of Veterans Affairs. *J Manipulative Physiol Ther.* 2016 Jun;39(5):381–386.

8. Nancarrow SA, Booth A, Ariss S, Smith T, Enderby P, Roots A. Ten principles of good interdisciplinary team work. *Hum Resource Health.* 2013;11:19.

CHAPTER THIRTEEN

Sports Chiropractic

Russ Ebbets, DC

Years ago, broadcaster Howard Cosell made his dismissive remark that "sport is the toy department of life." On one hand, his statement is surprising in that his broadcast vocation had given him a degree of notoriety that his study of law never did. On the other hand, while sport may never generate the level of concern warranted by religious strife or political acrimony, sport does have its own section in the newspaper.

For most chiropractors, involvement in sport is an opportunity to participate in a community event that may have local, regional, national, or even international exposure. The synergistic combination of the athlete and the chiropractor can produce a gestalt that is mutually beneficial. For the athlete, there is the enhanced performance and accelerated recovery. For the chiropractor, there is the nearly immediate feedback of a job well done.

The difficulty in defining sports chiropractic is that individual situations set parameters. Just as no two practices are alike, it is safe to say no two sports chiropractors will be exactly alike. They do have one thing in common, however: a background in, and love of, sports. At the end of this chapter is an interview with a sports chiropractor to illustrate this point.

Working Definition of Sports Chiropractic

One needs to develop a working definition of sports chiropractic that is general enough to be inclusive for most, yet restrictive to the point that it allows for definition of the services to be distinct and unique in its contribution to sports health care.

Parameter number one would be that the sports chiropractor deal with athletes. But even that can be open to debate. What exactly constitutes an athlete? Is an athlete someone who does something athletic? Do they need to be on a team? Are there age parameters that need to be met? Can an athlete be 7 or 70? Do they have to compete? What about a ballet dancer or someone who competes against style point tables?

Training and competition arise as two important qualifying criteria. The goal here is to be inclusive. An athlete is one who does something athletic that clearly demonstrates use of the five biomotor skills (speed, strength, endurance, flexibility, and the ABCs of agility, balance, coordination, and skill).

Therefore, the working definition of an athlete will be an individual who is involved in a physical activity that requires expression of the five biomotor skills and encourages regular training for the improvement or perfection of the skills involved in the discipline.

Thus defined, an athlete could be a ball sport person, an individual competitor in a road race or triathlon, a participant in an aesthetic activity (body building or dance), or the musician or martial artist whose discipline dictates movement perfection. Efforts to expand the definition to include all workers as athletes, although defensible, belabors the point.

With an athlete defined, the sports chiropractor becomes easier to define, as a practitioner who enhances and refines movement. Exactly how this is done will vary from one practitioner to the next, but it is safe to say that the successful sports chiropractor will possess adjusting (manipulation) skills for the spine and extremities, have a thorough knowledge of the role soft tissue plays in human locomotion, and include some flexibility techniques in the treatment arsenal. More than anything else, the treatments of the sports chiropractor will be a combination of all three.

It warrants mention that these three treatments will be hands-on and require no equipment other than one's hands and a treatment table. The reason for this is that mobile, on-site care often does not afford one access to the equipment of a private office.

Often the mobile site will not have electricity, which can preclude most treatment modalities. Even with the advent of battery-operated equipment, transport, security, and an 8-, 10-, or 12-hour day present equipment challenges that bring into question the wisdom, if not the feasibility, of most modalities.

One may counter with the suggestion of tool-assisted therapies that have recently shown great promise. While the evidence could not be disputed, the issue of transport and security arise again. Of even greater significance is the fact that most off-site treatments are "one and done" encounters without follow-up care. This care is frequently done on first-time, new patients for whom the usual bruising that accompanies tool-assisted work may prove troublesome without the benefit of follow-up care.

In current practice, the sports chiropractor will be defined as a trained professional possessing a unique set of skills that allows for the evaluation, treatment, and possibly management of spinal and extremity conditions using articular joint manipulation, soft tissue techniques, and flexibility work.

Athletic recipients of this care are individuals involved in activities that are characterized by movement-oriented training disciplines with one of the goals being an effective and efficient execution of technique. The goal of the training may be competitive or participatory, an aesthetic presentation, or achievement of a performance goal, with the common denominator being movement. The sports chiropractor facilitates that movement.

Force-Frequency-Duration

In the discipline of ergonomics, the mechanism used to describe how occupational injuries happen is neatly explained with the schematic diagram of force, frequency, and duration. Injury to the body is the result of too much force, too-frequent performance of the offending activity, or involvement in the activity for too long a time. It is no different in sport.

The pursuit of competitive excellence leaves no stone unturned. For the truly dedicated, this is a full-time 24/7 job. But the quest for the ever-elusive goal of excellence is not without its consequences. Daily training requires one to challenge physical, mental, and physiologic limits. While pain and the threat of injury may be ever present, the greatest challenge may be to strike a balance among the three.

Injury or susceptibility to injury can therefore be seen as an imbalance within the athlete. This is evident in the self-evaluations used to describe failed attempts ("I wanted it badly" or "I tried too hard"), hinting at an imbalance where one quality (mental, physical, or physiological) dominated to the detriment of the overall performance.

Interestingly, one of the biomotor skills is balance. While balance as a biomotor skill refers to a physical sense, this concept can be expanded to include the relationship of the mental, physical, and physiological. One of the true challenges becomes to maintain the triune balance while striving for perfection of the physical. Therefore, sport by its very design strives to create a situation that will be problematic, where success, on the one hand, creates an imbalance that must be addressed. The role of the sports health care team is to ensure that, as much as possible, individuals maintain balance as they pursue excellence. As with many things in life, this is easier said than done.

A foreshadowing of the problem or an early awareness can go a long way in designing programs that can help lessen the damage of superlative efforts. As the athlete moves through the ranks from novice to competitive to possibly an elite-level performer, he or she is not on this journey alone. There is often a team behind the team or the individual that helps ensure success along the way. The sports chiropractor is a member of that team.

In an effort to define this team, and in particular the contribution of the sports chiropractor, this chapter will tackle the process in three parts. The first part will endeavor to define the various aspects of sport that play a role in the development of the athlete. Defining the various components presents for the sports chiropractor aspects of sport that warrant attention. Training theory is the use of periodization and the programmed development that can be used to systematically develop an individual or team toward reaching their highest potential.

A second area of focus will be testing and research. While the individual solo practitioner may not have an interest or access to the technology to do either testing or research of any depth, it is critical to the larger process that she or he be well versed in the goals of such activities. Familiarity with testing protocols, their application, and interpretation of results is becoming critical in modern-day sport.

One of the themes that will be repeated here is that the "athletic life" of an athlete is short. The cliché "time is of the essence" is never truer. Poor decisions, misdirected thinking, or lost time due to injury individually or collectively can combine to shorten and even ruin careers. This is an unforgiveable circumstance, especially considering that these emerging innovative technologies allow the coach, athlete, and the support team to make qualified judgments based on scientifically supported literature.

The third and final area will be a discussion on the integration of the sports chiropractor into the larger health care team. Care documentation, standardization of procedures, the establishment of policies, and the integration of the various contributors of the health care team with the goal of providing the best care possible for the athlete needs to be clearly stated and understood. A prima donna role by any of the contributors is counterproductive and potentially disastrous, particularly in a finely tuned championship situation.

Providing care to athletes is a rich opportunity for all parties concerned. Throughout this process it must be underscored that this opportunity would necessarily have the interests of the athlete as a primary goal. To that end, we begin.

Training Theory and Elite Sport Science

Training theory will be defined as the use of periodic training loads with the goal of ever increasing the training load to improve work capacity and ultimately performance. Elite sport science is the application of science to sport for performance enhancement and accelerated recovery. Both these topics are multifaceted areas that encompass individual physiology, psychology, training theory, planning, and time management. The subtle combination and complement of these disparate disciplines makes for a challenge and hints at the complexity of modern-day athletic competition and training.

Time Management

The Russian training theorist Matveyev suggested that lack of time is the limiting factor in athletic development. While most high-level athletic careers last fewer than 10 years, and significantly less in some professional sports, it becomes incumbent on the coach, athlete, and the support staff to capitalize on the time available.

Use of the most effective training methods, emphasis on accelerated recovery, and preventive efforts to limit or eliminate the lost time of illness and injury all become components of a comprehensive time-management program.

Directed actions that use the time allotted for daily training, the achievement of seasonal goals, and the attainment of one's lifetime potential all loom as benchmarks for time used wisely. If a great life is made up of great moments, so is a great athletic career.

The Daily Training Plan

The daily training plan (DTP) is made up of components (drills, techniques, plays, actions) and may be completed with several groupings of these activities or several sessions over the course of a day. The DTP is the basic building block of a career; it is a single brick of a great wall.

Time and planning should take place so as to carefully integrate goals and objectives of the DTP with the larger goals and objectives of a weekly micro-training cycle, the monthly and seasonal plan, and ultimately the career plan.

Physical, Technical, Tactical, and Psychological Preparation

There is no doubt these four topics warrant their own paragraph, even chapter. What needs to be understood is that these topics should be integrated on both a vertical (daily) and horizontal (weekly, monthly, career) basis.

Physical preparation entails increasing the athlete's work capacity, the ability to handle ever-increasing training loads. An increased work capacity is seen as the most important quality in modern training. Sensible, directed training leads to the development of a broader base that would include not only the conditioning to successfully meet the physical demands of a sport but the development of the inventory of particular skills that characterizes each sport or discipline.

The refinement of technique and technical skills (i.e., basketball dribbling and shooting ability, football tackling techniques, sport power positions, etc.) are all dependent on the development or attainment of a level of physical conditioning. It would be unrealistic to expect a novice to dunk a basketball without the size, jumping ability, and maturity necessary to accomplish such a feat.

Tactical preparation and tactical execution is dependent on the ability to exhibit certain techniques in stressful game conditions. The ability of a distance runner to effectively employ surges midrace hinges on both the physiological qualities developed through hours and possibly years of training and the technical manipulation of running stride and arm carriage that allows for these surges to be physiologically efficient and repeated by the runner for an extended period of time.

Psychological preparation is the combination of will along with the development of such qualities as self-esteem, confidence, and a value system (honesty, integrity, hard work, etc.) that is fostered by a supportive environment, including teammates, the coaching staff, and the health care support staff.

Taken together, these four qualities should be promoted daily. It is the successful integration or blending of the four qualities that develops the whole athlete.

The Four Levels of Sport

Critical to this whole discussion is how one determines which level of athlete is being discussed. As noted above, there are many "athletic"-type activities. The reason for the distinction is that there are differing goals for the different athletes. Other areas of concern include the goals of training, the dangers and benefits of participation, and the potential types of injuries that may result from participation.

The entry level of most athletic activities is the *fundamental level* and is concerned with development. Movement patterns, physical skill development, interpersonal cooperation, and an understanding of the importance of managed growth characterize this stage. Note that when done correctly, winning and/or stellar individual efforts are of secondary concern.

The largest level that lasts the longest time is the *fitness level.* Athletic activities used at this level are to accomplish or maintain the perceived health benefits of athletic involvement (weight management, social outlet, cardiovascular fitness). Training is periodic (two or three times per week), and the activities are linear in nature with emphasis on the aerobic paradigm of fitness.

The *performance level* is competitive sport. Training may include five or more sessions per week. The stated goal is physical improvement and competitive effort. This improvement may approach the physical, mental, or emotional limits of the athlete. Overtraining, illness, and physical injury are ever-present circumstances. Although this level of sport may last only 10 years, the long-term consequences may be life altering. The Russians characterized work done in the performance level as not a natural or healthy thing to do with the body.

The final level of sport is split into two parts—*pre-hab and rehab work.* Pre-hab efforts are noncompetitive drills that condition the body for the stresses and strains of day-to-day training. Effective pre-hab work identifies weak links in an athlete through focused work of isometric, concentric, and eccentric movements strengthening and stabilizing joint complexes that allows for safer and smoother technical execution.

Rehab, or rehabilitation, efforts serve to restore the ill or injured athlete to a trainable state so that there can be resumption of activity, particularly to accomplish performance goals. It warrants note that rehab efforts are the result of previous work having gone "wrong," an inappropriate training load that the athlete is not prepared for. There has been an inappropriate amount of force, frequency, or duration. In the grand scheme, especially in the performance level, the problem with rehab efforts is that they represent lost time in the athlete's life that will never be recovered.

Progressive Overload

The mythological story of Milo and the bull has been used for ages to explain progressive overload. Milo was given a pair of calves, and every day he lifted the calves from the ground. Over time, the calves grew to bulls and Milo's strength grew proportionally. Eventually he was able to lift the two fully grown bulls off the ground.

Progressive overload as a training method consistently challenges the body by making physical feats incrementally more difficult. This gradually increases the work capacity, which is one of the requirements of modern training theory. Note that this increase must be gradual.

Attempts to subvert this process by accelerating development can result in overtraining, illness, and injury. The use of ergogenic aids, such as anabolic steroids, can result in unbalanced development between muscle and tendon, resulting in soft tissue rupture. Periodic physical testing, daily monitoring of sleep quality, and heart rate monitoring are methods that allow one to safely increase this work capacity.

Volume and Intensity

Volume and intensity are a classic training dichotomy that speaks to the necessary balance between how much work is being done (volume) and at what effort level (intensity).

With regard to the different levels of sport, the input of volume and intensity can vary greatly. At the fundamental level, volume is necessarily low, as is intensity. The thought is that the body's energies should be directed toward growth and development. Significant training volumes and intensities effectively steal energies that could be used for growth and development. The future is spent on the present.

At the fitness level, the routine of periodic exercise will dictate both volume and intensity. While there may be days where the perceived workload is "easy" and other days where the same workload is more difficult, the workload has essentially remained the same. With no immediate performance goal, the fitness level is generally characterized by a simpler, manageable, and repeating workload.

At the performance level, the complexities of training volumes and intensities come to the fore. Traditionally, these qualities are developed in a step pattern: the athlete performs a certain volume of work until his or her performance eventually plateaus, then the intensity is increased and the athlete performs the new workload until he or she again plateaus, at which point the volume is increased again, and so on. The process is repeated step by step.

Too rapid an increase in either volume or intensity can produce overtraining, illness, or injury. This overtraining has been further divided with too much volume resulting in parasympathetic nervous system overtraining and too much intensity resulting in sympathetic overtraining.

Growth and Development

While growth and development play a central role in the fundamental stage of sport, they also play a significant role in the fitness and performance levels.

The importance of growth and development is neatly summed up with the statement "all things only grow once." Carefully prescribed volumes and intensities combined with managed training and competition can create an inventory of skills that can serve the novice well as she or he progresses to the performance level. The converse is also true. Too much work, too soon, combined with excessive expectations of a "win at all costs" mentality and "no pain, no gain" advice can rapidly negate potential.

Growth may have slowed for many at the performance level, but there is nonetheless a period where exceptional changes may take place. The ability to capitalize on this final step of the maturing process and the subsequent adaptations can have a significant impact on ultimate performance.

At the fitness level, development may outweigh growth. In fact, exercise has been touted as an antiaging mechanism. The development these athletes undergo may be a combination of weight management, improved cardiovascular health, and general feelings of well-being.

Longevity

Longevity is defined as the time immediately past full maturity where one endeavors to delay the inevitable erosion of one's biomotor skills due to age, accidents, or the accumulated damage of athletic participation over a lifetime. Personal responsibility combined with a sensible and progressive training plan and a certain amount of luck come together to delay the inevitable progression of time.

In today's professional sports marketplace, longevity can be translated into millions, if not tens of millions of dollars. Attention to the refinement of personal habits and preventive measures can delay the onset of the erosion of one's biomotor skills and may help maintain a consistent level of performance.

Longevity is also a concern for the fitness athlete. Aging baby boomers who have had a lifetime of active lifestyles welcome the opportunity to sustain these activity levels. In fact, pithy statements such as "40 is the new 30" support this general intent.

Recovery

It is a simple fact that all improvement comes during recovery. Improvement is a direct result of recovery. Fully one-half of Yakolev's model is the recovery portion of the curve.

The unfortunate reality is that for most athletes and their support staff, recovery is a marginalized time period poorly regarded and misunderstood.

While recovery is a natural rebound process, most would agree that just as late hours, alcohol abuse, and a smoking habit could negatively affect recovery, consistent sleep patterns, proper nutrition, and adequate hydration all contribute positively to the restoration of the body's energy systems.

It stands to reason that if positive actions contribute to one's performance and directly contribute to one's longevity, there would be greater emphasis on the recovery efforts as opposed to letting natural processes simply unfold.

Athletes, coaches, and sports chiropractors in the know would argue that one needs to "recover as hard as one trains." Just as there is attention to detailed daily training plans, so there should be a time-management plan for the recovery time before the next bout of exercise.

A more complete recovery will allow one to increase one's work capacity over time, theoretically increasing performance potential. For the fitness athlete, a 10-minute warm down, a quick shower, and a satisfying meal may do the trick. For the performance athlete, it cannot be that simple.

Peaking

Peaking is a major concern for the performance-level athlete. It involves a reduction in the training workload for 10–14 days before a terminal or other important competition. This reduced workload allows the body's systems to rebound to a rested or even super-rested state that can allow for a stellar performance.

Peaking means different things to different sports. Ball sports teams can exhibit a peak performance by highly synchronous play. Aesthetic presentation activities (ballet, gymnastics, figure skating, etc.) exhibit peaking by the refinement and demonstration of technical elements and grand symmetric movements. Individual sports, such as track-and-field events or triathlons, exhibit peaking with both the refinement of technical (movement) execution and the efficiency of speed, power, and physiologic systems.

One of the common denominators for all sports in the peaking phase of a season is the emphasis on speed of execution of a particular activity. Viewed in this light, it should be evident that the team or individual athlete that is better able to execute desired actions more quickly and for a longer period of time has a greater probability of success.

Injury Prevention

It bears mentioning that no one participates in sport with the goal of becoming injured. Yet the reality is that on any given day, significant macro trauma may occur or the accumulation of a series of micro traumas may present that results in injury.

The role injuries play in the various levels of sport can be significant. In the fundamental stage, training should be of such short duration and low intensity that repetitive activities should not create overuse injuries. More recently, the wisdom of contact and collision sports for children has come into question. With these sports, macro traumas are inevitable and conceivably stifle development.

Fitness-based efforts within the aerobic paradigm tend to be linear activities. Running, stair climbing, cycling, and rollerblading all involve the repetition of movement in essentially a straight line. If the accumulation of micro traumas from workout to workout exceeds the body's ability for recovery and repair, an injury will result.

Often the injury that occurs is damage to the ligaments, tendons, or joint capsules due to the highly specific, linear movements. What is lacking in these linear movements are actions that create dynamic stabilization to the joint capsules and multilateral or multiaxial movements that are generally absent from most fitness-based programs.

For the performance athlete, injuries represent lost time in either development or participation and can negatively impact performance over a season or career. The health and well-being of an athlete necessarily becomes a preeminent goal of the coaching and support staff. But a large part of the responsibility for the athlete's health falls on the athlete. It is the athlete's conscientious preparation, attention to the details of warm-up and pre-hab efforts, and active role in recovery efforts that can help or hurt a team or career.

To that end, it becomes incumbent on all parties involved to work to identify problem areas or weak points in a training system or athletic physical makeup. Time spent devising means and methods to preempt or prevent injury from occurring is invaluable. This is where attention to pre-hab efforts can play a critical preventive role.

Pre-hab efforts need not take an extensive amount of time at the fundamental, fitness, or performance levels. Focus on problem areas (foot strength, ankle and knee stability, core stability, the rotator cuff, neck stability) may help to tone muscles with patterns that negate or lessen the damage of contact/collision or highly repetitive efforts.

One of the common denominators of all successful teams and individual athletes is the ability to avoid injury. Admittedly, there is an element of luck in this. But the more conscientiously one prepares, the more well thought out one's pre-hab efforts, the luckier one gets.

Sports Psychology

Sports psychology is a book unto itself. Nonetheless, it warrants a cursory mention as its import is that of a cornerstone, if not foundational quality, to sports performance.

Reduced to its most basic level, sports psychology is the role of self-esteem in an athlete's life. The core belief that "I can do this" is the starting point for all education, relationships, and performance. It is the responsibility of parents, coaches, and important others to instill this quality in the developing child right through to the most elite performer.

As one progresses through different levels of sport, the role and function of sports psychology changes. For the novice in the entry levels of sport, concepts such as personal responsibility, personal discipline, cooperation, and teamwork can, with maturity, allow the athlete to evolve into a teammate that can subjugate individual aspirations for team goals.

For the fitness athlete, the fostering of such qualities as dedication, goal setting, and personal discipline can enhance both the effectiveness and enjoyment of an athletic lifestyle. Personal improvement is incremental change, and while change can be intimidating, the only thing produced by the status quo is the status quo. The importance of accepting a challenge with an "I can do this" attitude cannot be overemphasized.

For the performance athlete, sports psychology can often mean the difference between victory and defeat. High-level concepts such as willfulness, controlled aggression, autogenic training, and the fostering of Duckworth's grit all have a role.

Core Stability

A stable core is one of the qualities that has come to be seen as necessary to safely produce power, acceleration, or something as seemingly mundane as quickly getting up off the ground. A stable core musculature, the muscles that stabilize the lumbar spine and pelvis, are closely linked to one's ability to dynamically stabilize the hips, which in turn allows one to generate power and acceleration.

As more time is dedicated to pre-hab efforts and exercises designed to focus on development of these muscles, the incidence of instability-related injuries will decrease.

Balance work on wobble boards or with exercise balls has proven to be a simple and effective means to address core stability. Rhythmic exercises with the reintroduction of minimally weighted objects addresses, in part, the timing and sequence of movements that can be both preventive in nature while also aiding performance.

Stationary isometric work, such as planks and back bridging, helps address the health of the holding elements, such as ligaments and tendons, and musculotendinous transition zones. Attention to these structures can help ensure healthy participation in both the long and short terms.

It has often been repeated that before one can be mobile one must be stable. Core stability is a training method that is easy to overlook in that it is a form of invisible training. Yet at whatever level of participation an athlete presents her or his enjoyment of sport, the recipient of the benefits of sport or his or her performance in sport will be enhanced with a history of core stability work.

Strength and Conditioning

Strength and conditioning as a professional discipline is approaching some 30 years of existence. Based on research, its incremental growth has moved the science of physical preparation away from anecdotal chatter and locker-room myth to the reproducible data of the science lab.

As the understanding and application of periodization has spread, there has also been a greater acceptance of the speed-strength or power paradigm. While the impact of strength and conditioning has been minimal in the fundamental levels of sport, it has made a significant contribution to both fitness and performance athletes.

The emphasis on proper techniques and the sequencing of the phases of training help to ensure safety and longevity of participation. Attention to flawless technical execution presents all athletes with a standard of preparation that helps promote safe participation.

Anatomical Adaptation

It would be difficult to pinpoint where the overreliance on the visual presentation gets its credence. No doubt this could be traced back to some archetypal action. We all like pretty things. While one's outward appearance may give clues, the adage of beauty being skin deep is true.

What is not apparent, even with a thorough visual inspection, is the functional integrity of the holding elements of the joints, ligaments, tendons, joint capsules, and the fascial planes that crisscross the body. Individually and in total, these tissues combine to form an invisible substructure that can be leveraged by the muscles and levers of the skeletal system to produce movements that are both graceful and powerful.

Davis's Law has long taught that the body adapts to the stresses placed upon it. Throughout the course of an athlete's life, the starts and stops, twists and turns have led to adaptations by the holding elements in and around a joint.

When the athlete's actions are balanced, and before the technical breakdown of fatigue, the holding elements strengthen in their abilities. Once training and competition has exceeded the ability of these tissues to withstand the strain, micro trauma can result, which can progress globally into aberrant movement patterns or present locally as ligament, tendon, or joint injury.

The aesthetic qualities of an athletic figure aside, it is the integrity of the invisible holding elements, this invisible substructure, that can work to ensure both short- and long-term health.

Multilateral Development

Fifty years ago, people spoke of the athletically gifted as "all-around athletes." Classically, these would be three-sport athletes throughout high school and even into college. Today, one can hear commentators speak of a player's "athleticism," but with increasing frequency the three-sport athlete has been replaced by the athlete that is solely a soccer player, basketball player, or runner on a year-round basis. Often this early specialization happens well before the age of 18, and this can present a problem.

Early specialization can negate multilateral development. This can be particularly problematic for the developing athlete in the fundamental level. One of the training goals with the novice athlete is to create an "inventory of skills." This inventory is a series of movement patterns that can be called upon to negotiate technical and tactical challenges presented by physical development, maturity, and the competitive nature of the performance level. Attaining these skills helps develop the neural pathways that can be refined throughout life.

The problem arises when this time for development is traded for an early and excessive competition schedule load. In the fundamental level, priority must be given to growth and development over training and competition.

Multilateral development is closely linked to anatomical adaptation. All-around development challenges the holding elements of the joint capsules, the ligaments, tendons, fascial planes, and musculotendinous junctions at a microscopic level. By developing the inventory of skills, these structures become better able to withstand the stresses and strains of training and competition.

In a very real sense, the multilateral development of the fundamental level is a pre-hab effort for the fitness and performance levels to come later in life. Early specialization often stifles multilateral development.

At the performance level, the import of multilateral development is lessened but still plays a critical role in the development and overall health of an athlete. At this stage, during early portions of a season or yearly plan, there is greater emphasis on multilateral development. It should be noted that pre-hab efforts on a daily basis should, however briefly, address multilateral development issues.

At the fitness level, multilateral development issues, although secondary, still play an important role in both daily enjoyment and exercise longevity. Due to the linear nature of most fitness programs, the dynamic stabilizers of the hip and foreleg atrophy, and their contribution to stability of the leg becomes compromised. The use of side planks, side lunges, foot drills, and other multiaxial movements can tone these muscles, better enabling them to handle the onslaught of repetitive motion.

Multilateral development is another form of invisible training, along with core stability, psychological preparation, and anatomical adaptation. While the importance of this quality shifts from level to level, its contribution cannot be denied and should not be ignored.

Testing and Research

The life of a high-performance athlete is short. Various professional sports track this statistic with startling results. Professional football players last on average a little more than three years. Professional baseball players last slightly more than five years. For many, a lifetime of preparation yields only moments of fleeting glory. All would agree that time is of the essence.

With these shortened life spans, the use of time in practice sessions on a given day or over longer periods (weeks, seasons) underscores the necessity managing this time intelligently. While the years of experience of a coach cannot be negated, there are limits to the accuracy of any human

sensory analysis, especially when success is often measured in hun-
dredths if not thousandths of a second. This fact becomes particularly
pertinent when one is faced with critical decisions, such as when to
increase or decrease training or whether a training method is working.

To that end, periodic testing can be an invaluable tool to a coach and
the athlete's support team. A rigorous, science-based testing program can
glean information that can be applied across a wide range of ability levels
that in turn will allow these athletes to safely and more thoroughly
approach their potential.

One cannot mention testing without discussing how testing can be
used to clarify the development of biomotor skills. Speed, strength,
endurance, flexibility, and the ABCs of agility, balance, coordination, and
skill are the fundamental building blocks of all athletic endeavors.

The ability of the coach to isolate and quantify the contribution each of
these skills make individually or in combination can be representative of
the efficacy of one's overall training regimen. Such questions as those
regarding improvement, health status, efficacy of training, overall development, and even long-term potential can be answered with the intelligent design of a series of simple test procedures that take 30 minutes or
less to execute.

There are currently multiple technologies available that can isolate
these qualities and interface with computers so that the data generated
can be interpreted, stored, and correlated so that future decisions are not
left to chance.

This possibility has far-reaching consequences at all levels of sport.
National governing bodies could accumulate this data as a means to identify, develop, and manage future talent. The widespread use of the information gleaned may help direct a child's choice of sport toward areas in
which he or she has the greatest potential to excel. If all things only grow
once, this circumvents the possibility of growing in the wrong direction.

The testing of fitness-level athletes allows these athletes the chance to
safely pursue the benefits of their lifelong fitness program by measuring
movement patterns and body symmetry with the ability to identify asymmetries and imbalances that, with the predominantly repetitive nature of
these activities, present the greatest injury risk.

Periodic testing would go a long way toward promoting longevity. A battery of simple tests using the Optojump system and a simple treadmill can
record ground contact times and document movement asymmetries that
could be addressed before these movements blossom into full-fledged injury.

For the performance athlete, the benefits of a comprehensive testing
program bear the greatest fruits. During the last few years, the National

Football League Combine Tests have generated significant press. The testing of athletes for performance dates back at least 50 years.

Soviet sport scientists recognized early on that certain correlations could be made between the performance of certain athletic activities and the ability to start quickly, accelerate, or jump. The Soviets came up with an inventory of tests, termed "stage control tests," that are able to translate into highly accurate predictors of athletic performance.

While these tests are admittedly low tech and unsophisticated by today's standards, they have nonetheless served their purpose well in terms of talent identification, monitoring health status, or quantifying the state of development. Data was produced that could be correlated and scrutinized over the short and long terms, all with the goal of perfecting the development of the athlete.

What constitutes a test? The list can begin with simple actions like a vertical jump, standing long jump, standing triple jump, or bounding for five steps for distance on one leg. More sophisticated tests could include bounding 100 meters while counting steps, bounding upward on right versus left leg (drift protocol), or timing and visual recording of a drop jump test.

With the evolution of the strength and conditioning profession, the ability to monitor development has greatly legitimized the use of testing as a means to identify talent, monitor changes and progress of a training plan, and finally monitor progress of rehabilitation efforts and a safe return to play.

Testing can also be used to place an athlete in an appropriate training group, predict performance, identify potential weaknesses, measure improvement, and serve as a motivational tool. Both in terms of assessing the efficacy of a current training plan or to chart a future direction, testing can offer a clearer, more documentable means to make logical decisions.

All major sports now pride themselves on the metrics or numerical data that practice sessions and individual athletes generate. While it is possible to effectively become paralyzed with all the data produced, it is also possible to gain a competitive advantage through a skillful application of this information and knowledge that may lead to a refinement of current practices and research design that pursues uncharted frontiers of human excellence.

Sports Health Care and Sports Outreach

A grounded understanding of training theory and the intricacies of elite sport science and an appreciation of testing and research can offer a significant and unique contribution to an athlete and his or her sports health care team.

The unifying thread in this process is the treatment rendered. The ability to effectively deliver an adjustment, identify and treat soft tissue dysfunction, and provide flexibility work constitutes a level of care that is unique and in demand.

The high level of clinical skills necessary for success in one's home office are no different than those needed on the field. There will always be the challenge of patient presentation. A sharpening of one's observational and palpatory skills is required for on-site care. As a rule, the sophisticated diagnostic equipment one may be accustomed to in the home office will not be available for on-site care.

The efficient performance of a range of examination procedures, including range-of-motion testing and neurologic, posture, soft tissue, and chiropractic exams, is critical to develop a standard of care that the public has come to recognize and expect.

The widespread use of set procedures and protocols would also help integrate chiropractic into the larger sports health care team. Paperwork and record keeping thus become a necessary component of care.

The remainder of this chapter will discuss a variety of topics germane to the treatment rendered to athletes. It should be noted that the topics discussed are within the paradigm of the athletic triage model. While there are sports chiropractors that can "do it all" in terms of offering emergency medical service, athletic training services, and chiropractic care for performance enhancement, this does not represent true integration of the profession into a larger health care team.

This reality becomes especially clear in larger events. The ability to manage hundreds or even thousands of athletes safely requires a well-coordinated health care support team whose fluid and coordinated actions save time but can also save someone's life. The coordination of these individual players begins with an emergency plan.

The Emergency Plan

Murphy's Law cynically states that if anything can go wrong, it will. While this may be an exaggeration, it speaks to the meticulous planning that must go into coverage for a sporting event.

It should be a given that at any time, anything can happen. Someone goes into anaphylactic shock from a bee sting, a broken bat lodges in a player's neck, a 17-year-old suffers a heart attack, a runner charges into a fire hydrant, a bomb goes off in the stadium—these may all be one-in-a-million shots, but modern coverage necessitates plans for all these eventualities. Today might be your day.

For the emergency medical service personnel, life-threatening situations are weekly if not daily occurrences. Taxonomies of thought and hierarchies of needs are part and parcel of the job. Calm under pressure, decisive, and action oriented, these professionals manage evolving and fluid situations with poise and aplomb.

The problem for many volunteers is that their duty may be an annual contribution to a community event. While no one hopes or plans for a catastrophic event, the reality may be only seconds away and may necessitate a response in less time than it has taken to read these four paragraphs.

For the annual volunteer, wishful thinking equates with poor planning. Having a functional emergency plan in which all parties involved understand their defined roles can make a dire situation unfold as seamlessly as possible and can mean the difference between life and death.

To ensure that this process unfolds in an orderly manner, pre-event meetings are essential. All parties must be on the same page as to responsibilities and their role in the larger plan. Their willingness to function in this capacity is essential to the success of the plan. Egotism is reckless. It is the true functioning of this team that can make the difference between life and death.

The team must establish communication channels and methods and consider a slew of seemingly mundane topics, such as who will have the keys to locked doors and gates, who will direct traffic for the incoming and outgoing ambulance, and who will manage crowd control and how. Set plans with practiced scenarios can bring order to seemingly chaotic situations.

An emergency plan is initiated by the individual who "first responds." Stabilizing the patient as possible and activating the emergency process are the first two orders of business. The activation of the emergency plan sets off a cascade of actions that ultimately provides a safety net for the ill or injured patient, rendering the necessary treatment as quickly as possible.

The nature of the sport may dictate different levels of precautions. To exclude or ignore planning simply because it is deemed unnecessary or because "that could never happen" is naive thinking at best and reckless thinking at worst. Although one hopes to never have to initiate the emergency plan, the time and planning that go into it are directly proportional to the timely actions that may save a life.

Credentialing and Travel to Treat

The days of the chiropractor practicing on athletes outside the fence are long gone. Most large events provide chiropractic care as a complimentary service to athletes, officials, and meet administrators as they progress through a day's event. That being said, credentialing has become one of the hallmarks of acceptance and recognition of the service by event directors. For security purposes, credentialing may entail badges hung from neck lanyards and strategic checkpoints that scan the badges. While one can view this whole process as a nuisance or an opportunity to obtain a souvenir, it is part of the price of admission for today's larger sporting events.

Within the United States, the scope of practice can vary significantly from state to state, depending greatly on the particular political climate within each state as the chiropractic profession achieved licensure and legislative recognition. Be that as it may, the overall intent is to ensure the services rendered by individual professions meet certain standards that protect the public's welfare.

Some state associations have a magnanimous stance on visiting professions, recognizing the levels of expertise and competence of visiting professionals. Other states do not. This can present a problem for the sports chiropractor who travels from one state to another as an individual's personal physician (e.g., a tennis player, boxer, or golfer) or as a team physician (e.g., basketball team, collegiate program).

While these traveling chiropractors do not offer their services to the general public, they are in effect practicing chiropractic in a jurisdiction where they are not licensed. Interpretations of this concept of "travel to treat" are the right and responsibility of the legislative body within each state. The problem may arise when a particularly conservative or parochial association practices in a very restrictive manner that presents a barrier for traveling athletes to receive the care they are accustomed to from favored team physicians.

While it could be argued that the standardization of care promoted above with specific practices (soft tissue, adjusting, and stretching) and the use of common paperwork intake forms would help standardize sports chiropractic, the reality is a different story.

The solution to this obstacle seems to lie with the national associations and their ability to align the various states and devise a national plan or procedure similar to that of a driver's license that would allow the traveling chiropractor the opportunity and right to provide care to individual athletes and teams without skirting any jurisdictional restrictions.

Paperwork

There is an old legal adage that states that if you don't write it down it never happened. It seems unconscionable that in this day and age someone would practice health care without keeping meticulous records. Yet in the not-too-distant past, records and record keeping were aspects of sports chiropractic that were not practiced and simply ignored.

While this old position is legally indefensible, it is equally unfortunate as it does not create a clear picture of the contribution a sports chiropractor can make. Record keeping produces a paper trail that in turn creates a clinical picture of not only individual athletes but also the services and treatments provided; it clarifies the unique skills the sports chiropractor brings to the treatment site.

The generation of treatment statistics produces solid evidence of the number of patients cared for, their presenting conditions, the techniques and skills necessary to treat those conditions, and, if used over time, the efficacy of treatments and services. For an event organizer, the generation of statistics helps justify the expense of a provided service and clarifies its use. For allied health care providers, treatment statistics clarify exactly what contribution the sports chiropractor makes to the larger sports health care picture. This awareness helps foster understanding, appreciation, and communication that would in turn foster intelligent referrals (as opposed to "dumping" a patient) and a stronger, cohesive support network for the athlete.

From an educational standpoint, the generation of statistics helps direct or redirect educational programs so that the efficacy of treatments can be refined, potentially accelerating and smoothing the learning curve of future sports chiropractors so that they are better prepared and more efficient in their actions.

In sum, modern-day health care demands the level of accountability thorough record keeping produces. In both the immediate and long terms, the generation of statistics serves the best interests of all parties involved in the event: organizer, fellow health care providers, current athletes, and future generations.

It bears mentioning that the records kept would most likely show significant differences if treatment is rendered in the home office versus an on-site treatment. Athletes presenting to one's office would be processed using the standard office paperwork. This practice makes sense on several levels. One would expect that athletes reporting to a private practice would have a longer-term relationship with the presenting physician. It would only make sense to process the athlete in the standard way. The athlete(s) come to the doctor. With on-site treatment, the doctor travels to the athlete(s). There are several other points that warrant mention. Frequently this doctor-patient relationship will be a one-time treatment. While the nature of the relationship will not change, the term of the relationship will. To that end, the use of lengthy exam forms, folders, and other standard practices of the home office would prove to be cumbersome and an obstacle to care.

Standard of Care

"Standard of care" is a medical-legal term that defines the level of knowledge, skills, and abilities a health care professional should possess. While it would be expected that the chiropractor by his or her very nature should be able to adjust the various areas of the body, this may not be the case.

An important determinant in the standard of care is the defined scope of practice. Scope of practice in the United States can vary slightly to significantly from one state to the next. Components that are included within the scope of practice are procedures and protocols, the use of various therapeutic modalities, the use of various diagnostic modalities, knowledge of the rules and regulations for a particular state, and even whether or not the chiropractor may use the designation "physician."

Standards of care for the sports chiropractor are loosely defined in the two postgraduate courses: the chiropractic sports physician certificate, and extensive study of its diplomate counterpart. While achievement of these certificate programs ensures a level of knowledge, the lack of a rigorous practical component can present an experience gap.

The standard of care within sports chiropractic dictates the chiropractor should possess exceptional skills adjusting the spine and extremities, a method to address the soft tissue, and a method of stretching various areas of the body. These three skills present a safe and effective means for treating the majority of athletes presenting for care.

Additional skills, such as tool-assisted work, functional movement taping techniques, and the knowledge of modalities can make an important contribution but may prove problematic due to the equipment necessary, its transportation, and the availability of electricity. It warrants mention that international travel may present with different power supply options, further complicating the use of modalities.

A third area that can significantly enhance the quality of care is the use of a standardized intake form. The form should concisely document an athlete's reason for seeking care, a focal history, and a review of systems. It should also provide space to record exam procedures, including orthopedic and neurologic findings, palpatory soft tissue and bony listings, a documented treatment plan, informed consent statement, and recommendations for further care or referral to another health care provider for follow-up care.

Not only does a consistent use of a standardized intake form allow for the abovementioned procedures to be documented event by event, using it allows the sports chiropractor to document the frequency of treatments rendered (adjusting, soft tissue, stretching, etc.). Other important information, such as age ranges, presenting conditions, the number of first-time patients, and the total number of patient visits, can be important information for future reference.

Through consistent record keeping, one can foster a standard of care that can be reproduced event to event. Additionally, good records provide a defensible form of risk management while also generating statistics, allowing for a more exacting postevent report that clearly details the use of services, which will help when planning future events.

Summary

Sports chiropractic is a subspecialty of the chiropractic profession with a unique set of skills and abilities. As with anything else, the knowing comes with the doing. Classroom education can only do so much to mimic the excitement, drama, and trying moments of a live, on-site experience. As sports chiropractors have gained greater access to sporting events through traditional avenues, their presence has become an integral contributor to the success of teams and individual athletes. An interview with a practicing sports chiropractor follows.

Interview with a Sports Chiropractor

Dr. Ira Shapiro is a sports chiropractor and two-time member of the U.S. Olympic team medical staff. He shares how he came to be a sports chiropractor and some of the highlights of his career.

How did you get into sports chiropractic?
"Sports chiropractic was a natural progression. Being an athlete all my life, I experienced sports injuries firsthand. Whether traumatic or overuse, the understanding of how and why injuries occur has greatly aided the evaluation, diagnosis, treatment, and rehabilitation of the sports injuries I experienced personally.

"As I treated athletes and they saw the benefits of sports chiropractic care, they realized I understood injuries from their point of view. My sports involvement and chiropractic education taught me the value of specific treatments designed to return them to the field of play ASAP."

What type of preparation did you have?

"I received my DC from Palmer College of Chiropractic in Davenport, Iowa. *However, graduating with a degree is not the end of an education, but only the beginning.* You are provided with a basic level of learning that must be continued in the field with real-world experiences. Chiropractic has many specialties. For me, it was sports chiropractic.

"My focus is on correcting athletes' biomechanical misalignments caused by faulty movement patterns and peripheral nerve entrapments that affect their performance. You need to keep up with advances in techniques and new methods for evaluating and treating sports injuries. The more you can evaluate a problem from different viewpoints, the better the chance of diagnosing and treating the more difficult cases. Not everything works on everyone. You have to be able to change your thought process if the treatment protocols are not correcting the cause of the biomechanical misalignments. That is why I pursued postgraduate certifications in a number of areas related to sports injury:

- CCSP (certified chiropractic sports physician)
- DACBSP (diplomate of the American Chiropractic Board of Sports Physicians)
- ICCSP (international certified chiropractic sport physician)
- EMT (emergency medical technician)
- CPR instructor
- Certified Active Release Technique (ART, for upper extremity, lower extremity, spine)
- Certified kinesio taping
- Certified functional and kinetic treatment with rehabilitation, provocation, and motion (FAKTR)"

What type of preparation did you wish you had but had to catch up on later?

"When I was in school, the emphasis was on the central nervous system and spinal biomechanics. In sports chiropractic, the extremities play an important role which were not part of the curriculum. I had to refocus my learning on movement patterns, peripheral nerve entrapments, soft tissue, and functional taping techniques. These additional certifications are supplemental and helped me excel in the field of sports chiropractic."

What do you find most fulfilling and inspiring about your career in sports chiropractic?

"There is nothing more fulfilling for a sports chiropractor than to represent your profession and your country at the highest level of athletic competition. Walking in the opening ceremonies of the Olympics as a member of the U.S. Olympic team medical staff was exhilarating for me as well as an accomplishment for the profession. Just as rewarding was my experience at the Pan American Games held in Guadalajara, Mexico. Due to my emergency procedures background, I was also assigned as a mat physician for the combat sports competitions held at the training center of the State Council for Sport Promotion and Youth Support (CODE) in Jalisco, just outside of Guadalajara. I worked alongside the facility's permanent medical staff, providing care to competitors engaged in approximately 50 daily matches of taekwondo, judo, and/or wrestling. I got to see Mexico from the point of view of the local doctors, not as a tourist. I ate in the local small cafe/bistro just like the locals. I saw where they lived and the types of houses they lived in and I was able to see things through their eyes. It was very rewarding to get to experience Mexico as a Mexican, not an American."

Do you have an experience that you feel captures the essence of this practice?
"At the Olympics in Turin, Italy, I was introduced to the skip of the U.S. curling team. I inquired about his right shoulder and left hip. He looked at me with a puzzled look and asked, 'Have we met before?' I said 'no.' 'Do you curl?' he asked. I replied I did not. Then he asked, 'How did you know about my shoulder and hip?' The movement patterns in the sport of curling are similar to those in bowling. I worked with the Pro Bowlers Tour for a number of years and was familiar with the sport's common overuse and repetitive motion injuries. This allowed me to transfer that knowledge to a sport with similar movement patterns—curling. Understanding these biomechanical and muscular movement patterns enabled me to better relate to their sport. I spent a lot of time working with the U.S. curling team at that Olympics. This was the first time a U.S. curling team ever won a medal in Olympic competition!"

What is your advice for other DCs who would like to become involved in this type of practice?
"They should begin with the sports they are most familiar with, including the ones they played. This knowledge will provide a deeper understanding of the biomechanics and injuries associated with that sport.

"Next, they must become proficient in not only spinal and extremity manipulation but also in soft tissue and functional taping techniques. There are postgraduate certification programs in sports injury that teach the basics. Chiropractors should be certified and then work actively in the field to further the principles taught in those classes. Start low. Aim high. As your skills and reputation for treating sport injuries grow, so will the opportunities for treating more diverse athletes and even those competing at the highest levels."

Summary

The ever-evolving nature of sport offers a tremendous opportunity but also a tremendous challenge for current and future sports chiropractors to remain on the cutting edge of their discipline. Just as coaches and athletes train relentlessly to sharpen their skills, the challenge for sports chiropractors is to remain on the cutting edge of their discipline through a thorough understanding of the dynamics of sport and the increasingly important role of testing and research and the ability to turn stumbling blocks into stepping-stones.

Note: Chapter 7 provides information on U.S. chiropractic colleges offering training in sports chiropractic, and Chapter 10 describes additional training and practice opportunities for sports chiropractors.

CHAPTER FOURTEEN

Future Directions for the Chiropractic Profession and Chiropractic Education[*]

Carl S. Cleveland III, DC; and
Michael R. Wiles, DC, MEd, MS

This concluding chapter presents perspectives ranging from those of highly experienced chiropractic educators to those of chiropractic students.

The Doctor of Chiropractic: An Emerging Role in the Future of Health Care

Carl S. Cleveland III, DC

Dr. Cleveland is the president of Cleveland University–Kansas City. His grandparents founded Cleveland Chiropractic College in 1922.

Increasingly, policy makers, third-party payers, and patients are seeking greater accountability from the health system and from individual physicians and care providers. This accountability is benchmarked by the

---

[*] Portions of this chapter have been reprinted from Carl S. Cleveland III, DC. "Chiropractic: Healing with a Human Touch." *The Advisor: The Journal of the National Association of Advisors for the Health Profession*, vol. 34, no. 4, December 2014, pp. 19–35. Reprinted with permission from the editor.

three goals of *improved outcomes*, *lower costs*, and *patient satisfaction*. For the profession of chiropractic, results related to these goals to date suggest an enhanced role in the future.

Trends including consumer interest in a nonpharmacological approach to health, public concern for side effects, the epidemic of opioid addiction, and an aging "boomer" population seeking to remain mobile and active in their golden years create opportunity for an expanding role for doctors of chiropractic (DCs). Couple these trends with over two decades of outcomes research demonstrating effectiveness, value, and cost savings of chiropractic spine care and chiropractic has an opportunity to position itself as the respected authority for conservative, first-contact, primary spine care for structural health and well-being.

Filling a Need for Conservative Spine and Musculoskeletal Care: Chiropractic's Role Looking Forward

Integrative Care for Low Back Pain: Chiropractic—A Nonopioid Approach to Care

The cover of *Time* magazine, June 15, 2015, described the issue of opioid overuse clearly: "They're the most powerful pain killers ever invented. And they're creating the worst addiction crisis America has ever seen."[1] Drug poisoning has become the leading cause of accidental death in the United States, surpassing car crashes. A person dies every 19 minutes, on average, from a prescription drug overdose. Since 2014, opioid analgesics were responsible for 40 percent of drug-poisoning deaths.[2] Most commonly, the scenario leading up to this is a middle-aged man getting a prescription for pain medication for his backache and dying several years later when he accidentally overdoses or mixes the drugs with alcohol.

In the face of this epidemic of opioid addiction, there is growing interest within health care in how to best blend conventional and complementary nondrug approaches in the management of musculoskeletal disorders. This is especially true for the costly and burdensome effects of low back pain, which has prompted increased research into the mechanisms, benefits, and risks of the complementary approach to spine care provided by DCs.[3] Chiropractic care today is gaining recognition as a cost-effective, conservative approach. For example:

- American College of Physicians/American Back Pain Society's 2007 "Guidelines on the Diagnosis and Treatment of Back Pain" recommended acupuncture, spinal manipulation, and massage therapy for low back pain.[4]

- In a 2016 review, the Agency for Healthcare Research and Quality (AHRQ) found several nonpharmacological approaches to be effective for improving low back pain and restoring function, and without serious harm, including spinal manipulation (what chiropractors identify as the spinal adjustment), acupuncture, and massage.[5]

- In 2011, the Institute of Medicine called for cultural transformation in pain prevention, diagnosis, and management, and recommended greater collaboration among the different clinical disciplines.[6]

- In November 2014, the Joint Commission (www.jointcommission.org) revised its Pain Management Standard for ambulatory care, critical access hospital, home care, hospital, nursing care centers, and office-based surgery accreditation programs. It stated that experts had concluded, based on extensive literature review, that both pharmacologic and nonpharmacologic approaches to pain management should be considered. They explicitly named chiropractic therapy, along with acupuncture, osteopathic manipulation, massage therapy, and physical therapy.

As a result of outcomes-effectiveness research and a long-standing record of consumer satisfaction, back pain patients are increasingly able to receive spinal manual adjustive procedures within integrative care settings.

Primary Spine Care Practitioner—An Emerging Model in Health Care Reform

It is widely recognized that the dramatic and increasing cost associated with spine-related disorders (SRDs) in the United States has not led to a corresponding improvement in patient clinical experience, nor in the clinical outcomes of medical care. The numbers of spine disorders continue to rise, and spine care costs continue to increase, with no evidence of improvement in quality of care.

An emerging model for the management of SRDs is training and credentialing primary spine care practitioners, a group of clinicians trained to function as primary care, first-contact providers for spine care. Early outcomes of pilot studies where trained primary spine care practitioners provided care compared to conventional medical treatment revealed patients received less spine surgery, less diagnostic imaging, lower episode costs, and reported high patient and provider satisfaction with strong clinical outcomes and annual overall per-patient costs 11 percent lower than traditional treatment.[7]

Managing Joint Function and Mobility: Tracking the Epidemic of Inactivity

Physical inactivity is considered the fourth leading risk factor for global mortality and the cause of an estimated 3.2 million deaths annually across the globe.[8] Inactivity is a fast-growing public health concern and contributes to a variety of chronic diseases and health complications.

Lack of motion within joints can result in disturbed biomechanics, even while not presenting with subjective pain or other symptoms. Disturbed joint biomechanics can reduce optimal performance, alter load distribution, increase risk of injury, and accelerate degeneration.

It is the role of the DC to identify dysfunctional joints and provide spinal and extremity adjustments to help restore normal biomechanics. Chiropractic adjustments specifically applied to joints can restore motion when the body's own muscles cannot. This helps relieve pain and restores and maintains normal movement, biomechanics, and function.

Simply stated, a joint that can't move can't nourish itself. Maintaining good motion is critical to the survival of discs and joints and may reduce the risk of future problems or injuries.

Joint Function and Motion in the Aging Patient

Senior citizens often experience structural problems, such as degenerative joint disease or osteoarthritis, and frequently present with pain and stiffness related to the spine and extremities. In the United States and across the globe, chronic back pain in the senior population (ages 65 and older) gives rise to increasing health care costs and is of increasing concern to third-party payers. The aging of the large baby-boom generation will lead to new opportunities for DCs.

Older adults are more likely to have neuromusculoskeletal and joint problems and are increasingly seeking treatment from DCs for these conditions as they lead longer, more active lives.[9] Doctors of chiropractic may outline a program of exercise that allows them to personally monitor the patient's progress, with a focused objective to rehabilitate and strengthen specific muscle groups. Alternatively, the chiropractor may recommend regular moderate-intensity physical activity, such as walking or cycling, as these activities can have significant benefits for health. This physical activity may include age-appropriate group activities or sports. It is well known that regular moderate-intensity activities can reduce the risk of cardiovascular diseases, diabetes, colon and breast cancer, and depression. Moreover, adequate levels of physical activity will decrease the risk of a hip or vertebral fracture and help control weight.

Simply stated, a solution for the growing physical inactivity problem in America is *movement*. DCs are well positioned to include guidance for exercise and physical activity when designing treatment plans for patients as it is well substantiated that exercise and mobility are integral to prevention and treatment of chronic disease.

Opportunities in Occupational Health, Ergonomics, and On-Site Workplace Health Clinics

The working American spends approximately 2,000 hours a year in the workplace. Understandably, the cumulative effects of the hours of sustained and repetitive activity can take a toll on the back, neck, wrists, hands, and other joints. In addition to cost-effective management of work-related neuromusculoskeletal injuries and participation with employer-funded on-site chiropractic care clinics, chiropractors have much to offer employers as consultants for worker safety and health, particularly relating to injury prevention and cost containment or reduction, workplace wellness, and ergonomics.

The science of ergonomics is a field of study that involves arranging the environment to fit the person. How the work environment is designed, and how it accommodates the individual's interface within his or her workplace, with the workstations, the controls, the keyboard, the height and angle of the computer screen and other equipment, and how it fits the worker's physical capabilities and limitations can be a key contributor to spine and extremity joint health.

Each day the body's joints, ligaments, and muscles experience repetitive motion, excessive force, mechanical stresses, awkward positioning, poor posture, and improper lifting, all activities that may occur in the workplace as well as at home as part of daily living. How the workstation is designed is fundamental to minimizing worker fatigue and discomfort and maximizing function and performance.

Selecting chairs for employees' work areas requires considering the degree of lumbar support and the seat height adjustability and ensuring the size is appropriate for the employee's body type.

Many of today's technological advances (computers, tablets, and wireless devices) may require the individual to perform repetitive procedures or work in sustained positions that put a great deal of stress on the musculoskeletal system. As an example, Americans are attached to text messaging on their cell phones, and DCs are starting to see the painful results in increasing numbers. "Text neck" is the term used to describe the distinct posture often seen in texting or staring downward at a cell phone, tablet, or other wireless device.

Tilting the head forward, as is typically done to view or create text messages, forces the neck muscles, tendons, and ligaments to strain to hold the head up. The human head weighs from 10 to 11 pounds. As the posture of the neck bends forward and downward, the weight on the cervical spine begins to increase, resulting in pain and spinal dysfunction, among other effects.

Box 14.1

Thoughts on the Future of the Profession: Dana Lawrence, DC, MMedEd, MA

Dr. Lawrence is professor and head of the Center for Teaching and Learning at Palmer College of Chiropractic. He was also the editor of the _Journal of Manipulative and Physiological Therapeutics_ (_JMPT_) for many years.

What are your thoughts on the future development of chiropractic education? Where is it going, and is that where it needs to go?

"This is an interesting and complicated question. Our future likely involves integrative approaches to the delivery of chiropractic care and adjustments, and in the transformation of learning through technology. We need to understand that our students learn in ways that fundamentally differ from how we learned 'back in the day.' They are more comfortable with technology, can take advantage of what it offers without fear, and are engaging in ways we need to learn, such as social media and in use of tablet and smartphone technology. Learning management systems are now in place, and faculty need to learn new skills to remain effective. The future is exciting!"

Chiropractic Inclusion in On-Site Corporate Health Clinics

Employers across the country are taking a more direct approach to improving the health and well-being of their employees. Employers are increasingly including DCs as part of on-site corporate health clinic services. Employer-funded on-site care programs that provide chiropractic services include companies such as Google, Cisco Systems Inc., Cerner Corporation, and Facebook, and studies support the value of this model of delivery.[10] This interest from the corporate community is driven by the favorable outcomes described in research demonstrating the effectiveness of chiropractic care in the management of the increasingly prevalent and costly neuromusculoskeletal conditions that represent a common cause of long-term pain and physical disability in the workplace today.

DCs are well trained to provide conservative, first-contact, drug-free, noninvasive approaches to care for neuromusculoskeletal care and pain management. Findings published in a 2012 issue of the _Journal of Occupational and Environmental Medicine_ suggest that chiropractic services offered at on-site corporate health clinics, contrasted to off-site physical therapy services, result in lower costs of care while improving neuromusculoskeletal

---

Box 14.2

Chiropractic Students' Thoughts on the Future of the Profession

"I feel the future of chiropractic is very exciting. In a time when we are all living longer and the NHS [National Health Service] is struggling to cope with meeting the health needs of the population, there is an opportunity for chiropractic to provide care to a greater number of the population and for chiropractic to work alongside other health care practitioners." *(Sharee, U.K.)*

"As a combat-injured veteran who regained my physical life through chiropractic care, I want to offer other veterans that same opportunity. As a chiropractic student, I am learning the skills not only to help my fellow veterans, but to improve the lives my own family members." *(Marco, United States)*

"I think the profession is blossoming around the world, but isn't without its political challenges. Whilst research is key in any profession, the future of chiropractic lies in relating the research to the patient. It's about ensuring the profession keeps its compassion in a world where everything is fast or brief and impersonal. It's also about ensuring we place ourselves in key places to help more people and grow the profession." *(James, U.K.)*

"I believe chiropractic will become a mainstream form of health care here in Australia, but it will take time, research, and the reorganization of health care." *(Yoshi, Australia)*

---

function.[11] Further, on-site chiropractic services in the workplace were directly connected with lower use of radiology services, lower use of outpatient and emergency settings, and lower use of physical therapy.[10]

DCs are being integrated within the on-site corporate health clinic in a variety of ways, ranging from part-time to full-time practitioners to executive positions responsible for leading key internal departments. On-site corporate health clinics are evolving to meet the specific needs of employers of various sizes and industries and are predicted to gain in popularity in the future.

Considerations on the Future of the Chiropractic Profession and Chiropractic Education

Michael R. Wiles, DC, MEd, MS

Dr. Wiles is currently dean of the new College of Chiropractic Medicine at Keiser University in West Palm Beach, Florida.

Today, the majority of chiropractors either have solo practices or are in small group practice with other DCs. However, with the evolution of complex health care systems within the United States and globally, and with a new and significant emphasis on teamwork and interprofessional collaboration, the chiropractic profession is now at an important point in its history. This is an unprecedented opportunity for the chiropractic profession to join with other health professions as part of multidisciplinary teams and to expand access to chiropractic care, serving greater numbers of people.

There are many new developments in support of this integrative role for the chiropractic profession. These include:

- increased opportunity with the Department of Defense and within the Department of Veterans Affairs medical and hospital system, as well as an increasing number of public hospitals offering chiropractic services
- a growing professional interest in expansion of services within interprofessional practice settings
- the development of the profession internationally
- a greater increase in scholarship, research, and interprofessional collaboration than at any time in the profession's history

Given these environmental factors, coupled with the urgency of the triple aim of improving cost effectiveness, patient experience, and population health, the chiropractic profession is well positioned to fill a need in team-based health care delivery. The future role of DCs will likely include the following:

- *Preventive and screening services to reduce the burden of musculoskeletal disorders.* The chiropractic profession has an opportunity to establish and refine valid screening processes for musculoskeletal dysfunction that might represent a "chiropractic check-up," analogous to the process established by dentistry for oral health. Research into the development of such a preventive approach, in accordance with accepted public health principles of health screening tests, would present an important service to the public and a great opportunity for chiropractic providers to move into a preventive role.
- *Practice in integrated health care environments.* As team members in an expanded health care system, chiropractors can expect to serve in a wide range of clinical settings, from small multidisciplinary or group practices to large community clinics and hospitals.

- *An expanded and more defined role in military health care.* There is a significant need for the conservative management of musculoskeletal conditions in all branches of the military, as evidenced by the growing popularity of chiropractic services within the VA health care system.

- *Formal postgraduate residency training.* With increasing opportunities for practice in multidisciplinary settings, chiropractic education is being positioned to expand and strengthen clinical training through residencies within these integrated settings. As described in Chapter 10, the profession has now established a VA residency, and such programs will likely use this as a model. Residency programs would also serve to expand interprofessional collaboration and to acculturate chiropractic providers to a wider range of practice settings.

- *An important role in public education regarding health promotion, lifestyle behaviors, and wellness.* The aging population is perhaps the most active and wellness oriented in history. There is a tremendous consumer interest in fitness and lifestyle management to preserve pain-free activity as long as possible. This interest seems to focus on musculoskeletal and nutritional fitness, both of which are traditional domains of the chiropractor.

- *A vastly increased participation in research, particularly publicly supported chiropractic research.* Chiropractic research has been consistently growing in recent decades. Possibilities for collaboration, particularly in multidisciplinary settings, will likely enable a quantum increase in research capacity and production, especially in areas of the prevention of musculoskeletal disability and dysfunction.

References

1. Calabresi M. Why America can't kick its painkiller problem. *Time* 2015;184(22):7–10.

2. National Center for Health Statistics. NCHS data on drug-poisoning deaths. NCHS Fact Sheet, March 2016.

3. Tsertsvadze A, Clar C, Court R, Clarke A, Mistry H, Sutcliffe P. Cost-effectiveness of manual therapy for the management of musculoskeletal conditions: a systematic review and narrative synthesis of evidence from randomized controlled trials. *J Manipulative Physiol Ther.* 2014;37(6):343–362.

4. Chou R, Qaseem A, Snow V, et al. Diagnosis and treatment of low back pain: a joint clinical practice guideline from the American College of Physicians and the American Pain Society. *Ann Intern Med.* 2007;147(7):478–491.

5. Chou R, Deyo R, Friedly J, et al. *Noninvasive Treatments for Low Back Pain.* Rockville, MD: Agency for Healthcare Research and Quality; 2016.

6. Institute of Medicine. *Relieving Pain in America: A Blueprint for Transforming Prevention, Care, Education, and Research.* Washington, DC: National Academies Press; 2011.

7. Murphy DR, Justice BD, Paskowski IC, Perle SM, Schneider MJ. The establishment of a primary spine care practitioner and its benefits to health care reform in the United States. *Chiropr Man Therap.* 2011;19(1):17.

8. World Health Organization. *Global Recommendations on Physical Activity for Health.* Geneva: WHO; 2010.

9. Bureau of Labor Statistics. *Occupational Outlook Handbook.* Washington, DC: U.S. Department of Labor; January 2014.

10. Kindermann SL, Hou Q, Miller RM. Impact of chiropractic services at an on-site health center. *J Occup Environ Med.* 2014;56(9):990–992.

11. Krause CA, Kaspin L, Gorman KM, Miller RM. Value of chiropractic services at an on-site health center. *J Occup Environ Med.* 2012;54(8):917–921.

Index

Academic careers, 231–232; academic
enhancement activities, 237–238;
and academic freedom, 240–241;
anywhere, anytime clinical
assessment, 249–250; anywhere,
anytime learning, 248–249; basic
premise, 241–242; and the
contemporary curriculum,
246–247; continuous learning
(professional development),
239–240; the evolving
environment, 255–256; fields of
research and scholarship, 250–251;
historical overview, 232–234; key
issues, 245–246; in large,
multidisciplinary university,
242–243; mentoring faculty,
251–252; peer review, 255;
qualifications, 239; research as
career path, 252–255; and the shift
to capability, 248; and social media,
248; terminology, 234–237; and the
term "subluxation," 243–244
Academic terminology, 234–237
Academy of Chiropractic Orthopedics
(ACO), 119, 216
Accountable care organizations
(ACOs), 260
Accreditation: advantages of, 85–87;
agencies overseeing, 85; new
directions in, 87; quantitative
approach to, 88
Accreditation standards, 5–6, 57; for
chiropractic colleges, 15; global,
85–88; number of patient
encounters required, 90; program
duration, 90–91
Activator Technique, 71, 207
Active Release Technique (ART), 143,
208–209, 298
Acupuncture, 13, 23, 24, 26, 27, 113,
114–115, 117, 124, 143, 210;
graduate degree programs,
128–130. See also Oriental
medicine
Acupuncture and Oriental Medicine
(AOM) programs, 128–130
Adjusting table, 144
Advanced clinical practice, 24
Advanced nutrition concepts, 71
Affordable Health Care Act, 7
Allied Health Professions Council of
South Africa, 34
Alternative medicine. See
Complementary and alternative
medicine (CAM)
American Academy of Pain
Management, 213
American Board of Chiropractic
Acupuncture (ABCA), 114

American Board of Chiropractic Internists (ABCI), 117, 221

American Board of Chiropractic Orthopedists (ABCO), 119

American Board of Forensic Professionals (ABFP), 117, 118

American Board of Independent Medical Examiners (ABIME), 227

American Chiropractic Association (ACA), 54, 57, 208, 216, 221; approved chiropractic specialty programs, 114–115

American Chiropractic Association Council of Chiropractic Rehabilitation, 110

American Chiropractic Board of Radiology (ACBR), 106, 116, 131

American Chiropractic Board of Sports Physicians (ACBSP), 109, 128, 132, 211

American Chiropractic Board on Occupational Health (ACBOH), 119, 226

American Chiropractic Neurology Board (ACNB), 116, 216

American Chiropractic Rehabilitation Board (ACRB), 110, 121, 212; courses offered by, 121–122

American Clinical Board of Nutrition (ACBN), 118, 126, 218

American College of Sports Medicine (ACSM), 109, 128

American Nutrition Association, 217

American Public Health Association, 217

American Society for Nutrition, 217

American Veterinary Chiropractic Association (AVCA), 228

Anatomical adaptation, 287–288

Anatomy courses, 16, 27, 34, 59–60

Andragogy, 57

Anglo-European College of Chiropractic (AECC), 36

Animal chiropractic, 227–228

Animal Chiropractic Certification Commission (ACCC), 228

Applied ergonomics, 115. *See also* Ergonomics

Applied kinesiology (AK), 71, 207. *See also* Kinesiology

Aquatic therapy, 69

Associated clinical topics, 66–67

Athletic performance management, 7

Athletic physicals, 143

Athletic trainer certification, 132

Athletic training, 24; anatomical adaptation, 287–288; core stability, 286–287; growth and development, 283; injury prevention, 285–286; longevity, 283; multilateral development, 288–289; peaking, 284–285; and progressive overload, 281–282; sports psychology, 286; strength and conditioning, 287; volume and intensity, 283. *See also* Sports chiropractic

Atlas orthogonal technique, 71

Australasian Council on Chiropractic Education (ACCE), 32

Australia, 29–30, 45, 101, 233; chiropractic clinics in, 195–198

Australian Health Practitioners Regulation Agency (AHPRA), 197

Back pain, 3, 8; chronic, 2; and disabled veterans, 7; epidemic nature of, 2; surgical response to, 3

Bahçeşehir Üniversity Chiropractic Program, 36

Balance training, 69

Barcelona College of Chiropractic (BCC), 34–35

Basic sciences, 81, 89

Billing, 77–78, 192–194

Biochemistry courses, 61

Biology, 25–26

Biomechanics, 71, 124

Biomedical sciences, 24

Biomedical technology, 34
Blackboard, 15
Blair Technique, 71
Board certification, 53, 57, 109, 110, 114, 212
Botanical medicine, 117
BPP University, 45
Bracing, 143
Branding, 173
Brazil, 30
Brigham & Women's Hospital's Osher Center for Integrative Medicine, 260
Bush, George W., 4
Business decisions, 138–139; financial considerations, 161–162; starting a practice, 160–161. *See also* Business plan
Business degree (MBA), 124
Business plan, 138, 161; appendix, 165; company description, 163; executive summary, 162; financial projections, 164; funding request, 164; how to make the business plan stand out, 164; market analysis, 163; marketing sales projection, 164; organization and management, 163; red flags, 165; services offered, 163; strengths and weaknesses, 164
Business skills, 12

Cambron, Jerrilyn, 252
Campus culture, 72
Canada, 30, 45, 232–233
Canadian Chiropractic Examining Board (CCEB), 53
Canadian Memorial Chiropractic College (CMCC), 30, 45, 107, 108, 110, 123, 232
Canvas, 15
Causation, 118
Central nervous system (CNS), 59–60
Central Queensland University, 101

Centro Universitario Feevale, Faculdade de Quiropraxia, 30
Certificate programs, 132
Certifications, 106
Certified Active Release Technique (ART), 298
Certified chiropractic extremity practitioner (CCEP), 132–133
Certified chiropractic sports physician (CCSP), 109, 128, 132, 211, 298
Certified clinical nutritionist (CCN), 126, 218
Certified health education specialist (CHES), 226
Certified independent chiropractic examiner (CICE), 227
Certified kinesio taping practitioner (CKTP), 134, 298
Certified medical examiner (CME), 227
Certified nutrition specialist (CNS), 126, 218
Certified personal trainer (NSCA-CPT), 128
Certified special population specialist (CSPS), 128
Certified sports nutritionist (CISSN), 126, 128, 218
Certified strength and conditioning specialist (CSCS), 109, 128, 133
Certified wellness practitioner (CWP), 226
Chile, 31
Chiropractic assistant (CA) programs, 21, 153, 155, 171, 201, 228
Chiropractic biophysics (CBP), 71
Chiropractic Board of Clinical Nutrition (CBCN), 118, 126–127
Chiropractic care: availability to military personnel, 4, 224, 309; as conservative approach, 302–303; holistic biopsychosocial philosophy of, 3; as pain-relief specialty, 141–142; as part of interdisciplinary

care, 6–7; patient satisfaction with, 2; as profession, 2; as a rewarding career, 7–8; and the VA system, 260–261, 267–270

Chiropractic Clinical Education: classroom level, 95–96; clinic level, 96–97; professional (practitioner) level, 97

Chiropractic clinics: in Australia, 195–198; direction, 182; doctor-patient relationships, 201; employee handbook/human resources, 167; in Indonesia, 200–202; insurance, record keeping, and billing, 192–194; leadership, 165–166; logo, 174; management, 166–167; marketing, 191–192; mission vs. vision statements, 173–174; organizing electronic information, 168; salary strategies, 168; sensory analysis, 176–177; staff size, 168; staff support, 182; strategic objectives, 174; successful practice, 194–195; in United Kingdom, 198–200; use of health education and health promotion, 187–189; website, 174–176. *See also* Business decisions; Chiropractic practice; Financial considerations; Patient management

Chiropractic colleges: academic rigor of, 12; accreditation standards for, 11–12, 15; application criteria, 43; application to, 39–40; availability of other degree programs, 13–14; campus culture of, 72; chiropractic students' perceptions of, 45–50; completing prerequisites for, 42; diversity of, 91–94; focused, middle, and broad philosophies, 14–15; information technology resources of, 14; location by country, international, 29–37; location by state, United States, 21–29;

questions to ask, 12–14; scholarships to, 45; selection of, 11–12, 43–44; tuition costs of, 44–45; U.S. enrollment standards, 40–42

Chiropractic curriculum, 232, 246–247; advanced clinical studies, 67–68; associated clinical topics, 66–67; basic sciences, 58–61; chiropractic principles and practice, 64–66; chiropractic techniques, 70–71; clinical sciences, 61–64; core programs, 58; elective course offerings, 71; other considerations affecting, 72; physiotherapy, 68–70; standard, 51–53

Chiropractic education: academic rigor of, 12; accreditation requirements for, 57; core curriculum, 58; coupled with business skills training, 12; coupled with other procedures, 13; evolution of, 101–102; evolution of curriculum, 54; full vs. limited, 12; historical context, 53–58; length of program, 12. *See also* Clinical education; Global chiropractic education

Chiropractic Education: Outline of a Standard Course (Nuget), 83

Chiropractic faculty, standards for, 54–55, 57

Chiropractic for children with special needs, 265–267

Chiropractic neurology, 215–216. *See also* Neurology

Chiropractic orthopedics, 106, 111–112, 216. *See also* Orthopedics

Chiropractic practice, 53, 137; clinical decisions, 138; day-to-day activities, 179–180; doctor-patient relationships, 180–181; financial considerations, 139; intake, 181; key business decisions, 138–139; management considerations, 139; marketing considerations, 138.

See also Chiropractic clinics;
Clinical decisions
Chiropractic principles and practice,
64–66
Chiropractic radiology, 108, 116,
214–215
Chiropractic Resident Training
Programs, 107
Chiropractic specialization, 205–206;
acupuncture and Oriental
medicine, 210; animal chiropractic,
227–228; diagnostic and internal
disorders, 221; ergonomics,
225–226; forensics, 226–227;
functional medicine, 219–221;
geriatrics, 222–224; integrative
pain management, 212–213;
manipulation under anesthesia,
224–225; manipulative (adjustive)
techniques, 206–208; military
medicine, 224; neurology, 215–216;
nonclinical career specialties,
228–229; nutrition, 216–219;
occupational health, 225–226;
orthopedics, 216; pediatrics,
222–224; personal injury, 213–214;
primary care, 221–222; radiology,
214–215; rehabilitation, 211–212;
soft tissue techniques, 208–210;
special populations, 222–224;
sports chiropractic, 211; women's
health, 222–224
Chiropractic sport science, 24
Chiropractic Sports Medicine,
108–109, 121–122. *See also*
Certified chiropractic sports
physician (CCSP)
Chiropractic students: on the future of
the profession, 307; global mobility
of, 100–101
Chiropractic technician (CT)
programs, 21
Chiropractic techniques, 53, 56;
coursework in, 70–71

Chiropractors. *See* Doctors of
chiropractic (DCs)
Chiropractors Association of Australia
(CAA), 197
Chronic disease management, 198
Chronic health conditions (CHC),
259
Chronic musculoskeletal disorders,
259. *See also* Musculoskeletal
disorders
Cleveland, Carl S., III, 301
Cleveland University—Kansas City,
College of Chiropractic, 14, 25–26,
123, 301–302
Clinical anatomy, 27
Clinical assessment, anywhere,
anytime, 249–250
Clinical decisions, 138; chiropractic
as pain-relief experts, 156–157;
doctor and staff attire, 147–148;
equipment list, 145–146; location
of practice, 139–140; marketing,
148–150; musculoskeletal issues,
144; new patient conversion,
151–155; new patient fulfillment,
157–158; new patient generation,
148–150; open vs. closed treatment
areas, 144, 147; patient education,
155–156; services and techniques,
142–143; summary, 158–159; type
or focus of practice, 140–142
Clinical education, 12–13, 27, 75;
additional clinically relevant
opportunities, 79; CCE competency
areas, 80–81; clinical oversight,
75–76; clinical rotations and
patient base, 76–77; diversity of
models, 98–100; documentation
and billing, 77–78; externships and
preceptorships, 79–80; graduation
requirements, 80–81; internships,
31, 53, 81; treatment approaches,
78–79. *See also* Chiropractic
education

Clinical neurology, 115, 115–116.
    See also Neurology
Clinical nutrition, 24, 27, 117. See also
    Nutrition
Clinical Nutrition Certification Board
    (CNCB), 126, 218
Clinical practice, advanced, 24
Clinical rehabilitation, 106. See also
    Rehabilitation
Clinical research, 111. See also
    Research
Clinical rotations, 76–77
Clinical sciences, 53, 89, 106,
    110–111
Clinical skills, 31
Clinical topics, associated, 66–67
Clinicians, overseeing, 75–76
Clinton, William "Bill," 4
Colegio de Profesionistas Cienctificos
    Quiropracticos de Mexico A. C., 33
College of Chiropractic Medicine
    (Keiser University), 307
Commission for Accreditation of
    Graduate Education in Neurology
    (CAGEN), 116
Community health, 229
Community health care, 112
Competencies, minimum, 89–91
Complementary and alternative
    medicine (CAM), 129, 221
Continuing professional development
    (CPD), 271, 39–240
Core stability, 286–287
Corrective exercise specialization
    (CES), 109, 128
Cost containment, 260
Council of Chiropractic Acupuncture
    (CCA), 114
Council on Chiropractic Education,
    234
Council on Chiropractic Education
    Australasia (CCEA), 32, 85;
    accreditation standards, 90
Council on Chiropractic Education
    USA (CCE-USA), 5–6, 12, 40, 54,
56, 57, 72, 83, 85, 108;
    accreditation standards, 90;
    meta-competencies, 80–81
Council on Chiropractic Extremity
    Adjusting (CCEA), 132
Council on Forensic Sciences (CFS),
    227
Council on Upper Cervical Care, 208
Councils on Chiropractic Education
    International (CCEI), 6, 11, 84, 85
Cox Flexion Distraction, 71, 207
CPR instructor, 66, 122, 132, 298
CPT codes (Current Procedural
    Terminology), 78
Cupping, 129
Current Procedural Terminology (CPT
    codes), 78

Daily training plan (DTP), 279
Denmark, 31
Department of Defense (DoD),
    224, 308
Department of Transportation (DOT)
    exams, 143
Department of Veterans Affairs (VA),
    4, 7, 106, 107, 198, 308
Department of Veterans Affairs Health
    Care Programs Enhancement Act
    (2001), 4
Desire2Learn, 15
Developmental Center for Research on
    Complementary and Alternative
    Medicine, 25
Diagnosis and management of
    internal disorders, 115, 117, 221
Diagnostic codes, 77
Diagnostic imaging, 27, 31, 63–64,
    106, 112, 115, 116–117, 124, 143,
    184, 198, 199, 214–215; graduate
    degree programs, 130–131;
    musculoskeletal, 36, 113. See also
    Radiology; Ultrasound
Diagnostic sciences, 81, 89
Diet, 28. See also Nutrition
Dietetics, 113

Differential diagnosis, 31
Digital X-rays, 20. *See also* X-ray technology
Diplomate certification as forensic examiner (DABFP), 227
Diplomate in chiropractic upper cervical procedures (DCUCP), 208
Diplomate in clinical chiropractic pediatrics (DICCP), 120
Diplomate of Gonstead Clinical Studies Society (DGCSS), 208
Diplomate of the American Board of Chiropractic Internists (ABCI), 117
Diplomate of the American Board of Forensic Professionals (DABFP), 118
Diplomate of the American Chiropractic Board of Neurology (DACBR), 116
Diplomate of the American Chiropractic Board of Sports Physicians (DACBSP), 122, 128, 211, 298
Diplomate of the American Chiropractic Neurology Board (DACNB), 216
Diplomate of the American Chiropractic Rehabilitation Board (DACRB), 121
Diplomate of the American Clinical Board of Nutrition (DACBN), 118, 127, 218
Diplomate of the Chiropractic Board of Clinical Nutrition (DCBCN), 126–127, 218
Diplomate of the International Board of Applied Kinesiology (DIBAK), 208
Diplomates, 106
Discharge to wellness system, 154
Distance learning, 119
Diversified technique, 70
Division of Federal Employees' Compensation, 4
Doctorate in public health (DrPH), 124, 229

Doctorate of acupuncture and oriental medicine (DAOM), 23
Doctorate of health professions education, 26
Doctor of medicine (MD), 124
Doctor of naturopathy (ND), 24, 124
Doctor of nursing practice (DNP), 124
Doctor of osteopathy (DO), 124
Doctor of physical therapy (DPT), 124
Doctor of veterinary medicine (DVM), 124
Doctors of chiropractic (DCs), 1, 5–6. 51; accreditation for, 4; day-to-day activities, 179–180; degree programs for, 26; education program, 5–6; employment outlook for, 2; favorable job ranking, 1; patient relationships, 180–181; as primary care physicians, 4, 112; on professional sports team staffs, 7, 211, 262; relationships with patients, 201; as sole proprietors, 12; state licensing standards for, 4; supplying conservative care, 2–3
Documentation, 77–78
Drop table method, 78, 207–208, 223
Dry needling, 143
Dual enrollment, 72
Durban University of Technology, Department of Chiropractic, 34
D'Youville College, 27, 123

Economics, 67
Education degree (EdD), 124
Electric stimulation, 78, 144
Electroacupuncture, 129
Electronic health records (EHR), 20, 181, 228
Electrotherapy, 69
Emergency medical care, 34, 113
Emergency medical technician (EMT), 298
Emergency procedures, 66–67, 132
E-Myth, The (Gerber), 137
Endurance training, 69

Ergonomics, 71, 115, 225–226,
    277, 305
Ethics, 67
European Council on Chiropractic
    Education (ECCE), 34, 35, 37, 85;
    accreditation standards, 90–91
Evidence-based practice (EBP),
    53, 112
Evidence-informed practice (EIP), 53
Exercise, 3, 13, 25–26, 69, 117;
    graduate programs in, 127–128.
    See also Physical activity
Exercise and lifestyle modification,
    143
Exercise and sports science, 24, 132
Exercise physiology, 69
Externships, 79–80

Faculty of Medicine of Veracruz, 33
Federal Motor Carrier Safety
    Administration (FMCSA), 227
Federation of Canadian Chiropractic
    (FCC), 85; accreditation standards,
    90–91
Fellow of Gonstead Clinical Studies
    Society (FGCSS), 208
Fellowships, 122
Fellows of the Academy of
    Chiropractic Orthopedics, 216
Financial aid, 44–45, 55
Financial considerations, 138,
    161–162; branding vs. marketing,
    173; business control systems
    (BCS), 170–171; financial basics,
    169–170; financial intelligence, 171;
    hiring, firing, and training staff,
    171–172; marketing, 172–173,
    191–192; setting goals, 172
Fitness-for-duty assessment, 118
Fitness testing, 69
Flexion distraction, 207, 223
Food supplements, 117, 143
Force Sensing Table Technology, 30
Forensics, 213, 226–227

Forensic sciences, 115, 117–118
France, 31
Fraud and abuse investigation, 118
Free Application for Student Aid
    (FAFSA), 44, 45
Functional and kinetic treatment with
    rehab (FAKTR), 133, 298
Functional capacity evaluations, 69
Functional medicine, 28, 117, 219–221
Fundació Privada Quiropràctica
    (FPQ), 35

General Chiropractic Council (GCC),
    36–37, 198–199
General diagnosis, 62–63
Gerber, Michael, 137
Geriatrics, 71, 113, 222–224, 304–305
Gliedt, Jordan, 267–269
Global chiropractic education, 83–84,
    103–104; advantages of
    accreditation, 85–88; chiropractic
    clinical education, 95; current
    status, 84–85; diversity of
    institutions, 91–94; futurist's view
    of chiropractic education, 101–103;
    globalization of learning manual
    skills, 87–88; global mobility of
    students, 100–101; importance of
    capability over competency, 94–95;
    industry engagement, 89;
    minimum competencies, 89–91;
    outcomes from first global
    conference, 95–100
Golden, Lorraine M., 265
Gonstead, 71, 207
Gonstead Clinical Studies Society
    (GCSS), 208
Graduate degree programs, 105–106;
    offered by chiropractic institutions,
    123; online storage capacity, 122
Graston Technique/Instrument-
    Assisted Soft Tissue Mobilization
    (IASTM), 208–210
Growth and development, 283

Ham, KeeSun, 32
Hanseo University, Department of
  Chiropractic (HUDC), 32–33
Headache, 3
Health care, use of technology in,
  20–21
Health care professionals, 119
Health care teams, collaborative, 93
Health clinics, on-site workplace,
  305–307
Health education, 187–189, 190, 309
Health fairs, 78–79
Health fitness specialist (HFS), 128
Health informatics, 26
Health professions, independent, 13
Health professions education, 26
Health promotion, 28, 25–26, 124,
  187–189, 190, 229
Health science degree (DHSc), 124
High-velocity, low-amplitude (HVLA)
  thrust, 70, 144
Homeopathy, 34, 117
Howard, John, 232
Human anatomy and physiology, 27, 34
Human biology, 25–26
Human resource directors, 119

ICD codes (International
  Classification of Disease), 77
Ice and heat, 78, 144
Inactivity, 303–304
Independent health professions, 13
Indonesia, chiropractic clinics in,
  200–202
Information literacy, 23
Information technology, 14
Infrared light therapy, 69
Injections, 110
Injury prevention, 285–286
Institut Franco-Européen de
  Chiropratique, 31
Instrument adjusting, 223
Instrument-Assisted Soft Tissue
  Mobilization (IASTM), 208–210

Insurance, 7, 192–194, 199
Integrative/Integrated clinical
  practice, 53, 106, 112
Integrative/Integrated medicine/health
  care, 112, 260, 270–273, 308
Integrative pain management,
  212–213
Interdisciplinary care, 6–7, 270–273
International Academy of Chiropractic
  Neurology (IACN), 116
International Board of Applied
  Kinesiology (IBAK), 208
International Board of Chiropractic
  Examiners (IBCEs), 53
International Board of Chiropractic
  Neurology (IACN), 116, 216
International certified chiropractic
  sports physician (ICCSP), 128,
  298
International Chiropractic Association
  Council on Chiropractic Pediatrics,
  120, 221
International Chiropractic Pediatric
  Association (ICPA), 120, 221
International Classification of Disease
  (ICD codes), 77
International College of Applied
  Kinesiology (ICAK), 208
International Federation of Sports
  Chiropractic (IFSC), 128
International Medical University, 33
International Society of Sports
  Nutrition (ISSN), 126, 128, 218
Internships, 31, 53, 81; research,
  71, 124
Interprofessional education (IPE), 53

Japan, 31–32, 233–234
Japanese Association of Chiropractors
  (JAC), 32
Joint fixation, 56
Joint function and mobility, 144,
  303–304
Jurisprudence, 4, 67

Keiser University, 307
Kinesiology, 25–26, 71, 78, 209
Kinesio taping, 134, 298
Kinesio Taping Association
    International (KTAI), 134
Korea (Republic of Korea), 32–33

Laboratory diagnostics, 143
Laboratory tests, 184
Lawrence, Dana, 251, 306
Leadership, in the chiropractic clinic,
    165–166
Learning, anywhere, anytime,
    101–102, 248–249
Learning Management Systems (LMS),
    15–16
Licensure, 14
Life Chiropractic College West, 14, 22
Life University, 14, 21, 24, 123
Location of practice, 139–140
Logan Basic, 71
Logan University, 14, 26, 107,
    108–109, 113, 123
Longevity, 283
Los Angeles College of Chiropractic
    (LACC), 23
Low-level laser therapy (LLLT), 69, 78

Macquarie University, Department of
    Chiropractic, 29, 233
Madrid College of Chiropractic-
    RCU, 35
Major League Baseball (MLB),
    211, 262
Malaysia, 33, 93–94
Management considerations. *See*
    Practice management
Manipulation under anesthesia
    (MUA), 224–225
Manipulative (adjustive) techniques,
    56, 206–208
Manual skills, globalization of
    learning, 87–88
Market analysis, 163

Marketing, 138, 148–150, 164,
    172–173, 191–192; logo, 174;
    social networking, 176; website,
    174–176
Massage therapy, 13, 24, 26, 143
Master's in health promotion, 25–26.
    See also Health promotion
Master's in nursing, 124. *See also*
    Nursing
Master's of acupuncture and Oriental
    Medicine (MAOM), 23, 24
Master's of public health (MPH), 111,
    124, 229. *See also* Public health
Master's of science (MS), 124
Maximum medical improvement, 118
MChiro, 37
McKenzie Institute International, 134
McKenzie Method, 69, 134
McTimoney College of Chiropractic
    (MCC), 36–37
Mechanical diagnostic technique
    (MDT), 134
Mechanotherapy, 69
Medical College of Wisconsin &
    Froedtert Hospital Spine Care
    Clinics, 260
Medicare and Medicaid, 4
Mental health, 113
Meta-Competencies, 80–81
Mexico, 33–34
Microbiology courses, 61
Military health care, 224, 309. *See also*
    Veterans Affairs (VA)
Minor League Baseball, 262
Mission statement, 173–174, 242
Mobile devices, 101–102
Modern medical diagnosis, 117
Moodle, 15
Moreau, Bill, 7
Morrison, Brian, 271–273
Motion palpation, 71
Motion Palpation Institute (MPI), 132
Moxibustion, 129
Multidisciplinary practice, 263–265

Multilateral development, 288–289
Murdoch University, School of Health Professions, 29
Muscle flexibility and strength, 144
Muscle rehabilitation, 69. *See also* Rehabilitation
Musculoskeletal diagnostic ultrasound, 36, 113. *See also* Ultrasound
Musculoskeletal disorders, 1, 2, 8, 81, 308; chronic, 259; of military personnel, 7; at VA facilities, 112

National Academy of Sports Medicine (NASM), 128
National Association of Nutrition Professionals, 217
National Basketball Association (NBA), 211, 262
National Board of Chiropractic Examiners (NBCE), 12, 55, 56, 60, 95, 130; exam part I, 58–62; exam part II, 64–67; exam part III, 67; exam part IV, 68; exam in physiotherapy, 68–70; national board exams, 55, 81
National Certification Commission for Acupuncture and Oriental Medicine (NCCAOM), 130
National College of Chiropractic, 232
National Commission for Certifying Agencies (NCCA), 216
National Commission for Health Education, 226
National Football League (NFL), 7, 211, 262
National Hockey League (NHL), 262
National Institutes of Health, 25
National Registry of Certified Medical Examiners, 227
National Strength and Conditioning Association (NSCA), 128
National University of Health Sciences (NUHS), 14, 21, 107, 111, 123, 131,
232; Chiropractic Medicine Program, 24–25; Florida site 23–24
National Wellness Institute, 226
Natural health care, 25, 27
Natural hormone replacement, 117
Natural therapeutics, 117
Naturopathy, 13, 24, 124
Network devices, 17–18
Networking, 78–79
Neuroanatomy, 59–60
Neurodiagnostics, 112
Neurology, 25, 71, 113, 115–116, 215–216
Neuromuscular rehabilitation, 69. *See also* Rehabilitation
Neuromusculoskeletal (NMS) diagnosis, 63
Neuromusculoskeletal medicine (NMSM), 3, 111–112
Neurosciences, 111
Neurosurgery, 113
New patient conversion, 151–155
New patient fulfillment, 157–158
New patient generation, 148–150
New York Chiropractic College (NYCC), 14, 27, 107, 113, 123, 131
New Zealand, 34
New Zealand College of Chiropractic, 34
NFL teams, 7, 211, 262
Nimmo technique, 208–209
Northwest Center for Lifestyle and Functional Medicine (NWCLFM), 28
Northwest Commission on Colleges and Universities (NCCU), 28
Northwestern Health Sciences University, 14, 26, 107, 108–109, 123, 226
Nugent, John, 232
Nurse practitioners, 124
Nursing, 34, 92, 94, 124; occupational, 119
Nutrition, 3, 4, 23, 24, 28, 115, 124, 216–219; certification in, 118;

clinical, 24, 27, 117; graduate
degrees in, 124–127; sports, 126,
128, 218
Nutrition concepts, advanced, 71
Nutritional counseling, 78–79, 143,
218–219
Nutrition and human performance,
26
Nutrition Council of the American
Chiropractic Association, 217

Objective structured clinical
examinations (OSCEs), 53
Occupational health, 115, 119–120,
213, 225–226, 305
Occupational nurses, 119. *See also*
Nursing
Occupational therapy assistants, 13
Office of Workers' Compensation
Programs, 4
Online storage capacity, 18
On-site workplace health clinics,
305–307
Opioid painkillers, 8, 272, 302
Optometry, 34
Oregon Collaborative for Integrative
Medicine (OCIM), 28
Oriental medicine, 13, 23, 24, 26, 27,
124, 210; graduate degree
programs, 128–130. *See also*
Acupuncture; Traditional Chinese
medicine (TCM)
Orthopedic clinic, 113
Orthopedics, 106, 111–112, 115,
119–120, 216
Orthotics, 4, 143
Osteopathy, 124
Outcome-based care, 260

Painkiller addiction, 8, 302
Pain management, 113, 141–142, 143,
156–157, 212–213, 303
Palmer, Daniel David (D.D.), 53, 232
Palmer Center for Chiropractic
Research, 25

Palmer College of Chiropractic, 14,
21, 110, 123; Davenport Campus,
25, 107; Florida campus, 23;
West, 22
Palmer's School of Magnetic Cure, 232
Parker Research Institute, 28–29
Parker University (Parker College of
Chiropractic), 14, 28–29, 107, 123
Passive care modalities, 69, 78
Pathology courses, 60
Patient base, 76–77
Patient-centered care, 112
Patient-centered medical homes
(PCMH), 260
Patient education, 4, 155–156
Patient management, 31; assessing
risk, 189–190; doctor-patient
relationships, 180–181;
examination, 184–185; following
up, 186; health education and
health promotion, 187–189, 190;
history, 183–184; intake, 181;
interview or review of systems,
182–183; report of findings,
185–186; setting up a treatment
plan, 186
Peaking, 284–285
Pedagogy, 57
Pediatrics, 25, 71, 115, 120, 222–224
Peer review, 255
Performance enhancement specialist
(PES), 109
Personal injury (PI), 213–214
Personal training, 78, 128
Pettibon Technique, 71
PGA Tour, 262
Pharmacologic counseling, 117
Pharmacology, 66
Phillip Institute, 233
Phototherapy, 69
Physical activity, 190. *See also* Exercise
Physical medicine, 113
Physical therapy, 4, 13, 78, 124
Physician's assistants, 13, 124
Physioball exercises, 69

Physiology courses, 16, 60
Physio-taping, 143
Physiotherapy, 68–70, 197
Podiatry, 34
Positive psychology, 24
Postgraduate residency training, 309
Post-Isometric Relaxation (PIR)/
    Proprioceptive Neuromuscular
    Facilitation (PNF), 208–209
Practice Based Research Network
    (PBRN), 120, 197
Practice management, 53, 67, 71, 138
Preceptorships, 79–80
Pre-employment screening, 143
Pre-health programs, 25–26
Preventive services, 308
Primary care medicine, 113, 221–222;
    for the chiropractor, 112
Primary spine care provider, 106,
    109–110, 303
Professional sports teams, 7, 211, 262
Progressive overload, 281–282
Public health, 53
Public health degrees: DrPH, 124,
    229; MPH, 111, 124
Public policy, 229

Radiography, 34, 63–64
Radiology, 25, 113, 214–215. *See also*
    Diagnostic imaging
Radiology reports, 77
Real Centro Universitario Escorial
    Maria Cristina (RCU), 35
Record keeping, 192–194
Recovery, 284
Reexamination system, 153–154
Rehabilitation, 3–4, 13, 25, 71, 78,
    110, 113, 115, 121, 143, 144,
    211–212, 281; clinical, 106;
    graduate programs in, 127–128;
    muscle, 69; neuromuscular, 69;
    sports, 26, 106
Rehabilitation practice, 262–263
Report of findings (ROF) system,
    152–153, 185–186

Research, 250–253; chiropractic, 309;
    clinical, 111
Research internships, 71, 124
Resident training programs, 105, 106,
    122; university affiliations for, 107
Rheumatology, 113
Risk assessment, 189–190
Roseen, Eric, 262–265
Royal Melbourne Institute of
    Technology (RMIT) University,
    Division of Chiropractic, 29–30, 33,
    45, 233; in Japan, 32

Sacro-occipital technique (SOT),
    71, 207
Schneider, Michael, 253
Scholarships, 45
Scoliosis screening, 143
Screening services, 308
Selective functional movement
    assessment (SFMA), 133–134
Seminars, 71, 78–79
Sexually transmitted diseases
    (STDs), 66
Shapiro, Ira, 297–299
Sherman College of Chiropractic,
    14, 28
Social media, 246–247
Social networking, 176
Social sciences, 89
Soft tissue techniques, 13, 69, 71, 78,
    144, 208–210
Somatology, 34
South Africa, 34
Southern California University of
    Health Sciences, 14, 22–23, 107,
    108, 109–110, 113, 123
Spain, 34–35
Special populations, 71, 128, 222–224
Spinal anatomy, 59–60
Spinal cord injury, 113
Spinal manipulation, 3, 4
Spine care, nonsurgical, 3, 8
Spine-related disorders (SRD), 1, 3,
    110, 303

Spondylotherapy, 233
Sport and movement studies, 34
Sport coaching, 24
Sport health science, 24
Sports chiropractic, 25, 211, 275; credentialing and travel to treat, 293–294; emergency plan, 292–293; force-frequency-duration, 277–279; four levels of, 280–281; paperwork, 294–296; and rehabilitation, 281; sports health care and sports outreach, 291–292; standard of care, 296–297; testing and research, 289–291; and training theory, 279–280; working definition, 275–277. *See also* athletic training
Sports injury management, 7, 24, 71
Sports medicine, 28, 106, 115
Sports nutrition, 126, 128, 218. *See also* Nutrition
Sports psychology, 286
Sports rehabilitation, 106. *See also* Rehabilitation
Sports science, 124
Sports science and rehabilitation, 26
Sports studies, graduate programs in, 127–128
Staff management, 166–167, 182; employee handbook, 167; hiring, firing, and training, 171–172; human resources, 167; salary strategies, 168; staff size, 168
Stafford student loans, 44–45
State licensing standards, 4
Strength and conditioning, 128, 287
Strength training, 190
Stress management, 3
Student loans, 44–45, 55
Subluxations, 3, 56, 64–65; use of term, 243–244
Surgery, orthopedic, 113
Surgical response, 3, 110
Switzerland, 35, 93
Sydney College of Chiropractic, 233

Tactical strength and conditioning facilitators (TSAC-F), 128
Teaching assistants, 111
Technology: biomedical, 34; in chiropractic training, 96; in the classroom, 16; computer access, 19; electronic testing, 17; Force Sensing Table, 30; mobile networks, 17–20; for modeling professional practice, 20–21; for printing, 19; for teaching and learning, 15–17; visual, 16
Temporomandibular (TM) joints, 133
Testing, electronic, 17
Texas Chiropractic College, 14, 45, 123
Text neck, 305
Therapeutic heat and ice, 78, 144
Therapeutic stretching, 69
Thermotherapy, 69
Thompson Technique (drop), 71, 207
Time management, 279
Toho University, 32
Tokyo College of Chiropractic (TCC), 31–32, 95
Tokyo University of Medicine, 32
Toxicology, 66
Traditional Chinese medicine (TCM), 129. *See also* Oriental medicine
Traditional Medicine Department of Technical Cooperation for Essential Drugs and Traditional Medicine (WHO), 11
Training theory, 279–280
Transcutaneous electrical nerve stimulation (TENS), 69
Treatment plan, 186
Tui na, 129
Tuition costs, 44–45
Turkey, 36

Ultrasound, 36, 78, 113, 144
Ultraviolet light therapy, 69
United Kingdom, 45, 233; chiropractic clinics in, 198–200; chiropractic colleges in, 36–37

United States, 45; chiropractic colleges in, 21–29
United States Olympic Committee (USOC), 262
Universidad Central de Chile, Chiropractic Program, Faculty of Health Sciences, 31
Universidade Anhembi Morumbi, Faculdade de Quiropraxia, 30
Universidad Esatal del Valle de Ecatepec, Chiropractic Program, 33–34
Universidad Estatal del Valle de Toluca, 34
Universitat Autònoma de Barcelona (UAB), 35
Universitat Pompeu Favra (UPF), 35
Université du Québec à Trois-Rivières, 30
University affiliations, for chiropractic resident training programs, 107
University of Bridgeport College of Chiropractic, 14, 23, 33, 107, 111, 113, 123
University of Glamorgan, Welsh Institute of Chiropractic, 37
University of Illinois Chicago (UIC), 111
University of Johannesburg, Department of Chiropractic, 34
University of Maryland School of Medicine Center for Integrative Medicine, 260
University of Southern Denmark, Institute of Sports Science and Clinical Biomechanics, 31
University of South Wales (USW), 37
University of Western States (UWS), 14, 28, 107, 108–109, 123, 131
University of Zurich, 35, 93
Upper cervical technique, 71, 207
U.S. Department of Labor, 4

Vallone, Sharon, 265–267
VA Reform Act, 7
Vertebral subluxation complex (VSC), 56
Veterans Affairs (VA): chiropractic care and, 260–261, 267–270; chiropractic clinics, 113; residency in integrated clinical practice, 112, 113
Veterans Affairs (VA) Health Care system, 7, 80, 260
Veterans Health Administration (VHA), 224
Veterinary medicine, 124
Virtual reality (VR), 102
Vision statement, 173–174, 242
Vitamin and mineral supplementation, 78–79, 117, 143, 220
Voice recognition, 102–103

Wakefield, Pamela, 269–270
Webinars, 78–79
Wellness education, 309
Welsh Institute of Chiropractic (WIOC), 37
Whedon, James, 254
WHO Guidelines on Basic Training and Safety in Chiropractic, 11
Wiles, Michael, 307–308
Women's health, 71, 222–224
World Federation of Chiropractic (WFC), 21, 32, 89
World Health Organization (WHO), 11, 89; accreditation standards, 91; acupuncture guidelines, 114; guidelines for chiropractic education and practice, 32–33

X-ray technology, 63–64, 143

About the Editor and Contributors

Editor

Cheryl Hawk, DC, PhD, CHES, is an author on over 100 publications in peer-reviewed scientific journals and is the lead author of the 2013 book *Health Promotion and Wellness: An Evidence-Based Guide to Clinical Preventive Services.* She received her doctor of chiropractic degree in 1976 from the National University of Health Sciences and practiced full time for 12 years. In 1991, she earned a PhD in preventive medicine from the University of Iowa and became a certified health education specialist. She is currently cochair of the Research Working Group of the Academic Collaborative for Integrative Health. She has been named Researcher of the Year by the American Chiropractic Association and the Foundation for Chiropractic Education and Research.

Contributors

Lyndon Amorin-Woods, BAppSci(Chiropractic), MPH, has practiced for more than 30 years and was named Chiropractor of the Year by the Chiropractors Association of Australia in 2013. He has practiced in various multipractitioner settings and at present maintains a private practice alongside his role as senior clinical supervisor at Murdoch University. He is a member of the steering committee of ACORN, Australia's chiropractic practice-based research network, and is actively involved in chiropractic research and advocacy.

David Anderson, DC, MS-HSA, has worked in administration for multiple chiropractic colleges throughout his career, holding positions of leadership in clinical education, strategic planning, admissions, and enrollment management. He was also an active member of the admissions working group for the Association of Chiropractic Colleges. He is a 1987 graduate of Palmer College of Chiropractic with an MS in health services administration from the University of St. Francis.

Carl S. Cleveland III, DC, is a fourth-generation doctor of chiropractic and serves as president of Cleveland University–Kansas City, home of Cleveland College of Chiropractic and College of Health Sciences. He has served as president of the Association of Chiropractic Colleges and the Council on Chiropractic Education and has contributed to numerous educational materials and textbooks over his 40 years in chiropractic education.

Christina Cunliffe, DC, PhD, is a professor and dean of BPP University School of Health and principal of McTimoney College of Chiropractic. She obtained her PhD from the University of Manchester. A chartered biologist, she is a fellow of both the Royal Society of Biology and the Royal College of Chiropractors. She has served on the U.K. regulatory body and the General Chiropractic Council and was a member of its education committee.

Clinton Daniels, DC, MS, DAAPM, is a staff chiropractor for the Veterans Affairs Puget Sound Health Care System in Tacoma, Washington. He was a member of the inaugural class of the Veterans Affairs chiropractic residency program. He is a diplomate of the American Academy of Pain Management, a member of the Scientific Commission of the Council on Chiropractic Guidelines and Practice Parameters, and holds faculty appointments with Logan University and the University of Western States.

Russ Ebbets, DC, is a level-three coach in U.S.A. Track and Field (USATF) Coaching Education. He has spoken at the High Performance Summits on improving distance running in America. Since 1999, he has edited *Track Coach,* the technical journal for USATF. He has presented at the International Federation of Sports Chiropractic World Conference on Sport and Training Theory. He has directed complimentary chiropractic care at 250+ events.

Phillip Ebrall, BAppSci(Chiropractic), PhD, is vice president of international affairs at Tokyo College of Chiropractic. Dr. Ebrall has restructured or established five chiropractic programs in four countries. His publication record is significant, and he continues to mentor, research, and facilitate new chiropractic programs globally. His main interest as a creative futurist is to redesign education in alternative and complementary health care to enhance its relevance and maximize its engagement with the Wi-Fi generation of learners.

Cathryn S. Evans is a support specialist and office assistant with the Mississippi State University College of Education. She has over 20 years of experience in higher education, association management, and office administration. She has experience as a research coordinator in chiropractic research as well as medical and chiropractic practice office management.

Marion W. Evans Jr., DC, PhD, MCHES, is professor and department head of Food Science, Nutrition, and Health Promotion at Mississippi State University. He holds a PhD from the University of Alabama in health promotion. He is a master certified health education specialist and a certified wellness practitioner with the National Wellness Institute. He is the author, with Cheryl Hawk, of a 2013 text entitled *Health Promotion and Wellness: An Evidence-Based Guide to Clinical Preventive Services.*

Ronald J. Farabaugh, DC, has been in practice in Ohio since 1982. Dr. Farabaugh was appointed by the governor to serve on the Ohio Chiropractic Board in 2010, serving as its president from 2012 to 2013. He has served on the Board of Advisors of the Official Disability Guidelines. He is founder and owner of Chiro Ltd., an evidence-based, patient-centered practice-management company dedicated to assisting doctors of chiropractic establish evidence-based, referral-driven offices.

Jordan A. Gliedt, DC, is a staff chiropractic physician currently serving within the Veteran's Affairs Health Care System in Phoenix, Arizona. He is a graduate of Logan University College of Chiropractic and has practiced in various integrative medical settings throughout his chiropractic career. Dr. Gliedt currently holds a faculty appointment with Logan University and is an active member with North American Spine Society and the Scientific Commission of the Council on Chiropractic Guidelines and Practice Parameters.

Shawn Hatch, DC, is a 2006 graduate of Western States Chiropractic College. He has practiced in a variety of settings, including multidisciplinary clinics and private practice in Peru. Since 2011, he has been working as an attending chiropractic physician in the Campus Health Center at the University of Western States. Having a lifelong interest in sports and exercise, he achieved certification as diplomate of the American Chiropractic Board of Sports Physicians in 2011.

Brad Hough, PhD, has worked in educational technology for over 20 years, earning a PhD from Vanderbilt University in 2000. Currently, he provides technology leadership as Logan University's chief information officer. In 2005, he helped launch one of the early MOOCs, providing educational content to millions of self-learners. He is a board member for Promise Christian Academy, a school for special needs, and works with local and state organizations to support technology in higher education.

Stefanie Krupp, DC, MS, completed her doctor of chiropractic and master's in applied clinician nutrition from New York Chiropractic College. She practiced chiropractic and functional medicine before becoming a clinician and assistant professor at Texas Chiropractic College. She also worked in academic assessment at the University of Western States. Dr. Krupp is now employed by the Oregon Health Authority and works as a data specialist for the Maternal and Child Health section.

Rachael Pandzik, DC, completed her doctor of chiropractic from University of Western States (UWS) in 2009. She currently works at UWS as the director of chiropractic curriculum and assessment, overseeing all benchmark exams and the university's standardized patient program. Dr. Pandzik enjoys working to improve the educational experience for the next generation of chiropractors.

Jesse Politowski, DC, is a native of St. Louis, Missouri. He received his doctor of chiropractic degree from Logan University in St. Louis, Missouri. Since then, he has practiced as a chiropractor both in the United States and in Southeast Asia. For the last two years, he has been practicing in Indonesia. His wife, Stephanie, is a native Indonesian and practices medicine as a general practitioner in Indonesia.

Ruth Sandefur, DC, MS, PhD, graduated from Cleveland Chiropractic College in 1968. She practiced in Leavenworth, Kansas, for 15 years prior to starting a teaching career at Cleveland Chiropractic College in 1983. She received a master's in clinical nutrition from University of Bridgeport in 1981 and a PhD in curriculum from the University of Missouri at Kansas City in 1991. She retired from Cleveland Chiropractic College in 2010.

Currently, she works part time in her son's chiropractic and law office in St. Petersburg, Florida.

Stacey Till, MSEd, works for the office of the president at Logan University. Stacey started her career as an admissions counselor and progressed to eventually lead operations for several chiropractic admissions offices. She has helped students enroll in chiropractic colleges across the country for almost 20 years. She holds an undergraduate degree in finance from St. Ambrose University and graduated from Western Illinois University with a master's of science in education in counseling in 2007.

John Weeks is an organizer, writer, speaker, consultant, and sometimes executive who for three decades has worked to transform the medical industry's reactive and reductive focus through advancing the movement for integrative health and medicine. Toward this end, he helped create and guide multiple interprofessional and multistakeholder initiatives. He is the publisher-editor of *The Integrator Blog News & Reports* and editor in chief of the *Journal of Alternative and Complementary Medicine.*

Michael R. Wiles, DC, MEd, MS, earned his doctor of chiropractic from Canadian Memorial Chiropractic College in 1976. He has a master's of education from Brock University and master's of science (medical education leadership) from the University of New England College of Osteopathic Medicine. He is currently dean of the College of Chiropractic Medicine at Keiser University in West Palm Beach, Florida.